Devinder Kumar · David J. Waldron · Norman S. Williams (Eds.)

Clinical Measurement in Coloproctology

W0106033

With 83 Figures

Springer-Verlag
London Berlin Heidelberg New York
Paris Tokyo Hong Kong

D. Kumar, PhD, FRCS
Senior Lecturer in Surgery, Department of Surgery,
Queen Elizabeth Hospital, Birmingham, B15 2TH, UK

D. J. Waldron, MCh, FRCS, FRCSI
Senior Registrar in Surgery, Cork Regional Hospital,
Cork, Republic of Ireland

N. S. Williams, MS, FRCS
Director, The Surgical Unit, The Royal London Hospital,
Whitechapel, London, E1 1BB, UK

Cover illustration: Fig. 12.3. A barium meal examination showing megaduodenum in a patient with familial visceral myopathy

ISBN-13:978-1-4471-1824-4   e-ISBN-13:978-1-4471-1822-0
DOI: 10.1007/978-1-4471-1822-0

British Library Cataloguing in Publication Data
Kumar, Devinder
Clinical measurement in coloproctology.
1. Man. Colon. Diseases 2. Man. Anus & rectum. Diseases
I. Title II. Waldron, David J. III. Williams, Norman S.
616.34
ISBN-13:978-1-4471-1824-4

Library of Congress Cataloging-in-Publication Data
Clinical measurement in coloproctology/[editors] Devinder Kumar, David J. Waldron & Norman S. Williams.
p. cm.
Includes index.
ISBN-13:978-1-4471-1824-4
1. Colon (Anatomy) – Diseases – Diagnosis. 2. Anorectal function tests. 3. Defecation disorders – Diagnosis.
I. Kumar, Devinder, 1952– .II. Waldron, David J., 1956–   III. Williams, Norman S., 1947–
[DNLM: 1. Colonic Diseases – diagnosis. 2. Rectal Diseases – diagnosis. WI 520 C641]
RC803.C58 1991 616.3′4075 – dc20 DNLM/DLC
for Library of Congress   90–10263
                                                                                                  CIP

Typeset by Wilmaset, Birkenhead, Wirral

2128/3830–543210 Printed on acid-free paper

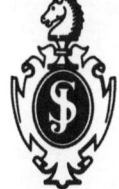

Preface

Our current understanding of the pathophysiology of colorectal disorders is dependent upon our ability to carry out an accurate assessment of colorectal function. The techniques employed in making such an assessment, such as manometry, electromyography, defaecography and scintigraphy, are generally regarded as research tools and are therefore looked upon with a degree of scepticism by the practising clinician. In recent years, with the advancement in technology, development of new methods has enabled us to carry out a much more accurate and meaningful assessment of colorectal function. So much so that important and crucial decisions like surgical intervention are based on the results of such an assessment. Nevertheless, many of these techniques still continue to be regarded as part of a research worker's armamentarium.

The principal aim of this book is to document fully the scope of useful investigations and to present them in a clear and simplified manner, so that not only specialists but also non-specialists are able to understand and set up tests for specific colorectal disorders. It reviews the basic anatomy, physiology and histology of the colon and anorectum. All available methods for the assessment of colorectal function except for conventional radiology and colonoscopy have been discussed and their role in clinical practice established so that the reader understands what is "ideal", what is optimal and what constitutes research. Areas which have made major advances in recent years, such as the neorectum, have been discussed in a separate chapter, particularly focussing on problems in function of ileal and colonic pouches and coloanal anastomosis. Colonic function and its integration with anorectal function has also been included where appropriate.

We hope that the text, explaining the value of established and new techniques in the management of colorectal disorders, will be helpful not only to the devoted coloproctologist but to all general surgeons, physicians, people in training and of course the research scientists who wish to increase their understanding of colorectal pathophysiology.

Birmingham, Cork, London
1991

Devinder Kumar
David J. Waldron
Norman S. Williams

Contents

Contributors

N. R. Binnie, FRCSEd
Surgical Registrar, Department of General Surgery, Western General Hospital,
Edinburgh EH4 2XU, UK

J. Christensen, MD
Professor of Internal Medicine, University of Iowa College of Medicine, Iowa City,
IA 52242, USA

R. I. Hallan, MA, MB BS, FRCS, FRCSEd
Registrar in Surgery and MRC Research Fellow in Anorectal Physiology, The Surgical
Unit, The Royal London Hospital, Whitechapel, London E1 1BB, UK

M. M. Henry, MB, FRCS
Consultant Surgeon, Central Middlesex Hospital, Acton Lane, London NW10 7NS, UK

D. Kumar, PhD, FRCS
Senior Lecturer in Surgery, Department of Surgery, Honorary Consultant Surgeon,
Queen Elizabeth Hospital, Birmingham B15 2TH, UK

V. Loening-Baucke, MD
Associate Professor of Paediatrics, University of Iowa College of Medicine, Iowa City,
IA 52242, USA

R. Miller, MB BS, FRCS
Senior Registrar in Surgery, Royal United Hospital, Bath BA1 3NG, UK

P. R. O'Connell, MD, FRCSI
Senior Lecturer and Honorary Consultant Surgeon, The Surgical Unit, The Royal
London Hospital, Whitechapel, London E1 1BB, UK

J. H. Pemberton, MD
Associate Professor of Surgery, Mayo Medical School, and Consultant in General, Colon
and Rectal Surgery, Mayo Clinic, 200 First Street SW, Rochester, MN 55905, USA

S. F. Phillips, MD
Professor of Medicine, Mayo Clinic, 200 First Street SW, Rochester, MN 55905, USA

D. S. Rampton, MA, BM, DPhil, FRCP
Consultant Gastroenterologist and Senior Lecturer, Royal London Hospital and Medical
College, London E11 B13, UK

A. N. Smith, MD, FRCSEd, FRCPEd, FRSE
Wade Professor of Surgical Studies, Royal College of Surgeons of Edinburgh, Reader in
Surgery, University Department of Surgery, Western General Hospital, Edinburgh
EH4 2XU, UK

C. J. Steadman, MB BS, FRACP
Gastrointestinal Unit, Mayo Clinic, 200 First Street SW, Rochester, MN 55905, USA

M. Swash, MD, FRCP, MRCPath
Consultant Neurologist, St. Mark's Hospital, City Road, London EC1V 2PS, and The
Royal London Hospital, Whitechapel, London E1 1BB, UK

D. J. Waldron, MCh, FRCS, FRCSI
Senior Registrar in Surgery, Cork Regional Hospital, Cork, Republic of Ireland

N. S. Williams, MS, FRCS
Director, The Surgical Unit, The Royal London Hospital, Whitechapel, London E1
1BB, UK

D. L. Wingate, FRCP
Director, GI Science Research Unit, The London Hospital Medical College, Whitechapel, London E1 1BB, UK

N. R. Womack, FRCS
Senior Registrar in Surgery, Bradford Royal Infirmary, Yorkshire, UK

MORPHOLOGY AND TECHNIQUES

Before obtaining any useful benefit from the measurement of various indices of function in the large bowel, the investigator must be familiar with its normal anatomical arrangement and the integration of the various tissues which allow it to function as a unit. The opening chapter of this text provides an explanatory framework which should not only be read as an introduction to the book, but also be referred to, as necessary, during the perusal of individual chapters when specific clinical problems arise or when introducing a new form of investigation to a department.

The following chapters summarize details of the techniques used in measurement of functional abnormalities of the large bowel including basic description of the apparatus itself and the manner in which it can best be used in the clinical laboratory. We would hope that the reader with an interest and background in coloproctology may be able to use this section of the book as a guide to setting up an investigative unit, whether serving an individual requirement or a more comprehensive service. Most of the chapters in this section deal with techniques appropriate to the anorectum and this, of course, reflects the fact that more work has been performed in this area than in the colon, as the former is much more accessible to study. However, Chapter 2, on the investigation of colonic function, gives an excellent up-to-date account of those techniques most likely to be of benefit in this difficult area. Although some techniques, such as measurement of anorectal sensation, colonic absorption and secretion may not have achieved prominence outside the research laboratory as yet, it is important to be aware of the patients most likely to benefit from assessment of these parameters and, if necessary, to refer appropriate patients to units where these facilities exist.

1 · Morphology of the Colon and Anorectum

J. Christensen

Introduction

Understanding the structure of an organ underlies understanding the function. This chapter is intended to present what is known of the structure of the colon and anorectum, to point out matters that are known but often passed over or neglected, and to indicate areas of deficient information.

Much of what is known comes from studies of the organ in species other than man. Physicians tend to think in terms of the human species alone. There are major variations in the structure of the organ among species, however, and so much of what can be said is subject to the caveat that species variations may exist. The existence of species variations means that further consideration of the human is needed. The subject of morphology is not closed, and one can plead for more study of the human organism in respect to morphology of the colon and anorectum.

Still, species variations in morphology seem to be more quantitative than qualitative, and the same is true of function. Thus, some generalizations about morphology among mammals are at least reasonable.

The morphology of the organ is, for the most part, in the realm of established facts and ancient history. The literature is well reviewed in standard textbooks: for this reason, the references used here constitute mainly such standard texts, rather than the primary literature of the subject, except where recent observations of importance have not yet been incorporated into the body of received knowledge.

Colonic and Anorectal Structure in Animals Other Than Man (Hume 1982; Stevens 1988)

When one surveys the large intestine in other animals than man, the most conspicuous variability found is in the extent and distribution of the part of the colon that is sacculated, and in the size of the caecum (Fig. 1.1).

The Relative Extent of the Sacculated Colon

In the human colon, a sacculated appearance characterizes nearly the whole organ from the apex of the caecum to the sigmoid colon. In contrast, when one inspects the colon of the dog, no part of the organ exhibits sacculation. Other common animals whose colons are devoid of sacculation include the rat, the mouse and the cat. Still other species have parts or segments of sacculation along the colon. These include the rabbit, the pig, the horse and most ruminants.

Sacculation of the colon, in whole or in part, is generally considered to be a characteristic of those

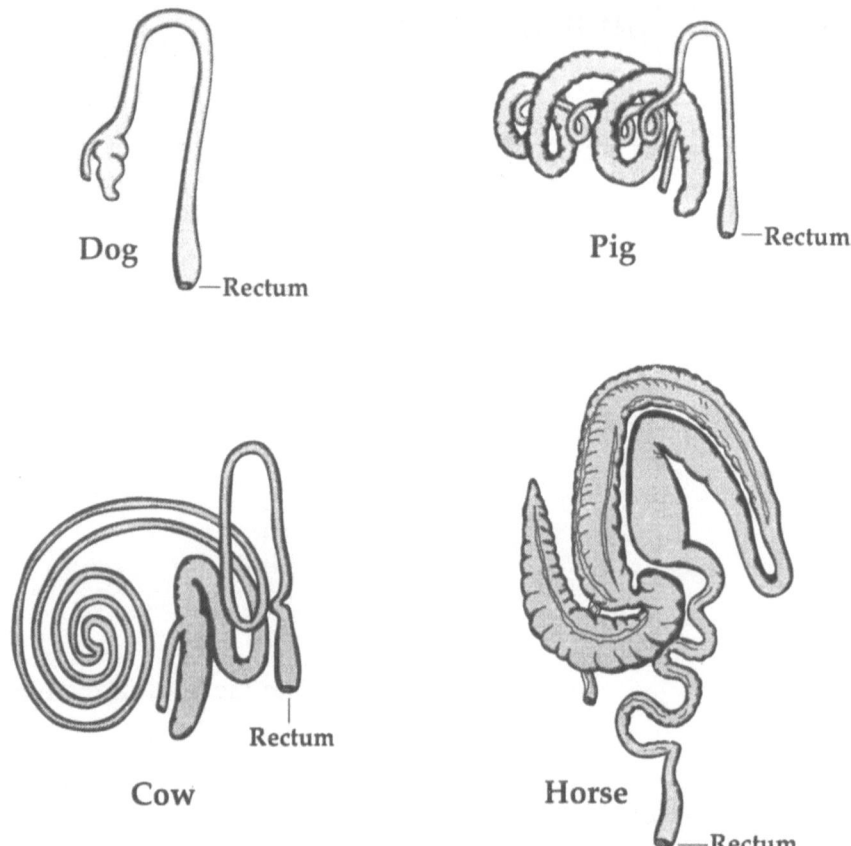

Fig. 1.1. The colons of four common animals compared.

species that are herbivores, and a consideration of the diets of the species with sacculations supports this view.

Sacculation is considered to be a morphological specialization that has occurred because of the greater content of nonabsorbed fibre reaching the colon with a vegetable diet, and is related to the occurrence of the bacterial fermentation that takes place to reduce the fibre to relatively simple chemical molecules that can be absorbed and utilized as a source of energy by the organism. The bacterial fermentation is slow, and so the sacculated parts of the organ should exhibit slow antegrade transit, a predominance of wall motions that mix the colonic content rather than propel it antegrade, and a capacity to hold a large volume. In support of this, some species with fantastically elongated and sacculated colons, notably the perissodactyls (horses and their relatives), have been found to receive a large proportion of their nutrition from bacterial fermentation of fibre in the cephalic end of the colon. Indeed, that part of the colon in such species has evolved to serve the same function as the complex stomach in ruminants (cows, sheep and similar animals).

The Relative Size of the Caecum

The caecum in man is rather small compared to the rest of the organ. It is even smaller in those species that lack a sacculated colon, and relatively large in those species with highly sacculated colons. Thus there is, in general, a parallel between the relative size of the caecum and the extent of sacculation. Man (and other primates) seem to be an exception to this rule, in having extensive sacculation without a very large caecum. A large caecum can therefore be considered to be a further adaptation to an herbivorous diet. In support of this, a caecum of any notable size nearly always exhibits sacculation. Indeed, it is the only sacculated part of the organ in the guinea pig and some other species.

Why Does Colonic Morphology Not Always Reflect Diet?

There are some apparent exceptions to the rule correlating a complex colon (a long colon with a large caecum and extensive sacculation) to the diet of the species under consideration. These exceptions are mostly among the omnivores. The pig, for example, possesses a complex colon and yet is not a strict herbivore; and rats and mice, as herbivores, have simple colons. Even more striking exceptions exist in birds: common domestic fowl have two very long caeca; hawks (carnivores) have only one long caecum; woodpeckers (mostly carnivores) have none; but parrots (mostly herbivores) have none either.

The answer to this paradox can only be guessed. It is possible that colonic morphology changes slowly in evolution while dietary practices can change rapidly, as animals must adapt to new environments. Thus, the possession of a complex colon may indicate only evolution from an herbivorous ancestor, and a simple colon may indicate evolution from a carnivorous ancestor. It seems clear, however, that in the most fantastically complex colons, like those of perissodactyls in which colonic fermentation has become a major source of nutrition, the organ commits the species to an herbivorous diet and adaptation to other diets is thereby impossible. The simple colon of carnivores is one that makes no such commitment, and so one sees simple colons in animals like some rodents and omnivores who may subsist on largely vegetable diets.

Gross Colonic and Anorectal Structure in Humans (Clemente 1985)

The Parts of the Organ

The human colon is about 1.5 m long. It arises at the end of the ileum in the right iliac region, extends cephalad to contact the caudal surface of the liver, then bends to the left to arch over the anterior protrusion of the lumbar spine, touches the spleen in the left hypochondrium, extends caudal to reach the left iliac region, then bends complexly to descend along the posterior wall of the pelvis, and ends at the anal opening.

This configuration has given rise to a set of terms that describe its gross parts. These terms are the *appendix*, the *caecum*, the *ascending colon*, the *transverse colon*, the *descending colon*, the *sigmoid colon*, the *rectum* and the *anal canal*.

These segments are continuous, and the

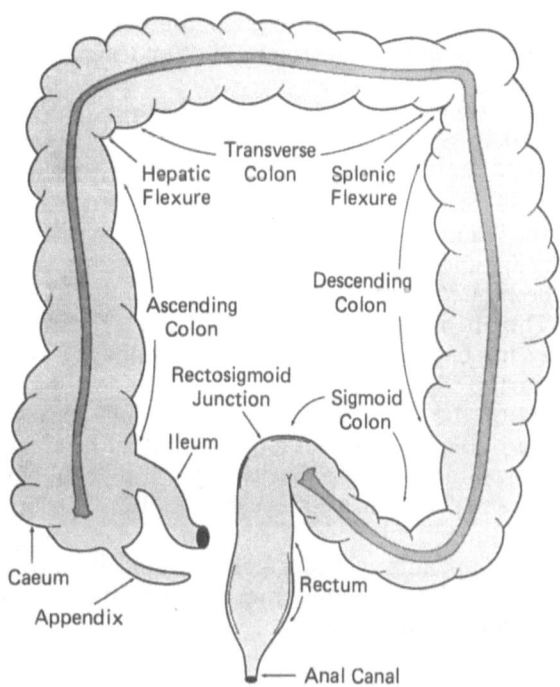

Fig. 1.2. The human colon, labelled to show the parts and loci as named in this chapter.

junctions between them receive appropriate terms that define specific loci along the large intestine. These loci are the *ileocaecal junction*, the *hepatic flexure*, the *splenic flexure* and the *rectosigmoid junction*. These parts, segments and loci are shown in Fig. 1.2.

These terms have become so firmly established that they are applied to the large intestine in nearly all species, even though the configuration of the colon in many species is such that the use of these terms is not really appropriate. Veterinarians, for example, have a different set of terms to apply to the complex colons of horses. Similarly, the smooth curvature of the colon of the cat hardly allows one to identify the hepatic or splenic flexures as distinct loci.

The Appendix, Caecum and Ileocaecal Junction in Humans

The *appendix* is a narrow blind tube, devoid of sacculation, up to 20 cm long and about 10 mm in diameter. It extends from the caecal apex, lying in a position that varies greatly among individuals.

The *caecum* is a sacculated blind pouch (except for its junction to the appendix) that extends from the ileocaecal junction into the right iliac fossa. Its position varies considerably among individuals. It usually touches the anterior abdominal wall and the right iliopsoas muscle and it often touches the rectum.

The *ileocaecal junction*, also called the ileocaecal valve, is a distinct structure that separates the ileum from the colon. Strictly, the junction, which usually occurs at an angulation between the axes of the ileum and colon, marks the line between the caecum and the rest of the colon. Thus, it is also called the *ileocolic junction*.

The opening between the small and large intestines lies between two lips that are demilunes, one lip on the edge toward the ascending colon and the other on the side toward the caecum. The narrow horns of these demilunes touch so that the opening is surrounded by a lip that is wider at its cephalic and caudal margins than it is laterally. The lips contain much fat.

The appendix, caecum and terminal ileum all possess a generous mesentery which gives them considerable mobility.

The Ascending, Transverse, Descending and Sigmoid Parts of the Colon

The *ascending colon*, extending from the ileocaecal junction to the *hepatic flexure* (where the colon touches the liver), is a sacculated tube. It has little or no mesentery so that its position is quite constant over the iliac and quadratus lumborum muscles, the aponeurotic origin of the transverse abdominal muscles and the anterior and lateral surfaces of the right kidney. Anteriorly, this part of the organ contacts the distal ileum and the ventral abdominal wall. At the surface of the liver, the organ touches the liver at its *colic impression* to the right of the gallbladder.

The *transverse colon* extends from the *hepatic flexure* to the *splenic flexure* as a sacculated tube. It must loop anteriorly to pass over the arch of the lumbar spine and it commonly loops some way caudad toward the pelvis. It possesses a generous mesentery, the transverse mesocolon, which arises along the caudal border of the pancreas. The mesentery gives this part of the organ a great deal of mobility. The breadth of the mesentery increases with age and the mobility of the segment increases correspondingly. At the splenic flexure, the mesentery is shorter, forming part of the *phrenicocolic ligament* that brings the splenic flexure into contact with the spleen.

The *descending colon* is a sacculated tube extending from the splenic flexure to the pelvic brim, the cephalic aperture of the lesser pelvis. This part of the organ has little or no mesentery, like the ascending colon. Consequently, the investing peritoneum holds the colon quite close against the anterior and lateral surfaces of the left kidney, the lateral border of the psoas muscles, the valley between the psoas and the quadratus lumborum muscles, the aponeurotic origin of the transverse abdominal muscles and the quadratus lumborum. The most caudal part of the descending colon loops medially, anterior to the iliopsoas muscle just above the pelvic brim.

The *sigmoid colon* is a loop of the colon merging indistinctly with the caudal end of the descending colon. This loop varies greatly in size and is suspended from a generous mesentery so that it can frequently move or extend from its normal position within the pelvis up into the abdomen. The mesentery tends to broaden with age, so that a long loop of sigmoid colon extending into the abdomen is more commonly found in the elderly than in the young. Dorsally, the sigmoid colon is usually in contact with the external iliac vessels, with the left piriform muscle and with part of the sacral plexus of nerves. It is usually separated from the urinary bladder by loops of the ileum. Its caudal limit lies at the level of the third sacral vertebra where it joins the apex of the rectum at the *rectosigmoid junction*.

The Rectum and Anal Canal

The *rectum* extends from the level of the third sacral vertebra to the anal canal. This part of the organ is relatively straight, hence its name. It really is not straight, for it exhibits two slight curvatures, both dorsoventral. It shows a slight ventral convexity just above the anal canal and a slight dorsal convexity as it curves along the sacrum. It is about 12 cm long, but its length varies considerably. A slight widening just above the anal canal is called the *rectal ampulla*. The *valves of Houston*, fixed transverse demilunar folds, indent the rectal lumen. There are usually three such valves, each 10–12 mm thick, spaced about 3 cm apart. Usually, the most cephalic fold projects from the right side, the middle fold from the left and the most caudal from the anterior surface, but the number and positions of these folds varies among individuals.

The rectum has no mesentery. The peritoneum is reflected from the rectum to other structures about 7 cm above the anal canal (a little less in females), so that most of the rectum is extraperito-

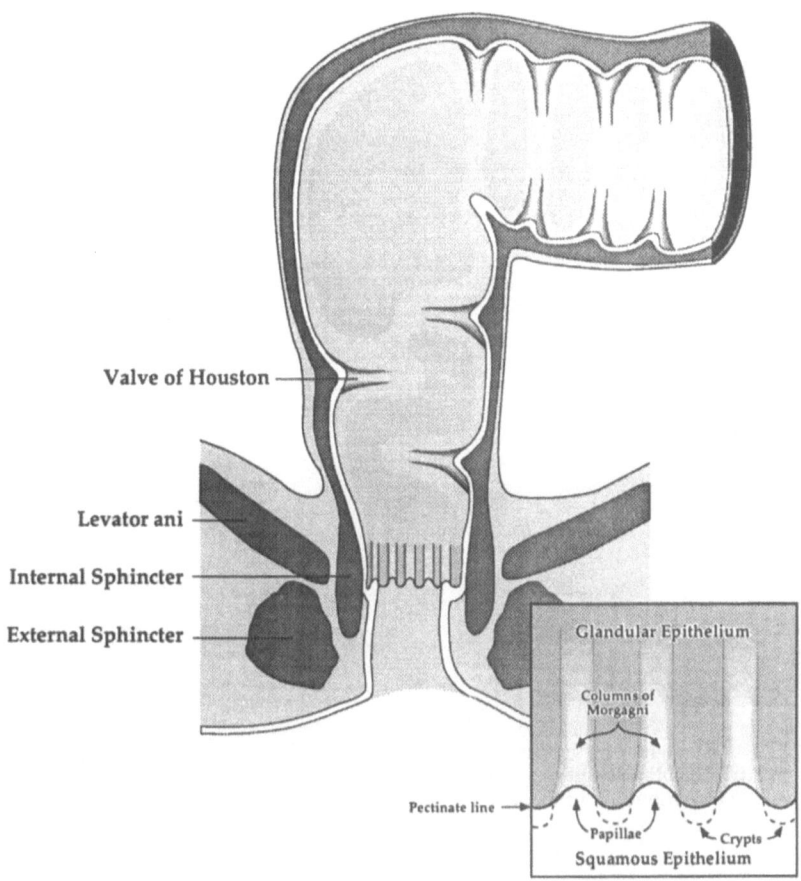

Fig. 1.3. The anal canal.

neal. It is held fast by connective tissue, lying upon the sacrum and coccyx posteriorly and approximating the urinary bladder, prostate, seminal vesicles and ductus deferens anteriorly in males, and the vagina in females.

The *anal canal* is a short segment, 2–4 cm long, extending from the end of the rectum to the external anal orifice (Fig. 1.3). This is the segment of the organ that traverses the pelvic floor. The anal canal is invested by the *external anal sphincter*, a specialized part of the striated musculature of the pelvic floor. The membranous urethra, the bulb of the penis and the urogenital diaphragm lie anterior to the anal canal in males, and the vagina in females. The *perineal body* and the *postanal plate*, structures of the pelvic floor respectively anterior and posterior to the anal canal, are fibromuscular structures fused to the *levator ani* muscles.

The mucosal lining of the anal canal is thrown into longitudinal or axial folds, the *columns of Morgagni*, which are separated by crevices, the *rectal sinuses*. The columns of Morgagni terminate

caudally in fleshy nipples, the anal papillae, covered by squamous epithelium. The squamocolumnar epithelial junction or border, the *pectinate line*, connects these anal papillae laterally, forming thin mucosal folds, the *anal valves*. Small blind pockets, the *anal crypts* or *sinuses*, lie behind these anal valves.

The Shape of the Colon and Anorectum in Cross-section

As pointed out above, most of the human colon has a sacculated appearance. This shape characterizes the caecum, ascending colon, transverse colon, descending colon and sigmoid colon, but the rectum and anal canal have a smooth cylindrical configuration.

The sacculated appearance of the colon arises from the fact that the outer longitudinal layer of the main muscular coat in this region is not uniformly thick in the circumference of the organ (Fig. 1.4). Rather, it is formed into three thick

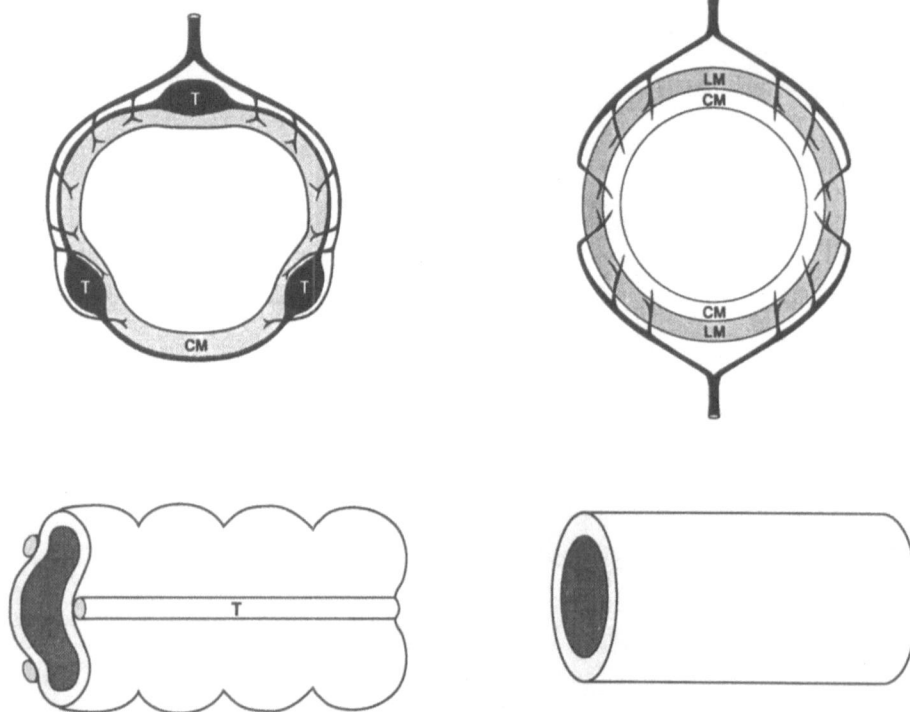

Taeniated Sacculated Part of the Large Intestine   Rectum

Fig. 1.4. The sacculated and cylindrical parts of the colon compared as to structure. Taeniae are indicated by T; CM, circular muscle layer; LM, longitudinal muscle layer. The distributions of the arteries are indicated.

bands, the three *taeniae coli*. One taenia lies along the line of the mesenteric insertion and the others lie approximately equidistant from the mesenteric taenia. Thus, the colon in the sacculated regions tends to have the cross-sectional shape of an equilateral triangle. The walls of the colon between the taeniae contain principally the circular layer of the main muscle coat, with a very thin layer of the longitudinal muscular layer over the outer surface. The muscle coats tend to bulge out in the spaces between the taeniae. These bulging intertaenial walls are interrupted at intervals by thin circumferential shelves that represent tonically-contracted bands of the circular muscle layer, the *haustral markings*. These bands are spaced a few centimetres apart. Their locations are not fixed, however, for bands of tonic contraction can form apparently at any level. At any single instant in time, and in fixed tissue, they appear to be quite uniformly spaced at intervals of 3–6 cm.

The axial indentations produced by the three taeniae and the circumferential indentations produced by the narrow circumferential rings of tonically-contracted muscle give the colon its sacculated appearance, as a chain of pockets. These

pockets are called the *haustra* (from the Greek term for the buckets on a water-wheel).

The three taeniae broaden and fuse at the level of the sigmoid colon, so that below the rectosigmoid junction there is no sacculation. The longitudinal muscle is uniformly thick in the circumference of the rectum.

The Construction of the Wall of the Colon and Anorectum (Fawcett 1986)

The Major Layers of the Wall

Like the rest of the gut, the wall of the colon is constructed of layers of different kinds of tissue. These layers are not separated but joined together by connective tissues and by the neural and vascular elements of the wall. Starting from the luminal surface, the following layers make up the wall.

The innermost layer is the *mucosa*; it consists of three subunits, the *epithelium*, the *lamina propria* and the *muscularis mucosae*. The next deeper layer is the *submucosa*. Peripheral to that lies the *muscularis propria*; it consists of three subunits, the inner *circular muscle layer*, the *intermuscular space* and the outer *longitudinal muscle layer*. The *serosa* lies outside the muscularis propria.

The Mucosa

The Epithelium

A glandular epithelium lines the whole organ except in the most caudal 1–2 cm of the anal canal, where the epithelium is squamous. The glandular epithelium is formed into glands, the *crypts* or *glands of Lieberkühn*, 0.5–0.7 mm deep, extending from the luminal surface nearly to the surface of the muscularis mucosae. The principal cell of the epithelium is the *columnar absorptive cell*, a typical columnar cell. *Goblet cells* are abundant among the sheet of columnar absorptive cells. There are very sparse *enteroendocrine cells* as well. The paneth cells which characterize the small intestinal epithelium are not found in the colonic epithelium.

The epithelial cells are constantly renewed, growing from undifferentiated cells located at the deepest points of the crypts of Lieberkühn. The cells newly formed at this level immediately differentiate into columnar absorptive cells, goblet cells or enteroendocrine cells and migrate up the sides of the crypts to the luminal surface. The oldest cells slough from extrusion zones that are spaced at uniform distances from the mouths of the crypts. Goblet cells and columnar absorptive cells of the colon have a half-life of about six days, considerably longer than that of the cells of the small intestinal epithelium. The half-life of the enteroendocrine cells is even longer. This means that the enteroendocrine cells must migrate more slowly than the two other kinds of cells, and independently from them. A thick basal lamina forms a plate under these epithelial cells. This basal lamina probably also moves from the depths of the crypts to the luminal surface, along with the epithelial cells.

The *columnar absorptive cell* resembles that of the small intestinal epithelium. It is a tall columnar cell with a nucleus located near the base, opposite the end of the cell that approximates the luminal surface. A well-developed Golgi apparatus, an abundant endoplasmic reticulum, free ribosomes and mitochondria fill the apical portion of the cell.

The apical surface (at the luminal surface) contains a few microvilli, but these are rudimentary. Junctional complexes connect these colonic enterocytes at their apical poles. These are occluding junctions, sealing the luminal space from the paracellular spaces between the colonic enterocytes. Thus, the colonic enterocytes resemble those of the small intestine.

The *goblet cells* also resemble those of the small intestine. A goblet cell has a basal nucleus, with the great bulk of the cell filled with a mass of mucinogen granules which compresses the organelles into a thin peripheral layer of cytoplasm. The goblet cells lie with a basal pole on the basal lamina and an apical pole at the luminal surface, discharging their contents through this apical pole.

The *enteroendocrine cells* of the colon are much rarer than they are in the small intestine. Considering these cells as a whole along the gut, one can distinguish some 17 types on the basis of the appearance of their secretory granules and the peptides that can be identified in them by immunohistochemistry. Only a few of these 17 types of enteroendocrine cells are to be found in the colon. These include Type D cells (containing somatostatin), Type D_1 cells (peptide unknown), Type EC cells (containing serotonin and various other peptides), Type L cells (containing glucagon), and Type PP cells (containing pancreatic polypeptide).

Aside from details of the appearance of their secretory granules, these cells all have a similar morphology. They tend to be solitary rather than aggregated into the small groups which occur in the small intestine. Most of the cell lies in the deeper half of the epithelium, but a thin apical protrusion may extend to the luminal surface. The rounded nucleus is surrounded by a cytoplasm that is filled mainly by secretory granules. The organelles otherwise are inconspicuous, and the endoplasmic reticulum is not prominent. The extensive contact of these cells with the basal lamina suggests that these enteroendocrine cells may discharge the peptides and other substances that they may produce into the lamina propria or into the paracellular spaces rather than into the lumen.

The Lamina Propria

This layer, as in the small intestine, fills the space between the epithelium and the muscularis mucosae. It is made up of a loose stroma of connective tissue fibres, principally collagen. This mesh is somewhat denser at the surface next to the basal lamina than it is next to the muscularis mucosae. Lymphocytes, plasma cells, eosinophils and macrophages lie in abundance in this stroma. The lymphocytes are the most prominent cells in this region, and some of them penetrate the basal lamina to lie in paracellular clefts within the epithelium. Lymphoid nodules are common in the colonic lamina propria, and some of them are so large that they bulge through the muscularis mucosae into the submucosa.

The Muscularis Mucosae

A thin layer of muscle cells, the *muscularis mucosae*, lies at the base of the lamina propria, separating it from the submucosa. These muscle cells are arranged with their long axes in both the longitudinal axis (mostly on the serosal side) and in the circumferential axis (mostly on the luminal side). A network of collagen and elastic fibres surrounds these cells and delimits bundles of smooth muscle cells within which the muscle cells are closely apposed. The sheet of muscle is thin, only about 30–40 μm, and contains no more than about six muscle cell thicknesses. Axons ramify among the smooth muscle cells.

The Submucosa

A thick space peripheral to the muscularis mucosae, the *submucosa*, makes up about one-half of the total thickness of the wall of the colon. This is largely an "empty" space, filled with a loose stroma of collagen and elastic fibres that contains fibroblasts and macrophages and a small proportion of lymphocytes and eosinophils. The submucosa also contains plexuses and arterioles, capillaries and venules from which branches extend into the adjacent mucosa and muscularis propria. The submucous plexus of nerves is also present in the form of ganglia, interganglionic bundles and the axons that branch from them. These axons also extend into the adjacent mucosa and muscularis propria. The "floor" of the submucosa, the surface that abuts the circular layer of the muscularis propria, is covered by a thin but dense plexus of axons derived from the submucous plexus. This plexus of axons also contains numerous fibroblast-like cells, interstitial cells of Cajal. The details of the submucous plexus are described more fully on page 17.

The Muscularis Propria

The Muscle Layers

The muscularis propria, the major muscular coat of the colon, lies in two layers. The muscle cells and bundles extend along the longitudinal axis in the outer (serosal) layer to form the longitudinal muscle layer. Those of the inner muscle layer are oriented along the circumference of the colon to form the circular muscle layer. Such an arrangement is the rule throughout the gut, of course, but a major specialization characterizes the colon, in that the longitudinal muscle layer is not uniformly thick about the circumference of the organ. Rather, the muscle is thickened to form the three taeniae, one of which lies along the line of the mesenteric insertion, with the other two spaced at uniform distances on the antitaenial surface. A very thin layer of the longitudinal musculature, discontinuous in places, covers the circular muscle layer. The circular muscle layer is much thicker than the longitudinal layer. It is particularly thickened in the anal canal to form the *internal anal sphincter*. This sphincter is surrounded by, but separate from, the striated muscle of the external anal sphincter.

The Intermuscular Space

The intermuscular space is a thin space, about 100 μm wide, that lies between the two coats of the muscularis propria. It contains principally the neural elements of the myenteric plexus and vascular plexuses of arterioles, capillaries and venules. The vessels are less abundant here than they are in the submucosa. The myenteric plexus consists of ganglia, interganglionic fascicles, axons that branch from them and numerous fibroblast-like cells that probably include interstitial cells of Cajal. The myenteric plexus is described in more detail on page 16.

The Serosa

A continuous sheet of squamous epithelial cells, the mesothelium, invests the outer surface of most of the colon. This mesothelium is separated from the underlying longitudinal muscle layer by a thin layer of loose connective tissue containing collagen and elastic fibres. There are localized accumulations of fat beneath the mesothelium which may be very large and so bulge from the surface of the colon. These are called the *appendices epiploicae*.

The Structure of Smooth Muscle in the Colon and Anorectum (Gabella 1987)

The contractions of the smooth muscle of the colonic wall create the forces that mix the colonic contents and propel them antegrade. This activity is a major function of the colon, making possible the optimal extraction of water from the faecal mass, facilitating bacterial proliferation and allowing controlled defaecation. Thus, it is appropriate at this point to provide a description of the morphology of gastrointestinal smooth muscle. This description is a general one, derived almost entirely from the examination of smooth muscle in other parts of the gut, mainly the small intestine. There may be certain morphological features that are specific to the muscle of the colon. If so, they are unknown. A specific study to seek special morphological features of colonic smooth muscle remains to be done.

Smooth Muscle Cells

Morphology at the Level of the Light Microscope

Smooth muscle cells in the gut, like those everywhere, are uninuclear fusiform cells, generally about 500–700 μm by 5–15 μm. There may be variations in these dimensions among organs and loci, but probably not great differences. Exact dimensions are obviously difficult to discover in cells whose boundaries are so hard to resolve at light microscopy and whose dimensions normally vary so much in the course of normal function.

The broadest part of the cell contains the single *nucleus*, an elongated or "cigar-shaped" body in which the chromatin forms a very delicate pattern of aggregation fairly uniformly dispersed in the nucleoplasm. At light microscopy, usually only the slightly thicker aggregates at the inner surface of the nuclear envelope are visible. There are usually two or more small nucleoli. The nuclear outline is often indented from passive distortion in contracted muscle.

In a sheet of muscle, the nuclei tend to be arranged in palisades. This is because the nuclei always lie in the central thick part of the cell and because the muscle cells are oriented in an orderly way, with the thick central parts adjacent to the thin extremities of adjacent cells.

The sarcoplasm appears at light microscopy to be nearly devoid of organelles. Some stains may reveal the myofibrils as faint longitudinal striations and some stains may show other organelles very faintly. In all cases, however, the organelles are inconspicuous, so that the sarcoplasm appears to be quite homogeneous. The cell membranes are also poorly seen, so that the muscle has the appearance of a uniform matrix, hence the name "smooth muscle".

The smooth muscle cells are aggregated into bundles in which they lie with their long axes in parallel. Connective tissue, mostly collagen fibrils with fibroblasts, bind the bundles together and fill the spaces between bundles, binding them together. Bundles branch and fuse irregularly to form a coarse network. Thus, the bundles and their confining collagen meshwork ensure that the force of contraction is uniformly distributed throughout the sheet of cells. There are about 180 000 smooth muscle cells per mm^3 in gut smooth muscle, and the volume of the extracellular space is 10%–30%, depending upon the method of determination. Within a bundle of smooth muscle, there are thin sheets of collagen fibres between adjacent cells. These do not, however, separate the muscle cells enough to interfere with cell-to-cell contacts between adjacent muscle cells.

Morphology at the Level of the Electron Microscope (Fig. 1.5)

Smooth muscle cells have a high surface-to-volume ratio because the cells are small, about 3500 μm^3. A single cell has a surface area of about 5000 μm^2. The amount of cell surface available for exchange with the extracellular space is about 1 m^2/g of tissue.

The cell membrane contains abundant flask-shaped invaginations, the *caveolae*. These conspicuous structures are about 70 nm across and about 120 nm deep, with the longer axis perpendicular to the surface of the cell. The basal lamina which surrounds the muscle cell does not enter the caveolae, but lies loosely over its opening to the extracellular space. Markers placed in the extracellular space readily enter the caveolae. The caveolae are arranged in rows oriented in the long

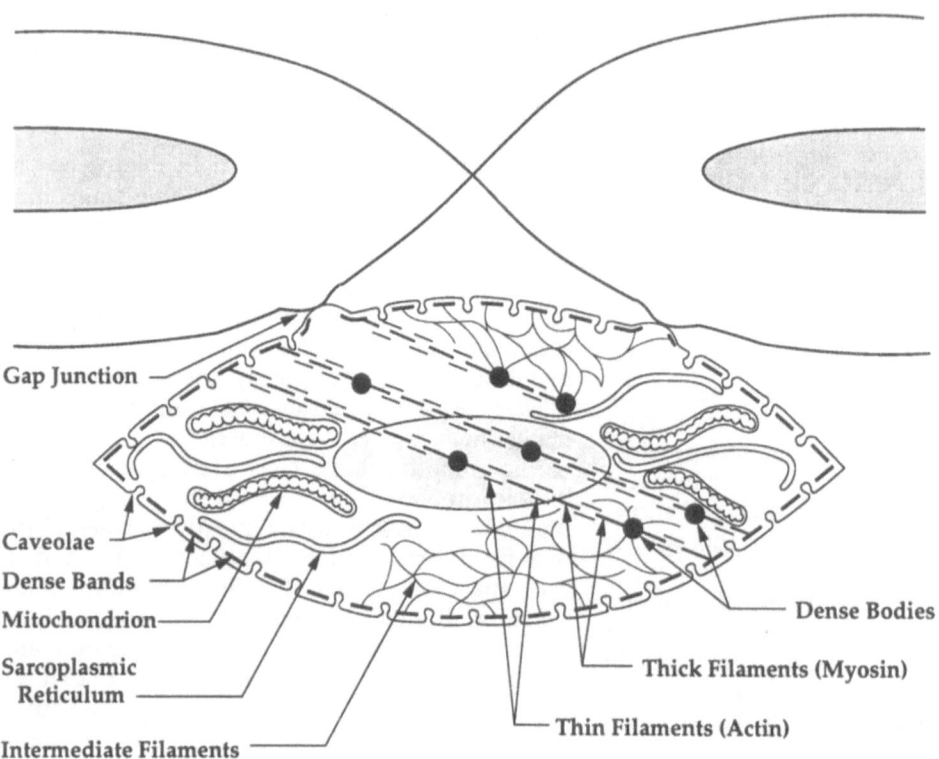

Gap Junction

Caveolae

Dense Bands

Mitochondrion

Sarcoplasmic
   Reticulum

Intermediate Filaments

Dense Bodies

Thick Filaments (Myosin)

Thin Filaments (Actin)

Fig. 1.5. A diagram of a smooth muscle cell.

axis of the muscle cell. These rows of caveolae alternate with *dense bands*, discussed below. A single cell contains about 170 000 caveolae (about 20–30 per μm^2 of all surface), and they can be calculated to increase the cell surface by 50%–70% over the area which would be calculated in their absence. That is, more than one third of the cell surface enters into the formation of the caveolae.

The *dense bands* are aggregates of electron-dense material on the inner surface of the cell membrane. These structures (also called *dense patches* or *membrane-associated dense bodies*) are about 0.2–0.4 μm × 1–2 μm, and they are about 30–100 nm thick. About 30%–50% of the cell surface is covered by the dense bands. The dense bands are anchor points attaching the cytoplasmic filaments to the cell membrane. Contractile and structural filaments terminate in these dense bands. Alpha-actinin is a major component of the dense bands. This same protein also occurs in the Z-lines of striated muscle, which are also anchor points for cytoplasmic filaments in such muscle.

Cisternae of the *smooth endoplasmic reticulum* lie throughout the smooth muscle cell. Some ramify near the cell membrane, lying very close to the caveolae and to the dense bands, often approaching as close as 10 nm to the cell membrane. Cisternae are also concentrated near the

two poles of the nucleus, and they are sparsely distributed among the myofibrils of the sarcoplasm. About 2% of the cell volume is occupied by the smooth endoplasmic reticulum.

Mitochondria are also concentrated near the two poles of the nucleus and just beneath the cell membrane. An estimated 5%–9% of the cell volume is occupied by mitochondria.

The other usual organelles are present in smooth muscle, but they are not prominent. These include *centrioles*, the *Golgi apparatus*, a *rough endoplasmic reticulum*, *lysosomes* and *microtubules*.

Sarcoplasmic Filaments in Smooth Muscle

Three kinds of filaments fill the sarcoplasm of smooth muscle. The thinnest filaments, 7 nm in diameter, are filaments of actin. They constitute the great majority of the sarcoplasmic filaments. Filaments of 10 nm are much sparser. They are filaments of desmin, and are the cytoskeletal filaments. The thickest filaments, 15–18 nm in diameter, are filaments of myosin.

The *thin filaments* of actin occur in a ratio of about 12:1 in proportion to the thick filaments. They are occasionally oriented in rosettes around the thick filaments, but they mainly occur in masses, organized into long bundles that split and merge irregularly.

The *thick filaments* of myosin are often poorly preserved in electron microscopic sections. In good preparations, these filaments closely resemble the myosin filaments of striated muscle. They never lie in groups. Rather, the occur as solitary fibres surrounded by thin filaments. They are quite uniformly distributed in the sarcoplasm. These filaments interact with the actin filaments as the *contractile proteins*.

The *intermediate filaments* of desmin are much sparser than the other two types. These occur as solitary filaments, occasionally as small bundles or groups. They form what is called the cytoskeleton. The function of the cytoskeleton is unknown but it is conjectured that the cytoskeleton provides some sort of organizing framework within the sarcoplasm.

All three types of filaments insert into the membrane-associated *dense bands*. They also are inserted into the *dense bodies* which are distributed irregularly throughout the sarcoplasm. The dense bodies are amorphous aggregates of electron-dense material resembling that which makes up the dense bands. The dense bodies also contain alpha-actinin. They are considered to be anchor points for the contractile and cytoskeletal filaments, uniting the sarcoplasm into a single functional mass.

Intercellular Junctions in Smooth Muscle

Adjacent cells in a sheet of smooth muscle make specialized contacts with one another. Actually, a great deal of variation exists in different smooth muscles in this respect: in some muscle tissues, such specialized junctions are abundant, and in others they are absent. There are several kinds of such junctions.

The *intermediate junction* is common. This junction has a characteristic form. In two adjacent cells, the portions of the two cell membranes that contain a dense band are matched or lined up so that the two dense bands lie side by side. The membranes of the two cells come very close, but a cleft remains that is 30–40 nm wide. The basal laminae of the two conjoined cells fuse to form a single condensed band of basal lamina that lies in this cleft. Since the dense bands function as anchor points for the contractile filaments within the cells, these intermediate junctions probably provide points of attachment that serve to transmit the force of contraction throughout the muscle mass.

A *modified intermediate junction* is recognized as a slightly different structure. It has a smaller diameter, a narrower intercellular cleft (15–20 nm) and symmetrical condensations of electron-dense material (resembling dense bands) at the conjoined surfaces that do not receive myofilaments and cytoskeletal filaments. Thus, these junctions seem to have some function other than a mechanical linkage. Their function is unknown.

The *gap junction* is a common structure having a very different morphology. Oval patches on the contiguous points of two adjacent cells are separated by an intercellular cleft of only about 2–3 nm. The area of contiguity is about 0.01–0.15 μm^2. In tissues where gap junctions are abundant, a single cell may have up to 250 such junctions, and they occupy about 0.22% of the surface area of the cell. Gap junctions are rare in the taenia coli (of the guinea pig) and virtually absent from the circular muscle layer of the rectum. Furthermore, they are labile structures, increasing or decreasing in number with various treatments of the tissue.

The function of gap junctions can be inferred from their detailed structure. The narrow gap is devoid of basal lamina and the two opposed surfaces are joined together by bridges, regularly-arranged subunits called *connexons*. There are channels that allow for the exchange of small molecules and ions between the conjoined cells.

The Innervation of the Colon and Anorectum (Furness and Costa 1987; Gabella 1976, 1979; Kuntz 1953; Mitchell 1953)

The Extrinsic Nerves (Fig. 1.6)

Three major pathways convey nerves between the central nervous system and the large intestine.

The *vagus nerves* provide fibres to the right colon, extending in distribution from the appendix to the midpoint of the transverse colon. This is a parasympathetic pathway making connections to the vagal nuclei of the brainstem. The vagi, in many species, also distribute some sympathetic fibres, but these are probably very few.

The *mesenteric nerves* arise from prevertebral ganglia that lie at the roots of the major arteries that supply the gut. These are the coeliac, superior mesenteric and inferior mesenteric ganglia. Each ganglion sends up to about six major nerve trunks

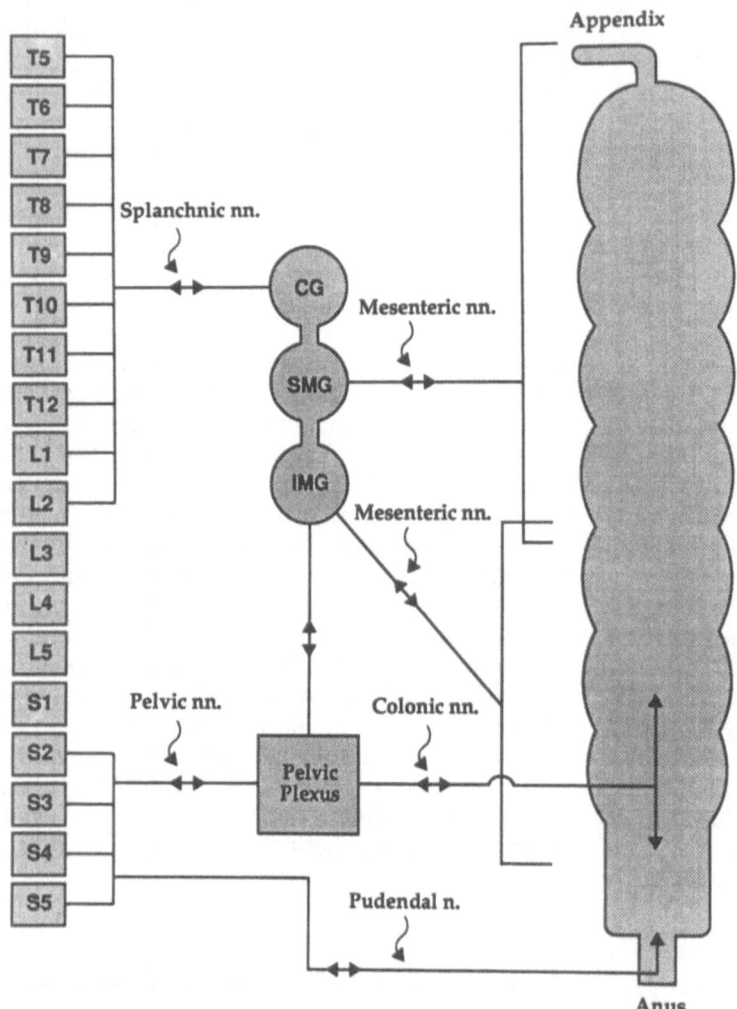

Fig. 1.6. The extrinsic innervation of the colon. The coeliac, superior and inferior mesenteric ganglia are indicated by CG, SMG and IMG respectively.

alongside the artery that it is associated with, and these trunks branch as the artery branches. The superior and inferior mesenteric ganglia are probably the major origin of the mesenteric nerves to the large intestine. The coeliac ganglion, however, is closely interconnected with the other two. Indeed, in some species the three ganglia are variably fused together. Thus, it should not be excluded from possibility that the coeliac ganglion also supplies some axons to the large intestine by way of the mesenteric nerves. These are sympathetic nerves, part of the thoracolumbar part of the autonomic nervous system. The prevertebral ganglia are connected to the thoracic and lumbar segments of the spinal cord through the splanchnic nerves.

The *pelvic nerves* supply the large intestine through the *pelvic plexus*. Nerve trunks from the sacral levels of the spinal cord form the pelvic plexus which lies about the organs above the pelvic

floor. The pelvic plexus gives colonic branches to the distal colon as well as branches to the urinary bladder and genital organs. The pelvic plexus also receives fibres from the inferior mesenteric ganglion and so (like the vagus) may be a minor pathway for the distribution of sympathetic fibres as well. The pelvic plexus contains some small ganglia.

The Intrinsic or Intramural Nerves
(Christensen et al. 1983, 1984; Christensen and Rick 1985, 1987a, b)

The Intramural Distributions of Extrinsic Nerves

Physiological evidence for the distribution of the extrinsic nerves confirms the anatomic descriptions given above. Similarly, physiological evidence supports the distribution patterns of the mesenteric nerves. In both cases, direct anatomical demonstration of these distributions is difficult to achieve because the fibres extrinsic in origin can be very few and difficult to find among the mass of nerve fibres in the intramural plexuses.

The *pelvic innervation*, however, can be traced more readily, as the *ascending nerves of the colon* (Fig. 1.7). These are extensions of the colonic branches from the pelvic plexus that run in the plane of the myenteric plexus cephalad up to the level of the mid-colon and caudad down to the anal canal. They have been mapped extensively only in various laboratory species.

They arise at the zone of the rectosigmoid junction where the colonic branches of the pelvic plexus penetrate the longitudinal muscle layer. They run in the plane of the myenteric plexus as gross nerve bundles mainly lying in the craniocaudal direction, but many oblique lateral branches join them together. They do not pass through the ganglia of the myenteric plexus but rather pass among them, giving branches to the ganglia that they pass. At their terminations they burst into many small branches that disappear among the ganglia of the myenteric plexus.

These ascending nerves of the colon have the structure of peripheral nerves. They are surrounded by a sheath of connective tissue cells and they have a specific blood supply in the form of a capillary plexus that surrounds them as well as a central vessel in the core of the fascicle. They contain both myelinated and nonmyelinated nerve fibres, the myelinated fibres representing the axons of nerve cells located outside the myenteric plexus. Thus, the ascending nerves, though they lie with the myenteric plexus in the intermuscular plane, are peripheral autonomic nerves that are superimposed upon the myenteric plexus, supplying its ganglia throughout their domains.

The myelinated fibres can be traced from the point at which they enter the colon at the zone of the rectosigmoid junction to the point where the myelin sheaths disappear. These myelinated fibres leave the ascending nerves in the branches that are given off to a ganglion, pass laterally only one or two interganglionic distances and then turn to run cephalad within the ganglionated plexus. Thus, the extrinsic nerves, represented by the myelinated fibres, tend not to run far in the circumference of the organ.

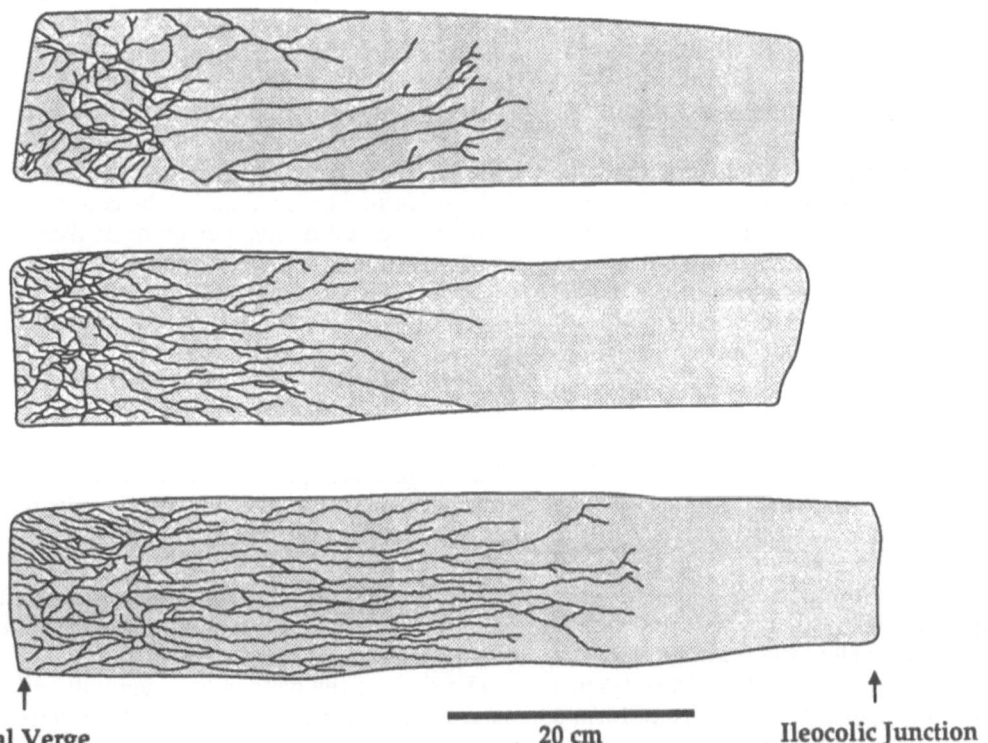

Anal Verge   20 cm   Ileocolic Junction

Fig. 1.7. The distribution of the ascending nerves of the colon in three cat colons.

Organization of the Myenteric Plexus of the Colon and Anorectum

The myenteric plexus in the large intestine resembles that in the rest of the gut, consisting of large *ganglia* joined together by *interganglionic fascicles*.

A *ganglion* is a compact disc containing principally two kinds of cells, *nerve cells* and *glial cells*, and a mass of the processes from these cells, the *neuropil*. These elements are encased in a coat of collagen with a surrounding thin basal lamina. There is no connective tissue sheath as such, and the coat of collagen and basal lamina is freely permeable.

The nerve cell bodies within a ganglion are only partly separated from one another by thin glial laminae. Nerve cell bodies come into very close apposition to one another, with no intervening glial elements, over quite considerable areas. Also, the surfaces of the nerve cell bodies have large areas of surface exposed to the extracellular space of the intermuscular plane. The ganglion is a densely-packed structure, a space of as little as 20 nm separating the membranes of the component cells. There is no conspicuous dedicated blood supply, but small blood vessels commonly ramify near ganglia.

Interganglionic fascicles connect the ganglia together. These are compact cylinders of axons with glial cells among them. They lack a connective tissue sheath, but they are surrounded by a thin basal lamina which is continuous with that of the ganglia.

The ganglia and interganglionic fascicles are organized to form a network, with the uniformly-disposed ganglia being joined by fascicles that extend in all directions to form a pattern of irregular polygons. The appearance of the plexus is much the same throughout the colon and anorectum, but there are minor variations. The ganglia tend to be a little more closely spaced along the line of the mesenteric insertion than they are remote from it, and a similar slight condensation of ganglia occurs beneath the taeniae coli. These are not marked or conspicuous differences. The ganglia become smaller and farther apart in the rectum, so that there are rather few in the rectal ampulla, at least in some species.

This polygonal mesh of ganglia and interganglionic fascicles is called the *primary plexus* of the myenteric plexus. Smaller fascicles branch from the major interganglionic fascicles to form a *secondary plexus* of fascicles within the polygonal interstices of the primary plexus. Still smaller axon bundles leave the fascicles of the secondary plexus to form a *tertiary plexus*, from which single axons depart to enter the layers of the muscularis propria. This pattern of primary, secondary and tertiary plexus tends to break down in the rectum. Here, the small ganglia, widely spaced, appear as appendages to an irregular network of coarse fascicles that seem to constitute, in large proportion, branches from the ascending nerves of the colon. The unique appearance of this plexus justifies it being called the *rectal myenteric plexus*, as distinct from the myenteric plexus of the rest of the colon.

The ganglia of the myenteric plexus in the colon are quite large. Quantitative studies have been done in only one species, the American opossum, to compare the density of the myenteric plexus among organs. The number of nerve cells in a single ganglion averages between 32 and 54 at various levels between the caecum and descending colon, and it falls to 13 in the rectum. In the rostral parts of the colon, some ganglia can be found that contain up to about 100 nerve cells. No such quantitative studies have been made in man. Not quite all nerve cell bodies are located in the ganglia proper. Solitary nerve cell bodies can be found occasionally buried in the interganglionic fascicles.

Just as the number and size of the ganglia diminish in the rectum, so also the density of distribution of nerve cells declines. In the opossum (again, where the only quantitative studies have been done), the number of nerve cell bodies per gram of tissue rises from 16×10^3 in the caecum to 35×10^3 in the ascending colon, and it declines from there to reach a nadir of 1.5×10^3 in the distal rectum. These values can be compared to 46×10^3 nerve cell bodies per gram of tissue in the small intestine in the same species.

Organization of the Submucous Plexus in the Colon and Anorectum

The submucous plexus differs considerably in arrangement from the myenteric plexus. The ganglia are smaller, further apart and much less uniformly distributed. The pattern of the ganglia and interganglionic fascicles is irregular and no secondary or tertiary orders of plexuses can be distinguished.

The sizes of the ganglia have actually only been determined carefully in the cat, where there are 13 to 31 nerve cells per ganglion, and in the opossum where there are 10 to 17. The number of ganglion cells in the submucous plexus of the cat was calculated at 1275 per cm^2 in the cephalic parts of the colon and 144 per cm^2 in the caudal part. Corresponding figures from the opossum are 206 per cm^2 and 61 per cm^2. These indicate a decline in the density of the submucous plexus toward the anus, just as the myenteric plexus density declines. These figures can be compared to the density of the submucous plexus of the small intestine in these same species, 3000–5000 cells per cm^2 in the cat and 1500–2200 cells per cm^2 in the opossum.

The description given above treats the submucous plexus as though it were a single structure. In fact it has three distinguishably separate layers. One is a layer of ganglia and fascicles lying close beneath the muscularis mucosae, sometimes called *Meissner's plexus* (a term that is also, confusingly, applied to the submucous plexus as a whole). A second layer of ganglia lies close to the circular layer of the muscularis propria. This is sometimes designated as *Henle's or Schabadasch's plexus*. These two layers are more distinctly separable in some species than in others. They are never completely separate structures, for they appear to be joined together by interganglionic fascicles.

A third laminar component of the submucous plexus is a very thin but very dense mat of axons with abundant interstitial cells of Cajal that covers the surface of the circular layer of the muscularis propria. The axons of this mat, called the *plexus submucosus extremus*, probably arise mainly from the ganglia of Henle's plexus. It was only described in 1971, but it has since been seen in many species including man. Its location implies that it represents some specialized innervation of the circular layer of the muscularis propria by the submucous plexus. It is not found in any other organ, and it is present in all parts of the colon. It is not clear how far it extends into the rectum. Its presence has been confirmed by electron microscopy in several species.

Interstitial Cells of Cajal (Thuneberg 1982)

The intramural nerves of the gut are intimately associated with certain cells that have the gross appearance of fibroblasts. These cells were long ago recognized at light microscopy as distinctive because of their special relationship to intramural nerve processes, and they were called, by Cajal, their discoverer, *interstitial cells*. These cells are not found with all nerves. In the colon they are particularly abundant in relationship to the myen-

teric plexus and in the plexus submucosus extremus. They are hard to find in the rest of the submucous plexus and in the ramifications of axons in the muscle layers.

These cells have the general form of fibroblasts with a single round or oval nucleus and long cytoplasmic processes. Their ultrastructure is different from fibroblasts, especially in the abundance of smooth endoplasmic reticulum. They always lie very close to axons, often as close as 20 nm, and their processes approach closely to smooth muscle cells and form gap junctions with them. These facts suggest that the interstitial cells are actively involved in the functional relationship between nerves and smooth muscle. Current evidence supports the idea that they are involved in the regulation of rhythmic activity in gastrointestinal muscle.

Nerve Terminals in the Wall of the Colon and Anorectum

Swellings or expansions all along the length of a terminal axon constitute the functional endings of such axons. These expansions, called the *varicosities*, are 1–2 μm in diameter and they are quite uniformly spaced, about 250–300 per mm of axonal length.

These varicosities contain several organelles characteristic of nerves, microtubules, neurofilaments, mitochondria and endoplasmic reticulum, but they are largely filled with structures that are uncommonly seen in other parts of the nerve cell, the *synaptic vesicles*. These vesicles vary a good deal in size, shape and appearance. The vesicles are packets of transmitter substances. Morphologic classifications have been made of vesicles in various types of axons in the hope of establishing a functional correlation of vesical morphology with the transmitter released. The validity of such correlations has been challenged, and so no firm correlations can yet be stated.

Most, if not all, of the varicose axons found in the muscle layers of the wall of the gut arise from nerve cell bodies in the ganglionated plexuses. Axons lie among the muscle cells running in bundles along the fibrous septa that separate muscle bundles and lying as triplet, duplet or singlet axons within the muscle bundles. Their density of distribution differs somewhat among the three muscle layers. They appear to be considerably less abundant in the longitudinal layer of the muscularis propria than they are in the circular layer of the muscularis propria. In these muscles, the larger nerve bundles are fairly completely surrounded by glial cells and their processes, but this wrapping becomes less complete as the bundles grow smaller. Singlet and doublet axons often lack a glial envelope. These terminal axons do not come into really close apposition to muscle cells. Generally, the closest approach of axons to smooth bundle cells is 40–100 nm. The muscle cells show no specialized structures at points where axons approach most closely.

Axons can be found in other parts of the wall as well. Arteries and arterioles are densely innervated with axons that are sympathetic, arising from the prevertebral ganglia. The venules are not innervated. Axons are also found in the lamina propria, but they are sparse at this level. The innervation of the epithelium is not conspicuous.

Problems in the Study of the Intramural Innervation of the Colon and Anorectum

Much of what is summarized above comes from studies of tissues other than the large intestine. Most of what is known about the morphology of the enteric nerves comes from the study of the small intestine of rodents. To the extent that the colon has been studied, however, the innervation generally conforms to the pattern of the small intestine, with the exceptions that have been noted above. The human organ, however, remains to be studied in such detail. For that reason, those concerned with function in the human colon and anorectum must keep in mind the possibility of unsuspected variations from the standard patterns.

References

Christensen J, Rick GA (1985) Nerve cell density in submucous plexus throughout the gut of cat and opossum. Gastroenterology 89:1064–1069

Christensen J, Rick GA (1987a) The distribution of myelinated nerves in the ascending nerves and myenteric plexus of the cat colon. Am J Anat 178:250–258

Christensen J, Rick GA (1987b) Intrinsic nerves in the mammalian colon: confirmation of a plexus at the circular muscle–submucosal interface. J Auton Nerv Syst 21:223–231

Christensen J, Rick GA, Robison BA, Stiles MJ, Wix MA (1983) The arrangement of the myenteric plexus throughout the gastrointestinal tract of the opossum. Gastroenterology 85:890–899

Christensen J, Stiles MJ, Rick GA, Sutherland J (1984) Comparative anatomy of the myenteric plexus of the distal colon in eight mammals. Gastroenterology 86:706–713

Clemente CD (1985) Gray's anatomy, 30th edn. Lea and Febiger, Philadelphia

Fawcett DW (1986) Bloom and Fawcett, a textbook of histology, 11th edn. Saunders, Philadelphia

Furness JB, Costa M (1987) The enteric nervous system. Churchill Livingstone, Edinburgh

Gabella G (1976) Structure of the autonomic nervous system. Chapman and Hall, London

Gabella G (1979) Innervation of the gastrointestinal tract. Int Rev Cytol 59:129–193

Gabella G (1987) Structure of muscles and nerves in the gastrointestinal tract. In: Johnson LR, Christensen J, Jackson MJ, Jacobson ED, Walsh JH (eds) Physiology of the gastrointestinal tract, 2nd edn, chap 11. Raven Press, New York

Hume ID (1982) Digestive physiology and nutrition of marsupials. In: Monographs on marsupial biology, chaps 2, 3, 4. Cambridge University Press, Cambridge, pp 27–109

Kuntz A (1953) The autonomic nervous system, 4th edn. Lea and Febiger, Philadelphia

Mitchell GAG (1953) Anatomy of the autonomic nervous system. Livingstone, Edinburgh

Stevens CE (1988) Comparative physiology of the vertebrate digestive system. Cambridge University Press, Cambridge

Thuneberg L (1982) Interstitial cells of Cajal: pacemaker cells? Adv Anat Embryol Cell Biol 71:1–130

2 · Measurement of Colonic Motor Function

C. J. Steadman and S. F. Phillips

Introduction

Overview of Colonic Function

The mammalian large intestine is a highly versatile organ that maintains fluid and electrolyte balance, salvages the products of intracolonic fermentation and stores faeces until elimination is convenient. These functions all depend ultimately on the colon's capacity to control the distal progression of contents. As chyme enters from the ileum, it is retained in the proximal colon, while colonic micro-organisms degrade indigestible food residues such as cellulose; water and electrolytes are absorbed actively at this time. The colonic contents are desiccated during further transit and solid faeces are formed, ready for defaecation. These processes are possible because colonic transit is much longer than is the time for movement through the rest of the gut.

Although these general statements are true for most mammals, colonic anatomy and function vary greatly among species. These differences largely reflect the composition of their diets. Monogastric herbivores, such as horses, have large sacculated or haustrated hindguts that accommodate large volumes of crude plant fibre, which are their major source of energy. In contrast, carnivores have short, narrow, poorly compartmentalized colons providing for only brief storage and rapid transit. Thus, the extent to which fibre residue is able to be fermented is related to retention (or transit) time (Van Soest 1988). Colonic motility and transit thus appear to be well matched to species specific differences in colonic anatomy and to the metabolic tasks that are necessary among the mammals.

Early Observations of Colonic Motility: Interspecies Differences

Much of the early information on colonic motility came from direct observations of colonic movements. At laparotomy, animals were studied after high obliterations of the spinal cord (Elliott and Barclay-Smith 1904); these were performed to increase the activity of the normally quiet colon.

In the rabbit, which has a large caecum, distension of the proximal colon with a vegetable paste caused churning contractions of the circular muscle and the caecum emptied by successive contractions of its wall. The guinea pig proximal colon exhibited antiperistalsis in response to distension, followed by swaying, oscillating sacculation of its wall; the caecum emptied by contraction of external longitudinal muscle bands which shortened the proximal colon. In the rat, which has a smaller caecum, antiperistalsis and less frequent, but simultaneous, aborad peristalsis was noted.

Carnivores, with smaller proximal colons, showed further differences. In cats, distension of the proximal third of the colon caused antiperistalsis, while distension in the intermediate and distal colons caused distally propulsive contractions. Fluoroscopy of the cat colon had previously shown antiperistalsis in vivo, both in the proximal colon, where it was the most common contractile event, and in the distal colon in response to water enemas (Cannon 1902). Antiperistalsis was never observed in the dog (Elliott and Barclay-Smith 1904) but the caecum was able to contract often and with great force "to [form] a hard white knob".

General Observations of Colonic Function in Man

Human colonic anatomy is adapted to an omnivorous diet; thus, like herbivores, the proximal colon is more voluminous and has more prominent haustration when compared to carnivores. The proximal colon in man contains fermentative bacteria which degrade organic material, principally fibrous complex carbohydrate, to short chain fatty acids. The predominant ionic species are acetate, propionate and butyrate. Short chain fatty acids are rapidly absorbed from the colon where they also augment sodium, chloride and water absorption (Ruppin et al. 1980); they are also a source of energy for human colonic epithelial cells (Roediger 1982). The fermentative and absorptive processes appear to be facilitated by proximal colonic contractile activity which stirs and mixes the colonic contents.

In man, the colon normally absorbs approximately 1.5 l ileal effluent each day (Phillips and Giller 1973), mainly in the proximal colon (Devroede et al 1971). Further desiccation of colonic contents occurs as they are propelled distally, and the end result is the convenient elimination of approximately 100–200 g formed stool in one or two bowel movements per day (Connell et al 1965; Rendtorff and Kashgarian 1967). When stressed by increased volumes of ileal effluent, the colon can absorb up to 4–6 l/d (Debongnie and Phillips 1978) before diarrhoea develops. The contribution of changes in colonic motility to the colonic absorptive reserve is uncertain; however faster rates of caecal infusion impaired the colonic capacity to reabsorb fluids (Debongnie and Phillips 1978).

The presence of haustral segmentation is an obvious difference between the small intestine and the colon. Haustration is not fixed, but results from frequent and variable muscular contractions of the colonic wall. However, direct observations of colonic contractile activity, haustrations and the volume of the colon, comparable to those made in animals under conditions of distension and altered nervous control, are clearly not possible in man. Instead, measurement of colonic contractile events in man depends on indirect observations with methods such as intraluminal manometry and electromyography. Both approaches have limited application because access to the colon in vivo is difficult. What has become clear is that the human colon has an extremely complex pattern of motility and few repetitive activities can be demonstrated reliably. This has meant that both the myogenic control activity of the colon, and its higher governing influences, have proven very difficult to dissect. In some persons, defaecation appears to be by "clockwork"; thus, colonic motility might best be summarized as the overall levels of activity that occur during each hour of the day. Such an approach did show diurnal rhythmicity in colonic contractility, with peaks occurring after waking in the morning and postprandially (Narducci et al. 1987).

Colonic Electromyography

The recording of electrical activity generated by the outer longitudinal and inner circular muscle layers of the colon is an important index of colonic physiology, but it has not yet achieved a significant role in clinical gastroenterology. In the small intestine, the basal electrical rhythm of the slow wave is a consistent finding and it is an index of physiology and pathophysiology. On the other hand, electrical activity in the colon is a complex and highly variable phenomenon (Huizinga and Daniel 1986); in addition, observations of colonic myoelectric activity in animal models show many differences from those made in man. Thus, the marked interspecies differences in the colon's anatomy and motility are also reflected by its neuromuscular structure and function (Christensen et al. 1984).

Neuromuscular Organization of the Human Colon

The human colonic muscularis propria is composed of (a) a continuous outer longitudinal layer thickened in three regions to form the taeniae coli, which are partially subdivided by incomplete longitudinal grooves (Daniel 1975) and (b) an inner circular muscle coat arranged in loosely packed bundles (Huizinga and Daniel 1986). The taeniae coli merge together in the distal sigmoid colon and rectum. The myenteric plexus (of Auerbach) lies between the circular and longitudinal muscle layers. Ganglion cells in this plexus lie mainly beneath the taeniae coli, are present in greater numbers in the proximal colon and are virtually absent in the lower anal canal. A deep muscular plexus lies within circular muscle, but it has only a few cell bodies and the submucous plexus (Meisner's plexus) has its major role in regulation of mucosal function (Furness and Costa 1980). Recently, the role of a plexus containing the interstitial cells of Cajal and found at the inner surface of the circular muscle layer (Christensen and Rick 1987) has been emphasized. These cells may be responsible for the generation of slow wave potentials (Thuneberg et al. 1982).

Relationship Between Neuromuscular Organization and Myoelectric Activity

Compared to that of the small intestine, colonic myoelectric activity is extremely variable in the basal state. In the small intestine, myogenic control mechanisms are tightly coordinated so that the oscillating electric potential in the muscularis propria (slow wave) is phase coupled, between the circular and longitudinal muscle layers, and circumferentially at any point (Daniel 1975). Gap junctions, which minimize electrical impedance between smooth muscle cells, provide a structural basis for synchronous electrical activity. A distally declining frequency gradient in the small intestine also allows the high frequency electrical oscillations of the proximal small bowel to function as a pacemaker and so to govern distal events. When the oscillating membrane potential depolarizes beyond the smooth muscle excitation threshold, bursts of rapid electrical oscillations or "spikes" occur in association with contractions. The frequency of electrical oscillation therefore determines the frequency of bursts of spikes and the associated contractions (Sarna 1985).

In the colon, the slow wave frequency is highly variable (4–48/min) and, indeed, is present only inconsistently (Huizinga et al. 1985). In vitro studies provide some insight into these diverse observations. The electrical activity of isolated, unstimulated, opened rings of human colonic circular muscle was synchronized only infrequently with the frequency of slow waves or with the electrical spiking. Cholinergic stimulation (carbachol) of these preparations evoked synchronized, periodic slow waves with superimposed spikes. Regular phasic contractions, at the fre-

quency of the bursts of electrical activity (approx 1/min), were blocked by atropine, but not tetrodotoxin (a nonspecific neurotoxin). This was thought to be consistent with a stimulus-induced pattern of myogenic activity resembling long spike bursts recorded in vivo (see Table 2.1 and Huizinga and Waterfall 1988). In longitudinal muscle, spontaneous electrical activity at a mean frequency of 26 cycles/min and an amplitude of 8 millivolts has been recorded, with spiking activity superimposed on the oscillations. Contractions in the longitudinal muscle corresponded to the frequency of bursts of oscillations, but not to the frequency of individual oscillations (Chow and Huizinga 1987).

Coupling appears to occur between the circular and longitudinal muscle layers in man, possibly by electrotonic spread of slow wave potentials through the smooth muscle cells (Huizinga and Chow 1988), however the anatomical basis for this interaction (e.g., intermingled smooth muscle fibres and intercellular connections such as gap junctions) is uncertain. In any case, resting membrane potentials are the same in the two muscle layers and spontaneous electrical activity showed similarities (Huizinga and Chow 1988). Possibly, slow waves spread towards the serosal surface from interstitial cells of Cajal located on the inner (mucosal) surface of the circular muscle layer (Smith et al. 1987).

In Vivo Recording of Human Colonic Myoelectric Activity

In vivo recordings of human colonic myoelectrical activity are characterized by variability over time, among subjects and between the results from different laboratories. Electrical control activity has been reported to be continuous (Sarna et al. 1981, 1982) or intermittent (Snape et al. 1976; Taylor et al. 1975) and to consist of two prominent frequency bands from 2–4 cycles/min and 6–12 cycles/min (Taylor et al. 1975; Snape et al. 1976) or a range of high and low frequencies. Spiking has been reported to be both unrelated or related to the slow wave, and contractions may or may not accompany spiking. Table 2.1 shows possible relationships between the in vitro and in vivo data on myoelectrical and contractile activity of the human colon.

There are a number of reasons why such variability could exist. Electrical activities arising from other parts of the gut may be recorded in the colon (Fioramonti et al. 1982); however, the intrinsic frequency of slow waves (electrical control

Table 2.1. Electrical and contractile activity in the human colon

In vitro observations			In vivo
Muscle	Electrical activity	Contractile activity	Electrical activity–potential correlations
Circular muscle Spontaneous	Low amplitude oscillation at 4.5–12 cpm		Slow waves (Taylor et al. 1974; Bueno et al. 1980) Electrical control activity (Sarna et al. 1982)
	With spike on oscillations	Contractions 4–12/min	Short spike bursts (Snape et al. 1976; Bueno et al. 1980) Discrete electrical response activity (Sarna et al. 1982)
	12–60 cpm	Summated (prolonged contraction)	Contractile electrical complex (Sarna et al. 1982)
Cholinergic stimulation	Continuous oscillations 12–24 cpm	Tonic contraction	
	Prolonged depolarizations (1–3 cpm) with spiking	Phasic contractions 1–3/min	Long spike bursts (Bueno et al. 1980; Schang and Devroede 1983)
Circular and longitudinal muscle			
	Bursts of oscillation at 14–24 cpm (circular) and 20–30 cpm (longitudinal) with superimposed spiking	Broad phasic contractions	Continuous electrical response activity (Sarna et al. 1982) Contractile electrical complex (Sarna et al. 1982) Long spike bursts

Modified from Huizinga and Daniel (1986); Huizinga et al. (1985, 1986).

activity) in vitro appears to vary more widely in man than in animals (Huizinga et al. 1985). Indeed, whether the circular and longitudinal muscle layers are consistently phase-coupled is unknown, even though in vitro studies suggest electrical communication between the layers (Huizinga and Chow 1988). From a technical sense, very low amplitude oscillations which occur in the absence of a stimulus may become indistinguishable from recording noise (Huizinga and Daniel 1986).

Technical factors are also germane to interobserver variability. Recording methods include bipolar electrodes on the serosal surface under the taeniae coli (Sarna et al. 1981; Taylor et al. 1975) and monopolar or bipolar electrodes attached to the colonic mucosa by suction. Electrodes have also been mounted on intraluminal tubes (Schang et al. 1986; Welgan et al. 1988) or clipped to the mucosal surface (Battle et al. 1980). These techniques all potentially record different electrical signals and poor mucosal contact by intraluminal electrodes appears to impair the recording of spiking activity. Most intraluminal recordings have been from the distal colon but more proximal segments have been sampled recently, by colonoscopic placement of electrodes (Dapoigny et al. 1988). Serosal electrodes probably record prefer-

entially activity from longitudinal rather than circular muscle.

The time of day, meals and the nature of the colonic contents all may affect colonic contractile and myoelectric activity. Thus, colonic myoelectrical activity is diurnal; there is little activity during sleep, but activity increases in the morning, after meals and during periods of stress (Dapoigny et al. 1988; Schang et al. 1988; Schang and Devroede 1983; Frexinos et al. 1985). Postprandial activity is influenced by the composition of meals such that a high calorie meal caused a greater increase in colonic activity than did a low calorie meal and ingestion of an amino acid mixture inhibited myoelectric activity (Battle et al. 1980).

Colonic myoelectric activity has also been scrutinized by a number of sophisticated techniques. Fast Fourier Transformations use samples of computerized recordings to identify dominant frequencies that may be present in what is, otherwise, irregular activity. This method was intended for the analysis of events in which overlapping frequencies remain constant throughout a recording. If frequencies change during a recording, the analysis may not reflect the true activity. Filtering the signal before analysis also affects results (Sunshine et al. 1985). Pattern recognition programmes have also been used to analyse myoelectric and contractile activity (Parker et al. 1987). Computerized pattern recognition has the advantage of greater test–retest reliability when compared with visual analysis, but it has produced results different from those of Fast Fourier Transformations. Thus, electromyography of the human colon must still be judged to be in a developmental stage.

Measurement of Colonic Contractile Activity (Colonic Manometry)

Pressure waves recorded manometrically are generally equated with contractile forces. In concordance with observations of myoelectrical activity, colonic contractions have also been found to be irregular, of varying frequency and amplitude and subject to many controlling influences. Individual emotional states, the types of meals that are eaten and the composition of chyme entering the colon from the ileum are all known to modulate colonic contractile activity, but they vary significantly in their importance in any person from hour to hour and day to day (Misiewicz 1984).

Techniques for Recording Colonic Motility

Colonic manometry has developed considerably from early attempts using compressible balloons

and open ended, air-filled tubes (Spriggs et al. 1951; Connell 1961a); today, high fidelity, internal strain gauges, electronic transducers, and pneumohydraulic capillary infusion systems linked to external transducers (Arndorfer et al. 1977) are available. Records can be retained for analysis by a variety of direct writing and computerized data storage systems. Current developments feature the refinement of ambulatory systems for prolonged recording that should allow motor patterns to be sampled day and night for several days outside the laboratory environment (Soffer et al. 1989).

Despite the improving quality of recording and analytical technology, records of colonic motility only provide general insights into the control of colonic contractile events. There are few recognizable patterns that occur within limited periods of observation, access to the colonic lumen is sometimes difficult and signals produced by the different types of pressure sensors vary. Thus, some intraluminal strain gauges may show directly opposite signals to serosal standards or capillary infusion manometry (Cook et al. 1988). Difficulties with access have up to now limited most studies of colonic motility to the rectum and distal sigmoid, the limit for insertion of a rigid sigmoidoscope. However, colonoscopy is now used to place motility sensors throughout the colon (Sugihara et al. 1983; Sasaki et al. 1986).

Basal Colonic Motility

Cyclical contractile activity with general similarities to the migrating motor complex of the small intestine was found in the colon of dogs (Sarna et al. 1984; Flourie et al. 1989; Fig. 2.1). Bursts of

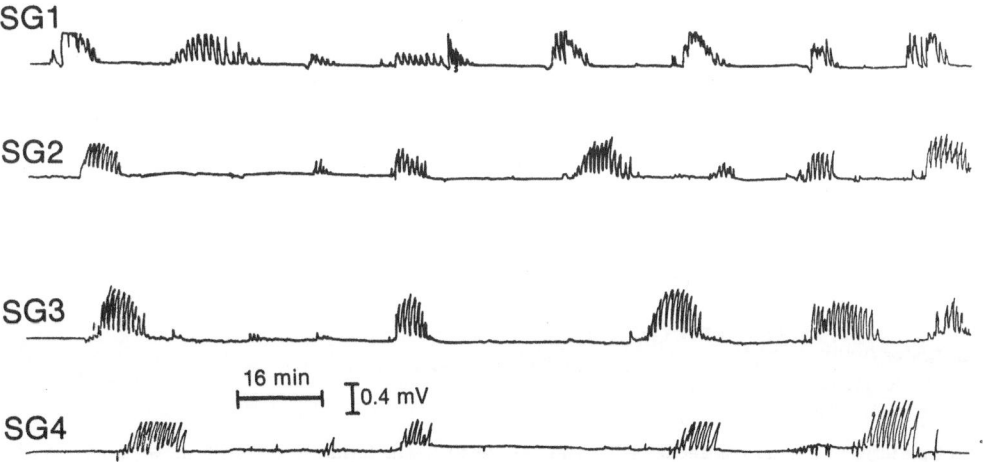

Fig. 2.1. Strain gauge (SG) recording from the proximal (1) to distal (4) canine colon showing cyclic bursts of contractions alternating with quiescent states at all recording sites. (From Sarna et al. (1984) with permission of the authors and publishers.)

contractile activity occur in the fasting and fed states; they migrate in orad and caudad directions. Stationary bursts also occur. However, in man, colonic cyclical contractile activity has not been reported.

Recordings of resting colonic motility made for short periods suggest that the colon is often "quiet" or that contractions are often isolated; sometimes, pressure waves are recorded in continuous bursts ranging in duration from 10 to 30 minutes (Kerlin et al. 1983). These bursts have a dominant frequency of approximately six contractions per minute in the right colon, but higher and lower frequencies have also been observed. In the distal colon, contractions are present in frequencies of 2.5 to 3.5 and approximately seven per minute (Kerlin et al. 1983; Fig. 2.2), but marked intra- and interindividual variation is the rule.

Phasic pressure waves are the most common pattern of activity but the role of phasic contractions in enhancing colonic absorption or facilitating propulsion is not well defined. Phasic colonic contractions are stimulated by meals, the response being characterized by increased numbers of pressure waves, usually expressed as a colonic motility index (a representation of the cumulative number and amplitude of pressure waves occurring in a predetermined period of time). Motility indices increase 20–30 minutes after a meal and they remain elevated for up to 3 hours, sometimes with a biphasic pattern when a peak of activity occurs at approximately 70–90 minutes (Holdstock et al. 1970; Holdstock and Misiewicz 1970). The response to eating remains despite absence of the stomach and after vagotomy (Duthie 1978). Thus, even in the absence of the stomach, food arriving in the small intestine elicits increased activity from the colon. If the stomach is intact, gastric distension and the chemical stimulation by nutrients elicits a comparable response. Lipids are the most potent nutrient (Wiley et al. 1988; Snape et al. 1979). The colonic response to eating occurs in all parts of the colon, but contractile events differ quantitatively from segment to segment (Kerlin et al. 1983; Kock et al. 1968).

Control of the colonic response to eating involves neural and, possibly, hormonal mechanisms. That part of the response mediated by gastric mechanoreceptors is very sensitive to blockade by atropine, but that mediated by the small intestine is only partially muscarinic. Cholecystokinin

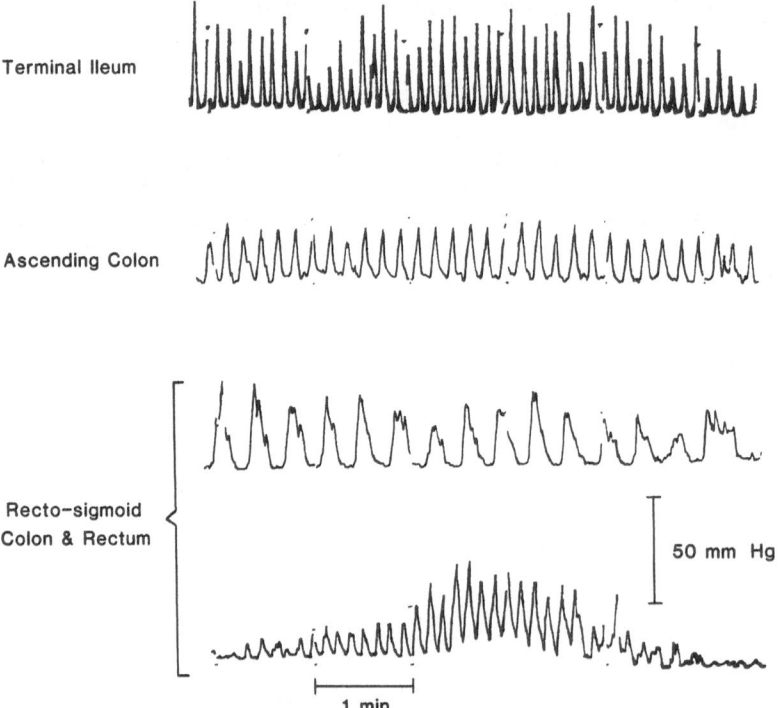

Terminal Ileum

Ascending Colon

Recto-sigmoid Colon & Rectum

50 mm Hg

1 min

Fig. 2.2. Compendium of patterns of regular contractile activity at various loci. The terminal ileal strip shows a portion of an activity front (phase 3) of the MMC; the ascending colon shows a burst of regular contractions of 5.6 contractions/min. The patterns of regular activity in the rectosigmoid colon and the rectum are shown in the lower two panels (from Kerlin and Zinsmeister (1983) with permission of the authors and publishers).

(CCK), which is normally secreted after meals, may have a role in the response since high blood concentrations of CCK stimulate contractile activity in both the small and large intestine (Kellow et al. 1987; Wiley et al. 1988). Increased phasic contractile activity also occurs in response to drugs, particularly morphine and prostigmine, but it is reduced by meperidine and largely abolished by anticholinergics (Painter and Truelove 1964a, b).

Longer periods of observation may well elucidate colonic motility, but there are still relatively few data of this type. Like pieces of a puzzle, data gained from shorter periods of study can be viewed as part of the overall diurnal cycle occurring in parallel with myoelectrical activity. Low amplitude contractions, appearing in bursts (at a frequency of approximately 3/min or 6–8/min) or singly, constitute most of each day's contractile activity.

Colonic Peristalsis

The early concept of categorizing intestinal contractile activity into segmentation and peristalsis is still useful in understanding colonic motility. Irregular phasic activity does not appear to propagate and equates with segmentation while high pressure, propagating waves are the peristaltic equivalent. In the dog, ricinoleic acid (the active principal of castor oil) instilled into the colonic lumen or drugs like guanethidine and neostigmine stimulate powerful, rapidly propagating contractions (giant migrating contractions) that propel colonic contents distally and cause defaecation (Karaus and Sarna 1987).

In man, manometry shows the diurnal pattern of propagated pressure waves more clearly than myoelectrical studies; unstimulated, isolated, high amplitude (up to 200 mgHg) peristaltic contractions, propagating at 1 cm/s over long distances, are uncommon but most frequently seen after waking and meals (Narducci et al. 1987). However, peristaltic waves occur reliably after instillation of irritants like bisacodyl and oxyphenisatin into the colonic lumen. Physical factors like distension of the resting colon, pH and the osmotic tonicity of colonic contents are not potent initiators of peristalsis, but may be important when the colon has been previously "primed" for peristalsis by other influences (Hardcastle and Mann 1968, 1970). Oleic acid (fat), infused into the colonic lumen to model steatorrhoea, stimulates powerfully propulsive contractile activity composed of high pressure (greater than 60 mmHg, range 60–95), long duration (greater than 10 s, range 10–48) propagating waves of contraction (Spiller et al. 1986). However, long-lasting, powerful contractions may not always be distally propulsive as the colon also generates high pressure (10–44 cm H_2O), low frequency (0.2–1.8/min) waves in the left colon during colonic perfusion with saline solution. These waves occur between the regularly-occurring, propagated and propulsive waves that come from the right colon during perfusion, and they appear to interrupt distal flow and cause retention of perfusate in the right colon (Chauve et al. 1976).

Future Directions

The future will see manual analysis of colonic contractile activity largely replaced by computerized analysis. Although manual analysis can provide an overall perspective easily lost in computerized approaches, automated analysis is more rapid and reproducible. It not only generates motility indices (as done by older electronic integrators) but can dissect the components of motility indices such as pressure peak counts and amplitude means or spectra (Rogers and Misiewicz 1989). Objective computer analysis is free from interobserver bias; however, it retains an observer based weakness in that it is extremely dependent on the arbitrarily-set programming instructions used to analyse the raw manometric record. Computer software will need to focus on the aperiodicity of pressure events and on determining propagation of pressure waves within complexes of activity. These new approaches may predictably define patterns of response to varying stimuli, such as different meals, where Fast Fourier and pattern recognition methods have been unsuccessful. Further impetus to computerization comes from the evolving technology being applied to 24-hour ambulatory monitoring (Soffer et al. 1989). The scientific advantages gained by freedom from laboratory-based data gathering are countered by the practical problems of analysing very long records unless computers are used to store and analyse data coming from portable electronic recorders.

Measurement of the Transit of Colonic Contents

Historical Perspectives

As early as Cannon's (1902) observations on the movement of bismuth subnitrate in the feline colon, it has been clear that colonic contents do not leave the colon in the same order in which they enter. Thus, in healthy man, glass beads of different colours given on successive days appear in the stool around 24 to 72 hours from the time of ingestion, but they are mixed together (Alvarez and Freedlander 1924). Many different types of markers have been tried ranging from knots of cellulose thread to gold and silver shapes (Hoelzel 1930). Differences in passage of these different particulate markers, as judged by their appearance in the stool, appeared to be proportional to their specific gravity; heavier material passed more slowly than did lighter contents. Cinefluorography of barium impregnated colonic contents (Ritchie 1968; Ritchie et al. 1971) has demonstrated mixing, storage and propulsion of colonic contents. Interhaustral shuttling, propulsion, retropulsion and movements to and fro mix the colonic contents. Propulsion and retropulsion appear to occur in similar ways. Contents move from one haustrum to the next, through multihaustral segments and by interhaustral propulsion. During multihaustral propulsion, three or more haustral segments become contiguous and the mass of contents moves onto the next segment, while the original haustration is reformed. Interhaustral propulsion and peristalsis are similar, but peristaltic contractions usually start as interhaustral constrictions, travel further along the colon, and are able to propel faeces distally. Defaecation invariably empties the distal colon, but colonic contents orad to those that are emptied may be relatively unaffected at the end of defaecation. The rectum is usually the only region which empties although, at times, material from the distal transverse colon can be eliminated (Edwards and Beck 1971; Halls 1965).

Rationale of Measures of Colonic Transit

Although cinefluorography describes the movements of contents, it does not quantify colonic transit. Quantification requires the use of a marker, the appearance of which in the faeces, or its imaging in segments of the colon, can be analysed mathematically. Marker substances can be taken orally or introduced directly into the caecum and can be given as a single bolus, repeated boluses or continuously. Observing the appearance and disappearance of markers in stools (mouth to anus transit) quantifies total colonic transit, but it does not assess changes in transit through colonic segments (segmental transit). Whole gut or segmental colonic transit can be expressed simply as the time taken for a proportion of the marker to pass by the location of interest (e.g. 80% emptying of a colonic segment). A better approach is to describe transit in terms of segmental or whole colonic half-emptying times ($T\frac{1}{2}$). The latter method takes into account the exponential emptying of marker materials from one colonic segment to the next.

The common principle underlying marker methods is to observe the time taken by any marker to reach a particular location or to reach the stool. If it were possible to observe continuously the movement of many distinct markers, the exact moment that each marker passed the location of interest could be precisely timed. An average of these times takes into account the variations in propulsion and retropulsion (mixing) to which each marker is subjected. Clearly, such variations are important, or all markers taken at the same time would appear at any point together. Variations in transit time can theoretically by controlled in several ways. Any system which delivers markers to the colon as a bolus minimizes the effects of gastric emptying and small intestinal transit on arrival of markers in the colon. If a large number of markers is used, then their mean transit should be more representative of the true transit time; moreover, administration of markers over increasingly long periods should minimize sampling error caused by day-to-day variation in bowel function. Frequent observations are more precise because markers may be lost in the stool before their transit time has been measured and, from the interpretive viewpoint, more widely spaced observations reduce the resolution of the test.

Which Transit Marker Is Best?

Barium

The widespread use of barium in contrast radiography of the gut led to trials of barium as a marker of intestinal transit (Alvarez and Freedlander 1924). When barium is ingested with food, the arrival of the head of the column and disappearance of all barium from the colon can be used to quantify transit from the mouth to the colonic segments or anus. After 24 hours, barium appeared in the rectum of 60% of normal subjects, 84% of patients with diverticulosis and 90% of patients with irritable bowel syndrome (Manousos et al. 1967). Approximately 4 or 5 days are necessary for 70%–80% of the barium to leave the colon. Barium has major disadvantages as a marker as it may influence the transit of contents through the gut (Alvarez and Freedlander 1924) and repeated x-rays are required. As only the progress of the head of the barium column and disappearance of contrast can be observed, transit times probably reflect the mixing as much as aborad propulsion of colonic contents.

Chemical Markers

Dyes (e.g. carmine red) and chemicals (e.g. chromium sesquioxide, copper thiocyanate) have been used but they have no advantages and quantitation of their recovery in faeces is sometimes difficult. Orally administered radioactive chromium-51, given as chromic oxide powder or sodium chromate solution, can be measured in the stool by scintillation counting (Hansky and Connell 1962). This method allowed three parameters of colonic transit to be measured, i.e. time to initial appearance, time to maximum counts and time of disappearance from stool. The method did not allow any assessment of the movement of contents through the colonic segments and recovery of chromate in the stool can be compromised by absorption and urinary excretion of the isotope (Donaldson and Barreras 1966).

Radio-opaque Marker Techniques

Whole Gut Transit. Discrete, barium impregnated polythene markers move with the colonic contents. Halls (1965) followed markers with abdominal x-rays, and estimated shifts of bowel content during defaecation. Later, Hinton et al. (1969) measured gastrointestinal transit times using solid, 2–5 mm polythene pellets, containing barium sulphate 20% (W/W), and small (2.7–4.5 mm diameter) pieces of radio-opaque polythene tubing. These inert, nonabsorbable markers were completely recoverable in the stool and had a specific gravity similar to gut contents. Markers appeared in the stool at similar times to orally administered liquid ^{51}Cr and powdered carmine red. When followed by either abdominal radiographs or stool radiography, the movement of such markers was taken to represent the transit of meal residues through the gut. No significant differences were found in the transit of markers when they were given immediately before or with a meal. In 25 normal male subjects, all but one had passed 80% of the markers by the fifth day after ingestion but none had passed 80% by the end of the first day (Hinton et al. 1969). All subsequent work with radio–opaque markers has been directed at refining this range of normality, reducing x-ray exposure and minimizing inconvenience (such as stool collections).

Methods involving many radio-opaque markers (15/day) taken over a long period (6 weeks) were compared to Hinton's single dose method (Cummings et al. 1976). This technique depended on the appearance of markers in stool and used a simple mathematical transformation to convert the number of markers in stool to a time in hours, by taking into account the period between marker ingestion and appearance of markers in the stools. Calculation of the colonic transit time utilized the turnover of markers accumulated in the colonic pool at "equilibrium", i.e. when daily elimination equalled the number ingested. Comparison of continuous and single dose marker methods showed a good correlation. A test for whole gut transit requiring collection of only a single stool was also developed (Cummings and Wiggins 1976).

Segmental Colonic Transit. The rate of disappearance of radio-opaque markers from colonic segments can be monitored with daily abdominal x-rays after a single dose of 20 radio-opaque markers (Martelli et al. 1978a, b). Right and left colonic, sigmoid and rectal segments can be defined by simply drawing lines between bony landmarks of the vertebral column and pelvis and confirming the validity of the segments using gas shadows (Arhan et al. 1981; Fig. 2.3). Two days after administration, markers may be found in all colonic segments; over two to eight days markers move from the right to the left colon with exponential emptying of markers from each segment. In a study of 114 healthy adults and children, none retained markers after eight days (Martelli et al. 1978a).

The French and Canadian groups (Martelli et al. 1978a) who began segmental analysis of colonic transit went on to develop a method that allowed calculation of actual segmental transit times,

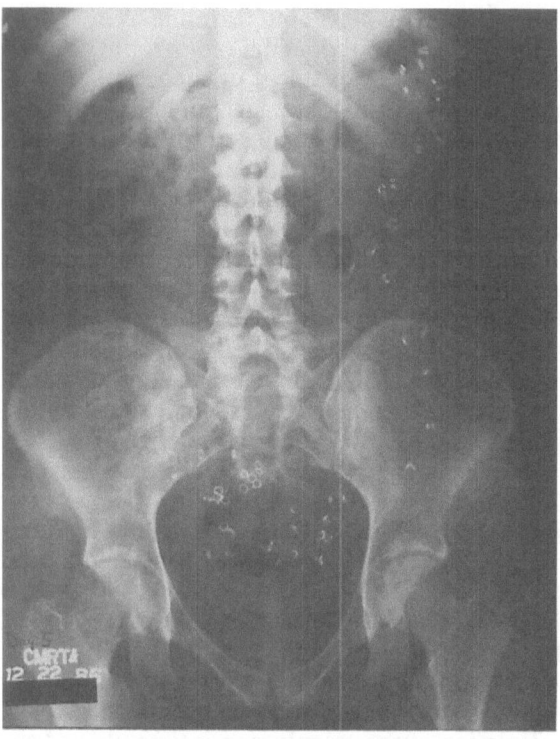

Fig. 2.3. Plain radiograph of the abdomen showing 3 types of radio-opaque markers. In the absence of clear outlines of the colon, markers to the right of the vertebral spinous processes above a line from the fifth lumbar vertebra to the pelvic outlet can be assigned to the right colon, those to the left of the processes and above a line from the fifth lumbar vertebra to the anterior superior iliac spine, to the left colon, and the remainder to the rectosigmoid colon and rectum.

rather than the rate of disappearance of markers from colonic segments (Arhan et al. 1981). A mathematical expression based on the time interval between serial abdominal x-rays describes the continuous change in numbers of markers at any location in the colon. Unfortunately, this method involves repeated abdominal x-ray exposure and the accompanying inconvenience of repeated visits to the hospital. Metcalf et al (1987) simplified this method so that only one x-ray with a fast film, high-kilovoltage technique is necessary and radiation exposure is minimal. Radio-opaque markers are taken in fixed numbers (20/d) at the same time (arbitrarily, 9:00 a.m.) each day for three days. Instead of having daily x-rays, on the fourth day, again at the same time, a radiograph is taken. Assuming that the colon handles all the markers the same way, the number of markers present on a single radiograph taken on the fourth day is equivalent to the total number of markers present on the first three sequential x-rays after a single bolus of markers. The results obtained from this technique correlate well with the daily x-ray approach, and are shown in Table 2.2 and Fig. 2.4. Both this method and the repeated x-ray method work on the assumption that a 24-hour sampling interval (either daily x-rays or markers) approximates continuous observation. Although distinctive markers can be used to estimate day-to-day variability in transit and mixing of contents (Becker and Elsborg 1979; Metcalf et al. 1987), they are not necessary for transit calculations (Chaussade et al. 1986, 1987). Rapid transit can cause all the markers to be lost in the faeces before

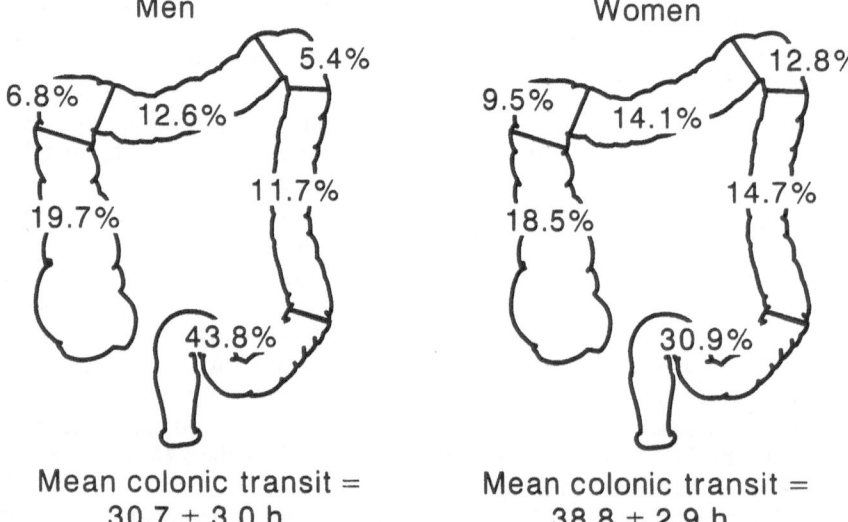

Fig. 2.4. Proportion of total colonic transit time spent in caecum and ascending colon, hepatic flexure, transverse colon, splenic flexure, descending colon, sigmoid colon and rectum in 73 healthy persons who had colonic transit assessed by the single abdominal x-ray technique. (From Metcalf et al. (1987) with permission of the authors and publishers.)

Table 2.2. Mean colonic transit times in 73 healthy persons estimated from a single fourth day abdominal x-ray that followed 3 days on which 20 radio-opaque markers were taken each morning

Variable	Colonic transit (h)			
	Right colon	Left colon	Rectosigmoid	Total colon
Gender				
Men (*n*=34)	8.9±1.1	8.7±1.5	13.0±1.7	30.7±3.0
Women (*n*=39)	13.3±1.6	13.7+2.1	11.8±1.6	38.8±2.9
Fibre				
Supplemented (*n*=39)	10.9±1.6	11.0±1.6	12.9±1.7	34.7±2.9
Not supplemented (*n*=34)	11.7±1.1	11.9±2.2	11.7±1.5	35.3±3.1
Age				
>40 yr (*n*=21)	9.4±1.6	11.8±2.8	11.8±1.6	33.0±3.9
<40 yr (*n*=52)	12.0±1.3	11.2±1.5	12.6±1.4	35.8±2.5

From Metcalf et al. (1987), with permission of the authors and publishers.
Men had significantly shorter whole colonic transit times compared with women but no effect of age or dietary fibre was detected.

radiography and, conversely in slow transit, all 60 markers may be present on the single radiograph. A day 7 film can then give more information. At present, the technique of Metcalf et al. (1987) is the safest and most practical way of reproducibly measuring segmental and total colonic transit within the limits of intra- and interindividual variation.

Radio-isotope Methods

The progress of gamma emitting radio-isotopes through the colon can be measured using a gamma camera linked to a computerized recording and processing system.

In contrast to x-ray methods, continuous observation of the isotope, or isotope-labelled material, is possible for long periods without increasing radiation exposure. Images can be quantified using scintillation counts; the transit of solids and liquids can be measured simultaneously if different isotopes are used to label liquid and solid bowel contents and intestinal regions of interest can be easily studied. Importantly, (a) the volume of radio-isotopes needed for satisfactory images is negligible, (b) when bound to suitable carrier molecules (e.g. diethylene triamine pentacetic acid (DTPA)) isotopes are poorly absorbed and biologically inert and (c) there is no patient discomfort in their use.

Although gamma scintigraphy has been applied successfully to the quantification of gastric emptying, where the method is in regular clinical use, its use in the large intestine is not so straightforward. Thus, if isotopes are given by mouth, one consequence of oro-caecal transit of the marker will be its dispersion within ileal contents and (probably) a prolonged period of ileo-caecal transfer. There may also be practical problems of isotope in jejuno-ileum overlying regions of interest in the colon. On the other hand, direct instillation of isotope into the colon requires oro-caecal intubation or colonoscopy.

Krevsky et al. (1986) and Spiller et al. (1986) instilled liquid isotope directly into the colon and Camilleri et al. (1989) followed labelled solids from the stomach, through the small bowel and across the ileocolonic junction. Colonic filling often included bolus movements of isotope separated by "plateaux" during which little isotope moved from small to large bowel (Camilleri et al. 1989). This finding raised the possibility that if a bolus of isotope could be delivered to the distal ileum it might be possible to define a "zero-time", when essentially all isotope entered the most proximal segment, e.g. the caecum–ascending colon. Such a starting time could then serve as a suitable base from which emptying curves could be constructed.

A pH sensitive polymer which dissolves at the pH of the ileum has been used to coat capsules containing isotopically labelled beads (Proano et al. 1990). By this approach, it has been possible to image the unprepared colon, without the use of intubation; it is hoped that such methods will allow more physiological measurements of colonic transit. Important questions still need to be addressed, such as the possibility of differential transits of solids and liquids, and the effects of particle size on transit as well as the quantification of transit in disease.

Finally, some have placed isotope into capsules or tablets that are designed to pass intact through the small intestine and colon (Kirwan and Smith 1974; Waller 1975; Hardy et al. 1987). Gastric retention of larger capsules (Mojaverian et al. 1985) and possible differences in how the colon handles large capsules as compared to food residues (Parker et al. 1988) probably limit the usefulness of such approaches.

The best approach to the analysis of colonic scintigraphy is still debated. Dividing the colon into regions of interest and producing time–activity graphs for each region is generally accepted methodology, but the best way to describe segmental transit is uncertain. Averaging of counts from different colonic regions of interest is an alternative; this yields a "geometric centre" of radio-activity which can be followed along the colon in sequential images (Krevsky et al. 1986). However, if the distribution of isotope in the colon is uneven, distal progression of the geometric centre may not represent the transit times through different colonic segments. The physics of scintillation counting must also be considered; factors include the decay of isotopes, tissue attenuation (absorption) of radiation (Collins et al. 1984) and overlap between radiation energies when two isotopes are used.

Combined Measurement of Motility and Transit

Only a few studies have attempted to correlate colonic motility and transit. When myoelectrical activity, intraluminal pressure and flow of an infused fluid were recorded together in the distal colon, rhythmic short (3 s) bursts of spiking electrical activity were associated with small rises in intraluminal pressure but no increase in flow. Sporadic, long spike bursts (range 3–120 s; mean 12) were associated with higher intraluminal pressures and flow to the rectum was greatest when the long bursts propagated distally (Schang et al. 1986). Although slow distal transit has been associated with increased phasic pressure activity, the particular pressure patterns that propel colonic contents (or those that retard flow) are uncertain. Phasic activity may often result in interhaustral shuttling of colonic contents and little aboral movement.

The most clear relationship between colonic motility and transit is seen when distally propagating, high pressure waves (colonic peristalsis) propel boluses of colonic contents towards the rectum (mass movements). Instillation of oleic acid into the ascending colon induced high pressure waves (>60 mmHg) which moved colonic contents distally over several minutes and resulted

in daefecation (Spiller et al. 1986; Fig. 2.5). However, propagating waves do not always move colonic contents distally. Radio-isotope instilled at the splenic flexure moved away from the flexure in both directions during the recording of propagating pressure waves (Moreno-Osset et al. 1989). Radio-labelled enemas also undergo retrograde spread to the hepatic flexure during increased colonic pressure activity induced by their instillation (Hardy et al. 1986).

Clinical Measurement of Colonic Function

Measurement of colonic motor function is of most immediate clinical importance in disorders such as the irritable bowel syndrome and idiopathic constipation. It is only when the symptoms of functional bowel disease can be related to objective data that a pathophysiological basis can be developed for rational therapy.

Basic Assessment

Departure from orderly stool production causes many patients to seek medical care, but frequency of defaecation, stool consistency, faecal volume, weight and dry weight are highly variable within and among individuals (Wyman et al. 1978; Cummings et al. 1976). Thus, altered bowel habit has little specificity for any particular diagnosis and is only a very limited index of colonic transit. When faced with altered bowel habit as the primary symptom, the high incidence of disease arising in the colonic mucosa (e.g. neoplasia, inflammation), and manifested by diarrhoea or constipation, obliges the clinician first to investigate symptomatic patients for structural organic disease. If organic intestinal or a general medical disease (e.g. hypothyroidism) resulting in colonic dysfunction is not detected, then functional diagnoses such as idiopathic constipation or irritable bowel syndrome can be entertained.

Standard investigations add little to the assessment of colonic dysfunction. The distribution of faecal shadows in the abdomen is extremely variable and gives little or no indication of the movements or function of the colon (Connell and Lennard-Jones 1964). Radiological contrast studies (e.g. with barium or soluble contrast

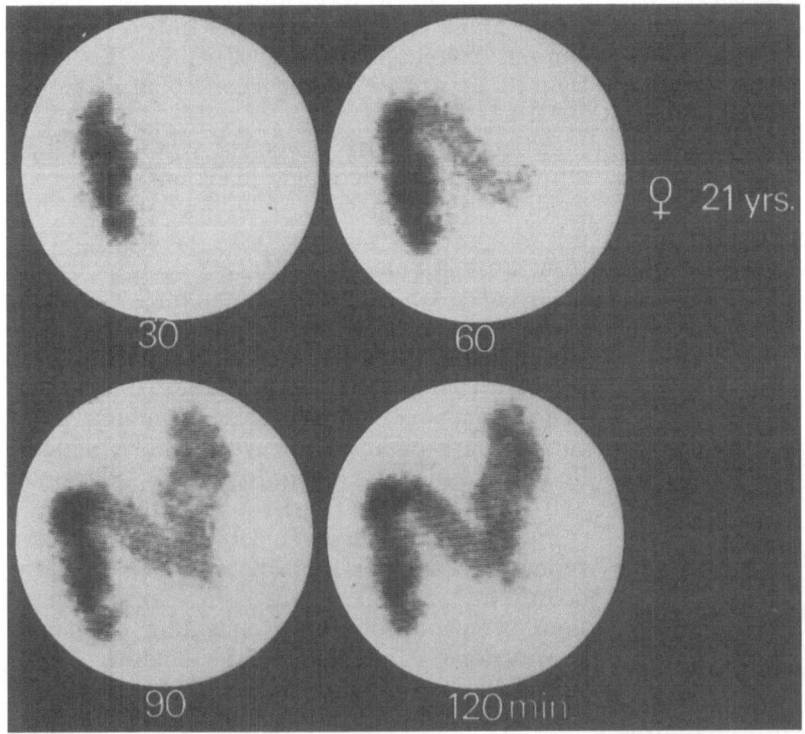

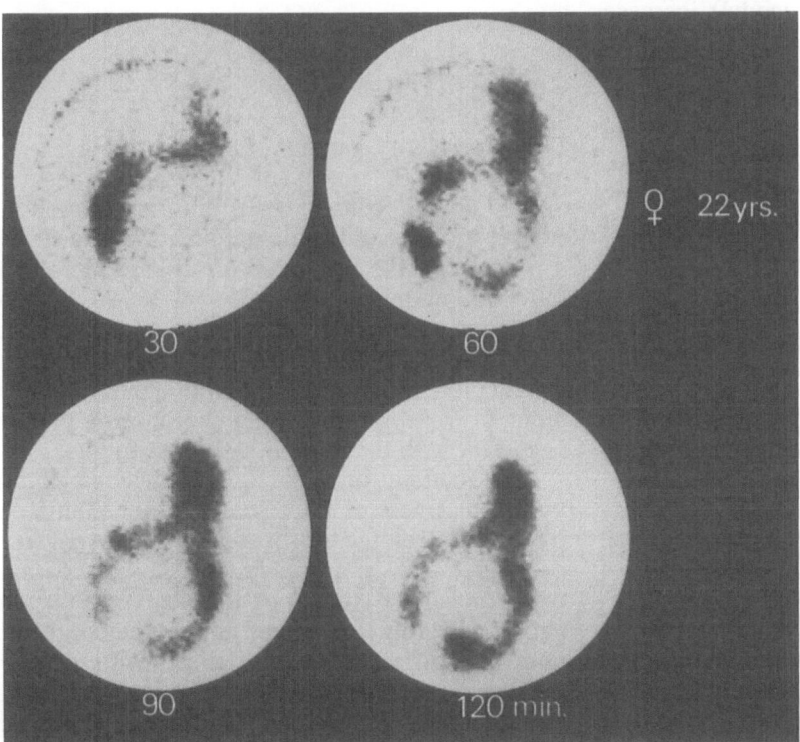

Fig. 2.5. Abdominal scans obtained 30, 60, 90 and 120 minutes after commencing colonic infusion with either saline (a) or oleic acid (b). During saline infusion, significant amounts of isotope did not enter the transverse colon before 60 minutes and remained confined to the ascending and transverse colons at 120 minutes. During oleic acid infusion, isotope had entered the descending colon and rectosigmoid by 60 minutes, and by 120 minutes there was a substantial amount of isotope in the rectosigmoid. (From Spiller et al. (1986) with permission of the authors and publishers.)

agents) in the prepared colon allow measurement of segmental colonic diameters but are unhelpful unless major changes are present (e.g. megacolon) (Patriquin et al. 1978). Moreover, clinical measurements of colonic motor function need to be considered only in a few circumstances (e.g. intractable constipation) and should, therefore, be considered very selectively. However, measurement of colonic transit is important in many areas of clinical research, though they are probably best reserved for specialized centres.

Colonic Electromyography

Investigation of myoelectrical activity in the irritable bowel syndrome has not yielded consistent results, but the best documented finding is of increased 3 cycles/min basal electrical rhythm (Snape et al. 1976) and increased postprandial, migrating, long spike bursts in patients with painless, irritable bowel syndrome (IBS) with diarrhoea (Frexinos et al. 1987). Mental stress also caused higher motor and spike potential activities in IBS patients, when compared to controls (Welgan et al. 1988).

Laxatives (sennosides and bisacodyl) increase propagating spike bursts (Staumont et al. 1988; Schang et al. 1985) and sporadic spiking activity (Schang et al. 1985). The resolution of postoperative ileus is associated with stabilization of the colonic slow wave, followed by bursts of spike activity that, though random at first, later become propagating and associated with the passage of flatus or defaecation (Condon et al. 1986).

Colonic Manometry

"Paradoxical motility" has been described in patients with diarrhoea and constipation; those with active diarrhoea had significantly fewer pressure fluctuations than did normals but many patients with constipation had more (Connell 1962; Murrell et al. 1966). Recent studies of patients with severe constipation have shown patterns of colonic motility characterized by reduced contractile activity that could not be stimulated by edrophonium, a short-acting anticholinesterase drug which normally causes increased colonic activity. Alternatively, a reduced colonic contractile response to food, but with retention of the response to edrophonium was noted (Reynolds et al. 1987). The distal rectum has also been shown to have a reduced contractile response to morphine

in some patients with constipation (Waldron et al. 1988). These changes are similar to those seen in chronic colonic pseudo-obstruction (Loening-Baucke et al. 1987) and megacolon (Connell 1961b).

Patients with irritable bowel syndrome (IBS) may have more frequent, high amplitude contractions during periods of abdominal pain but otherwise their resting records are not different from normal controls. The colonic response to meals may be excessive in patients with IBS (Holdstock et al. 1969) and be associated with abdominal pain, perhaps due to high intracolonic pressure (Stokes et al. 1988). However, the evidence remains conflicting, since postprandial pressures in the sigmoid colon have also been found to be both normal and low or high in IBS (Trotman and Misiewicz 1988; Rogers et al. 1989).

Patients with quiescent ulcerative colitis display reduced intraluminal distal pressures in the distal colon but, when the disease is active, they have more frequent, distally propagating propulsive contractions (Chaudhary and Truelove 1961). Intracolonic pressures are high in diverticular disease of the right or left colon (Sugihara et al. 1983; Trotman and Misiewicz 1988).

Colonic Transit

The transit of contents through the colon is influenced by the rate of entry and the composition of ileal chyme, colonic absorption and secretion, colonic motility and anorectal function. However, it is arguably the best overall measure of colonic function, at least in the clinical arena. Unlike manometry and electromyography, measurement of colonic transit is not limited to the proximal and distal colon, and it has the advantage of measurement over days rather than the shorter periods necessary with the more invasive techniques.

Many patients judge the severity of constipation by the hardness of their stools rather than stool frequency. Colonic transit studies will reveal truly prolonged transit; moreover, the severity of constipation can be gauged by the degree of prolongation. Severely constipated patients can be placed into two different groups, those with delayed passage of markers through all colonic segments and another that accumulates markers principally in the rectosigmoid region. Colonic dysfunction in the former group has been termed idiopathic slow transit constipation (Preston and Lennard-Jones 1986). In the latter, anorectal manometry showing anal dysfunction supports the concept of outlet obstruction causing retention of stool (Martelli et al. 1978b). Therapies for constipation which focus on one or other of these two groups are still evolving but assessments combining anorectal manometry and transit studies have shown an objective basis for symptomatic constipation in many patients (Ducrotte et al. 1986; Wald 1986; Waldron et al. 1988). Colonic transit studies have also been used to measure colorectal dysfunction resulting from spinal cord injury (Menardo et al. 1987) or multiple sclerosis (Weber et al. 1987).

The colonic response to changes in dietary fibre intake (Harvey et al. 1973; Kumar et al. 1987) has had a major impact on gastroenterological practice. Usually, an increased intake of dietary fibre results in reduced colonic transit times and a softer stool. However, the relationship between the irritable bowel syndrome and changes in colonic transit remains uncertain (Oettle and Heaton 1987; Cann et al. 1983). Radio-isotope methods have been applied in similar clinical situations to radio-opaque marker methods. In constipated patients, colonic transit of an intraluminal radio-isotope is not markedly shortened by caecal instillation of a laxative (Bisacodyl) when compared to healthy controls (Kamm et al. 1988). Patients with irritable bowel syndrome may show more rapid movement of isotopes through the colon but results are inconsistent (Hardy et al. 1986; Trotman and Price 1986).

In contrast to radio-opaque marker methods, radionuclides have been used to measure the patterns of colonic transit associated with diarrhoea caused by colonic irritants (Spiller et al. 1986), ulcerative colitis (Rao et al. 1987) and hormonal diarrhoea (Rambaud et al. 1988). Oleic acid, which is present in ileal chyme in malabsorption syndromes, not only caused rapid aboral transit of colonic contents (Spiller et al. 1986) but, on two-plane colonic scintigraphy, reduced the volume of the ascending colon (Kamath et al. 1990).

Of emerging clinical interest is the use of radionuclide transit measurements to assess the effects of drugs on colonic motor function. In the above study of oleic acid effects on the colon (Kamath et al. 1990), the reduction in volume of the ascending colon could be prevented by prior administration of intravenous morphine. Morphine also prolonged proximal colonic transit (Kaufmann 1988). In contrast, colonic transit was shortened by the new, prokinetic drug, cisapride (Krevsky et al. 1987).

In general, radio-opaque marker measurement of colonic transit is easy to perform, of minimal risk to patients and has direct clinical relevance.

At present, although radionuclide techniques are potentially useful, they demand too much technical expertise for widespread application.

To summarize, motor function of the human colon appears to involve more complex phenomena with perhaps more levels of control than does motility in the small intestine. Perhaps this reflects a more varied set of functions performed by the large bowel; overall transit is certainly slower but the colon still maintains the capacity to empty quickly. Moreover, there are storage phenomena to facilitate intraluminal bacterial metabolism and a predictable, ordered mechanism of evacuation. Thus, while still an area of much active research, the practical applications of measurements of colonic motor function to clinical practice are limited.

References

Alvarez WC, Freedlander BL (1924) The rate of progress of food residues through the bowel. J Am Med Assoc 83:576–580

Arhan P, Devroede G, Jehannin B et al. (1981) Segmental colonic transit time. Dis Colon Rectum 24:625–629

Arndorfer RC, Stef JJ, Dodds WJ, Linehan JH, Hogan WJ (1977) Improved infusion system for intraluminal esophageal manometry. Gastroenterology 73:23–27

Battle WM, Cohen S, Snape WJ (1980) Inhibition of postprandial colonic motility after ingestion of an amino acid mixture. Dig Dis Sci 25:647–652

Becker U, Elsborg L (1979) A new method for the determination of gastrointestinal transit times. Scand J Gastroenterol 14:355–359

Bueno L, Fioramonti J, Ruckebusch Y, Frexinos J, Coulom P (1980) Evaluation of colonic myoelectrical activity in health and functional disorders. Gut 21:480–485

Cann PA, Read NW, Brown C, Hobson N, Holdsworth CD (1983) Irritable bowel syndrome: relationship of disorders in the transit of a single solid meal to symptom patterns. Gut 24:405–411

Cannon WB (1902) The movements of the intestines studied by means of the roentgen rays. Am J Physiol 6:251–277

Chaudhary NA, Truelove SC (1961) Human colonic motility: a comparative study of normal subjects, patients with ulcerative colitis, and patients with the irritable colon syndrome. Gastroenterology 40:1–17

Chaussade S, Roche H, Khyari A, Couturier D, Guerre J (1986) Mesure du temps de transit colique (TTC): description et validation d'une nouvelle technique. Gastroenterol Clin Biol 10:355–389

Chaussade S, Guerre J, Couturier D (1987) Measurement of colonic transit (correspondence). Gastroenterology 92:2053

Chauve A, Devroede G, Bastin E (1976) Intraluminal pressures during perfusion of the human colon in situ. Gastroenterology 70:336–340

Chow E, Huizinga JD (1987) Myogenic electrical control activity in longitudinal muscle of human and dog colon. J Physiol 392: 21–34

Christensen J, Rick GA (1987) Intrinsic nerves in the mammalian colon: confirmation of a plexus at the circular muscle-submucosal interface. J Autonomic Nervous System 21:223–231

Christensen J, Stiles MJ, Rick GA, Sutherland J (1984) Comparative anatomy of the myenteric plexus of the distal colon in eight mammals. Gastroenterology 86:706–713

Colemont LJ, Human gastric emptying and colonic filling of solids characterized by a new method. Am J Physiol 257:G284–G290

Collins PJ, Horowitz M, Shearman DJC, Chatterton BE (1984) Correction for tissue attenuation in radionuclide gastric emptying studies: a comparison of a lateral image method and a geometric mean method. Br J Radiol 57:689–695

Condon RE, Frantzides CT, Cowles VE, Mahoney JL, Schulte WJ, Sarna SK (1986) Resolution of postoperative ileus in humans. Ann Surg 203:574–581

Connell AM (1961a) The motility of the pelvic colon. 1. Motility in normals and in patients with asymptomatic duodenal ulcer. Gut 2:175–186

Connell AM (1961b) Colonic motility in megacolon. Proc R Soc Med 54:1040–1043

Connell AM (1962) The motility of the pelvic colon. II. Paradoxical motility in diarrhea and constipation. Gut 3:342–348

Connell AM, Lennard-Jones JE (1964) The distribution of fecal x-ray shadows in subjects without gastrointestinal disease. Proc R Soc Med 57:894–895

Connell AM, Hilton C, Irvine G, Lennard-Jones JE, Misiewicz JJ (1965) Variation of bowel habit in two population samples. Br Med J ii:1095–1099

Cook IJ, Reddy SN, Collins SM, Daniel EE (1988) Influence of recording techniques on measurement of canine colonic motility. Dig Dis Sci 33:999–1006

Cummings JH, Wiggins HS (1976) Transit through the gut measured by analysis of a single stool. Gut 17:219–223

Cummings JH, Jenkins DJ, Wiggins HS (1976) Measurement of the mean transit time of dietary residue through the human gut. Gut 17:210–218

Daniel EE (1975) Symposium on colonic function: electrophysiology of the colon. Gut 16:298–306

Dapoigny M, Trolese JF, Bommelaer G, Tournut R (1988) Myoelectric spiking activity of right colon, left colon and rectosigmoid of healthy humans. Dig Dis Sci 33:1007–1012

Debongnie JC, Phillips SF (1978) Capacity of the human colon to absorb fluid. Gastroenterology 74:698–703

Devroede GJ, Phillips SF, Code CF, Lind JF (1971) Regional differences in rates of insorption of sodium and water from the human large intestine. Can J Physiol Pharmacol 49:1023–1029

Donaldson RM, Barreras RF (1966) Intestinal absorption of trace quantities of chromium. J Lab Clin Med 68:484–493

Ducrotte P, Rodomanska B, Weber J et al. (1986) Colonic transit time of radiopaque markers and rectoanal manometry in patients complaining of constipation. Dis Colon Rectum 29:630–634

Duthie HL (1978) Colonic response to eating. Gastroenterology 75:527–529

Edwards DAW, Beck LR (1971) Movement of radiopacified feces during defecation. Dig Dis 16:709–711

Elliott TR, Barclay-Smith E (1904) Antiperistalsis and other muscular activities of the colon. J Physiol 31:272

Fioramonti J, Bueno L, Sarna SK, Ruckebusch Y (1982) Origin of high slow wave frequency in the dog colon. Reprod Nutr Dev 20:983–990

Flourie B, Phillips SF, Richter H, Azpiroz F (1989) Cyclic

motility in canine colon: responses to feeding and perfusion. Dig Dis Sci 34:1185–1192

Frexinos J, Bueno L, Fioramonti J (1985) Diurnal changes in myoelectric spiking activity of the human colon. Gastroenterology 88:1104–1110

Frexinos J, Fioramonti J, Bueno L (1987) Colonic myoelectrical activity in IBS painless diarrhea. Gut 28:1613–1618

Furness JB, Costa M (1980) Types of nerves in the enteric nervous system. Neuroscience 5:1–20

Halls J (1965) Bowel content shift during normal defecation. Proc R Soc Med 58:859–860

Hansky J, Connell AM (1962) Measurement of gastrointestinal transit using radioactive chromium. Gut 3:187–188

Hardcastle JD, Mann CV (1968) Study of large bowel peristalsis. Gut 9:512–520

Hardcastle JD, Mann CV (1970) Physical factors in the stimulation of colonic peristalsis. Gut 11:41–46

Hardy JG, Wood E, Clark AG, Reynolds JR (1986) Colonic motility and enema spreading. Eur J Nucl Med 12:176–178

Hardy JG, Healey JNC, Lee SW, Reynolds JR (1987) Gastrointestinal transit of an enteric-coated delayed-release 5-aminosalicylic acid tablet. Aliment Pharmacol Therap 1:209–216

Harvey RF, Pomare EW, Heaton KW (1973) Effects of increased dietary fibre on intestinal transit. Lancet i:1278–1280

Hinton JM, Lennard-Jones JE, Young AC (1969) A new method for studying gut transit times using radiopaque markers. Gut 10:842–847

Hoelzel F (1930) The rate of passage of inert materials through the digestive tract. Am J Physiol 92:466–497

Holdstock DJ, Misiewicz JJ (1970) Factors controlling colonic motility: colonic pressures and transit after meals in patients with total gastrectomy, pernicious anemia or duodenal ulcer. Gut 11:100–110

Holdstock DJ, Misiewicz JJ, Waller SL (1969) Observations on the mechanism of abdominal pain. Gut 10:19–31

Holdstock DJ, Misiewicz JJ, Smith T, Rowlands EN (1970) Propulsion (mass movements) in the human colon and its relationship to meals and somatic activity. Gut 11:91–99

Huizinga JD, Chow E (1988) Electrotonic current spread in colonic smooth muscle. Am J Physiol 254:G702–G710

Huizinga JD, Daniel EE (1986) Control of human colonic motor function. Dig Dis Sci 31:865–877

Huizinga JD, Waterfall WE (1988) Electrical correlate of circumferential contractions in human colonic circular muscle. Gut 29:10–16

Huizinga JD, Stern H, Chow E, Diamant NE, El-Sharkawy TY (1985) Electrophysiological control of motility in the human colon. Gastroenterology 88:500–511

Huizinga JD, Stern HS, Chow E, Diamant NE, El-Sharkawy TY (1986) Electrical basis of excitation and inhibition of human colonic smooth muscle. Gastroenterology 90:1197–1204

Kamath PS, Phillips SF, O'Connor MK, Brown ML, Zinsmeister AR (1990) Colonic capacitance and transit in man: modulation by luminal contents and drugs Gut 31:443–449

Kamm MA, Lennard-Jones JE, Thompson DG, Sobnack R, Garvie NW, Granowska M (1988) Dynamic scanning defines a colonic defect in severe idiopathic constipation. Gut 29:1085–1092

Karaus M, Sarna SK (1987) Giant migrating contractions during defecation in the dog colon. Gastroenterology 92:925–933

Kaufman PN, Krevsky B, Malmud LS·et al. (1988) Role of opiate receptors in the regulation of colonic transit. Gastroenterology 94:1351–1356

Kellow JE, Miller LJ, Phillips SF, Haddad AC, Zinsmeister

AR, Charboneau JW (1987) Sensitivities of human jejunum, ileum, proximal colon and gallbladder to cholecystokinin octapeptide. Am J Physiol 252:G345–G356

Kerlin P, Zinsmeister A, Phillips S (1983) Motor responses to food of the ileum, proximal colon, and distal colon of healthy humans. Gastroenterology 84:762–770

Kirwan WO, Smith AN (1974) Gastrointestinal transit estimated by an isotope capsule. Scand J Gastroenterol 9:763–766

Kock NG, Hulten L, Leandoer L (1968) A study of the motility in different parts of the human colon. Resting activity, response to feeding and to prostigmine. Scand J Gastroenterol 3:163–169

Krevsky B, Malmud LS, D'Ercole F, Maurer AH, Fisher RS (1986) Colonic transit scintigraphy. A physiologic approach to the quantitative measurement of colonic transit in humans. Gastroenterology 91:1102–1112

Krevsky B, Malmud LS, Maurer AH, Somers MB, Siegel JA, Fisher RS (1987) The effect of oral cisapride on colonic transit. Aliment Pharmacol Therap 1:293–304

Kumar A, Kumar N, Vij TC, Sarin SK, Anand BS (1987) Optimum dosage of ispaghula husk in patients with irritable bowel syndrome: correlation of symptom relief with whole gut transit time and stool weight. Gut 28:150–155

Loening-Baucke VA, Anuras S, Mitros FA (1987) Changes in colorectal function in patients with chronic colonic pseudo-obstruction. Dig Dis Sci 32:1104–1112

Manousos ON, Truelove SC, Lumsden K (1967) Transit times of food in patients with diverticulosis or irritable colon syndrome and normal subjects. Br Med J iii:760–762

Martelli H, Devroede G, Arhan P, Duguay C, Dornic C, Faverdin C (1978a) Some parameters of large bowel motility in normal man. Gastroenterology 75:612–618

Martelli H, Devroede G, Arhan P, Duguay C (1978b) Mechanisms of idiopathic constipation: outlet obstruction. Gastroenterology 75:623–631

Menardo G, Bausano G, Corazziari E et al. (1987) Large-bowel transit in paraplegic patients. Dis Colon Rectum 30:924–928

Metcalf AM, Phillips SF, Zinsmeister AR, MacCarty RL, Beart RW, Wolff BG (1987) Simplified assessment of segmental colonic transit. Gastroenterology 92:40–47

Misiewicz JJ (1984) Human colonic motility. Scand J Gastroenterol 19 (supp 93): 43–51

Mojaverian P, Ferguson RK, Vlasses PH et al. (1985) Estimation of gastric residence time of the Heidelberg capsule in humans: effect of varying food composition. Gastroenterology 89:392–397

Moreno-Osset E, Bazzochi G, Lo S et al. (1989) Association between postprandial changes in colonic intraluminal pressure and transit. Gastroenterology 96:1265–1273

Murrell TG, Wangel AG, Deller DJ (1966) Intestinal motility in man. IV. Effect of serotonin on intestinal motility in subjects with diarrhea and constipation. Gastroenterology 51:656–663

Narducci F, Bassotti G, Gaburri M, Morelli A (1987) Twenty four hour manometric recording of colonic motor activity in healthy man. Gut 28:17–25

Oettle GJ, Heaton KW (1987) Is there a relationship between symptoms of the irritable bowel syndrome and objective measurements of large bowel function? A longitudinal study. Gut 28:146–149

Painter NS, Truelove SC (1964a) The intraluminal pressure patterns in diverticulosis of the colon. Part III: The effect of prostigmine. Gut 5:365–373

Painter NS, Truelove SC (1964b) The intraluminal pressure patterns in diverticulosis of the colon. Part I: Resting patterns of pressure. Part II: The effect of morphine. Gut 5:201–213

Parker R, Whitehead WE, Schuster MM (1987) Pattern-recognition program for analysis of colon myoelectric and pressure data. Dig Dis Sci 32:953–961

Parker G, Wilson CG, Hardy JG (1988) The effect of capsule size and density on transit through the proximal colon. J Pharm Pharmacol 40:376–377

Patriquin H, Martelli H, Devroede G (1978) Barium enema in chronic constipation: is it meaningful? Gastroenterology 75:619–622

Phillips SF, Giller J (1973) The contribution of the colon to electrolyte and water conservation in man. J Lab Clin Med 81:733–746

Preston DM, Lennard-Jones JE (1986) Severe chronic constipation of young women: idiopathic slow transit constipation. Gut 27:41–48

Proano M, Camilleri M, Phillips SF et al. (1990) Transit of solids through the human colon: regional quantification in the unprepared bowel. Am J Physiol 258:G856–862

Rambaud JC, Jian R, Flourie B et al. (1988) Pathophysiological study of diarrhea in a patient with medullary thyroid carcinoma. Evidence against a secretory mechanism and for the role of shortened colonic transit time. Gut 29:537–543

Rao SSC, Read NW, Brown C, Bruce C, Holdsworth CD (1987) Studies on the mechanism of bowel disturbance in ulcerative colitis. Gastroenterology 93:934–940

Rendtorff RC, Kashgarian M (1967) Stool patterns of healthy adult males. Dis Colon Rectum 10:222–228

Reynolds JC, Ouyang A, Lee CA, Baker L, Sunshine AG, Cohen S (1987) Chronic severe constipation. Prospective motility studies in 25 consecutive patients. Gastroenterology 92:414–420

Ritchie JA (1968) Colonic motor activity and bowel function. Part I. Normal movement of contents. Gut 9:442–456

Ritchie JA, Truelove SC, Ardran GM, Tuckey MS (1971) Propulsion and retropulsion of normal colonic contents. Dig Dis 16:697–704

Roediger WE (1982) Utilization of nutrients by isolated epithelial cells of the rat colon. Gastroenterology 83:424–429

Rogers J, Misiewicz JJ (1989) Fully automated computer analysis of intracolonic pressures. Gut 30:642–649

Rogers J, Henry MM, Misiewicz JJ (1989) Increased segmental activity and intraluminal pressures in the sigmoid colon of patients with the irritable bowel syndrome. Gut 30:634–641

Ruppin H, Bar-Meir S, Soergel KH, Wood CM, Schmitt MG (1980) Absorption of short chain fatty acids by the colon. Gastroenterology 78:1500–1507

Sarna SK (1985) Cyclic motor activity; migrating motor complex: 1985. Gastroenterology 89:894–913

Sarna SK, Waterfall WE, Bardakjian BL, Lind JF (1981) Types of human colonic electrical activities recorded postoperatively. Gastroenterology 81:61–70

Sarna S, Latimer P, Campbell D, Waterfall WE (1982) Electrical and contractile activities of the human rectosigmoid. Gut 23:698–705

Sarna SK, Condon R, Cowles V (1984) Colonic migrating and nonmigrating motor complexes in dogs. Am J Physiol 246:G355–G360

Sasaki D, Kido A, Yoshida Y (1986) An endoscopic method to study the relationship between bowel habit and motility of the ascending and sigmoid colon. Gastrointestinal Endoscopy 32:185–189

Schang JC, Devroede G (1983) Fasting and postprandial myoelectric spiking activity in the human sigmoid colon. Gastroenterology 85:1048–1053

Schang JC, Hemond M, Hebert M, Pilote M (1985) Changes in

colonic myoelectric spiking activity during stimulation by bisacodyl. Can J Physiol Pharmacol 64:39–43

Schang JC, Hemond M, Hebert M, Pilote M (1986) Myoelectrical activity and intraluminal flow in human sigmoid colon. Dig Dis Sci 31:1331–1337

Schang JC, Devroede G, Hebert M, Hemond M, Pilote M, Devroede L (1988) Effects of rest, stress, and food on myoelectric spiking activity of left and sigmoid colon in humans. Dig Dis Sci 33:614–618

Smith TK, Reed JB, Sanders KM (1987) Interaction of two electrical pacemakers in muscularis of canine proximal colon. Am J Physiol 252:C290–C299

Snape WJ, Carlson GM, Cohen S (1976) Colonic myoelectric activity in the irritable bowel syndrome. Gastroenterology 70:326–330

Snape WJ, Wright SH, Battle WM, Cohen S (1979) The gastrocolic response: evidence for a neural mechanism. Gastroenterology 77:1235–1240

Soffer EE, Scalabrini P, Wingate DL (1989) Prolonged ambulant monitoring of human colonic motility. Am J Physiol 257:G601–G606

Spiller RC, Brown ML, Phillips SF (1986) Decreased fluid tolerance, accelerated transit, and abnormal motility of the human colon induced by oleic acid. Gastroenterology 91:100–107

Spriggs EA, Code CF, Bargen JA, Curtiss RK, Hightower NC (1951) Motility of the pelvic colon and rectum of normal persons and patients with ulcerative colitis. Gastroenterology 19:480–491

Staumont G, Frexinos J, Fioramonti J, Bueno L (1988) Sennosides and human colonic motility. Pharmacology 36 (Suppl 1):49–56

Stokes MA, Moriarty KJ, Catchpole BN (1988) A study of the genesis of colic. Lancet i:211–214

Sugihara K, Muto T, Morioka Y (1983) Motility study in right-sided diverticular disease of the colon. Gut 24:1130–1134

Sunshine A, Ouyang R, Baker PL, Reynolds J, Cohen S (1985) Colonic slow wave analysis: limitations of the fast fourier transform (FFT). Dig Dis Sci 30:797

Taylor I, Duthie HL, Smallwood R, Brown BH, Linkens D (1974) The effect of stimulation on the myoelectrical activity of the rectosigmoid in man. Gut 15:599–607

Taylor I, Duthie HL, Smallwood R, Linkens D (1975) Large bowel myoelectrical activity in man. Gut 16:808–814

Thuneberg L, Rumessen JJ, Mikkelsen HB (1982) Interstitial cells of Cajal-an intestinal impulse generation and conduction system? Scand J Gastroenterol 17 (supp 71):143–144

Trotman IF, Misiewicz JJ (1988) Sigmoid motility in diverticular disease and the irritable bowel syndrome. Gut 29:218–222

Trotman IF, Price CC (1986) Bloated irritable bowel syndrome defined by dynamic ^{99m}Tc bran scan. Lancet ii:364–366

Van Soest PJ (1988) Fibre in the diet. In: Blaxter K, McDonald I (eds) Comparative nutrition. John Libbey, New York, pp 215–224

Wald A (1986) Colonic transit and anorectal manometry in chronic idiopathic constipation. Arch Intern Med 146:1713–1716

Waldron D, Bowes KL, Kingma YJ, Cote KR (1988) Colonic and anorectal motility in young women with severe idiopathic constipation. Gastroenterology 95:1388–1394

Waller SL (1975) Differential measurement of small and large bowel transit times in constipation and diarrhea: a new approach. Gut 16:372–378

Weber J, Grise P, Roquebert M et al. (1987) Radiopaque markers transit and anorectal manometry in 16 patients with multiple sclerosis and urinary bladder dysfunction. Dis Colon Rectum 30:95–100

Welgan P, Meshkinpour H, Beeler M (1988) Effect of anger on colon motor and myoelectric activity in irritable bowel syndrome. Gastroenterology 94:1150–1156

Wiley J, Tatum D, Keinath R, Owyang C (1988) Participation of gastric mechanoreceptors and intestinal chemoreceptors in the gastrocolonic response. Gastroenterology 94:1144–1149

Wyman JB, Heaton KW, Manning AP, Wicks ACB (1978) Variability of colonic function in healthy subjects. Gut 19:146–150

3 · Measurement of Anorectal Function

D. Kumar, R. I. Hallan, N. R. Womack, P. R. O'Connell and R. Miller

Manometry
D. Kumar

Introduction

The measurement of intraluminal pressures is the most direct available method for the assessment of gastrointestinal motor function. Manometry is a technique employed for recording pressure changes within the bowel lumen caused by contractions of the gut wall. In coloproctological assessment this technique has mainly been applied to the study of the anorectum and the sigmoid colon. Anorectal manometry has now become a standard clinical test for the assessment of the internal as well as the external anal sphincter. Assessment of anorectal function is generally made separately from measurement of colonic activity. Such studies must be interpreted with caution because an apparently normal anal canal may have associated motor abnormalities of the rectum and colon above.

Methods of Recording Anorectal Manometry

Anorectal pressure measurements are the commonest means of assessment of anal sphincter function. The existence of a high pressure zone in the anal canal is accepted by most workers but the choice of the most appropriate method of measuring this pressure still remains controversial.

Anorectal pressures can be recorded for short periods of time in a non-ambulant manner with the subject in the left lateral position or for prolonged periods of time using ambulant techniques.

Short Non-ambulant Anorectal Recordings

Conventionally, anorectal manometry is performed in the left lateral position using balloon systems (Ihre 1974; Frenckner and Von Euler 1975; Lubowski et al. 1988), low compliance perfused tube systems (McHugh and Diamant 1987a; Rao et al. 1987) and manometry sleeves (Dent 1976).

Balloon Systems

Fluid or air filled microballoons are connected to pressure transducers by a catheter. Balloons measure the resistance to distension of the anal canal. It has been argued that balloon systems are more sensitive than perfused tube systems (Duthie and Watts 1965). The size of the balloon determines the pressure recorded; the resistance to distension of the anal canal increases with an increase in the diameter of the balloon. Another limitation of the balloon systems is that they do not allow simultaneous recording of a length of anorectum to study coordinated activity. A station pull-through technique has to be employed to record pressures in different parts of the anal canal (Lubowski et al. 1988). Balloons have the advantage that they maintain a fixed spatial relationship between the catheter and the anal canal.

Perfused Catheters

Perfused Tube System

The principle of perfused tube manometry for the assessment of anorectal function is the same as that described for colonic manometry. The tube assemblies are usually custom made with a varying number of side holes for perfusion. The distance between perfusion ports also varies between studies. Thus data from different laboratories using such systems must be compared with caution. Pressures within the anal canal are measured either by a rapid pull-through technique (Kielmann and Bonnesen 1985; McHugh and Diamant 1987b) or more commonly a station pull-through technique (Taylor et al. 1984). The station pull-through technique uses fixed points starting within the rectum and if the sphincter is long then the stations assessed will differ in comparison to those of a short anal canal. In addition there are technical difficulties in doing station pull-throughs, especially in subjects with large buttocks. McHugh and Diamant (1987b) studied 12 healthy volunteers using a 4-quadrant pressure measurement and a mechanized rapid pull-through technique, and compared the results of rapid pull-through with those of the station pull-through technique. They concluded that the station pull-through technique gave reliable resting pressure measurements in the anal canal but the rapid pull-through technique allowed a more appropriate assessment of the anal sphincter profile. In a separate study the same authors have evaluated the effect of age, gender and parity on anal canal pressures to study the contribution of impaired anal sphincter function to faecal incontinence (McHugh and Diamant 1987a). They mea-

sured resting anal pressures and maximum squeeze pressures in 157 healthy subjects and 143 patients with faecal incontinence and concluded that ageing affects the resting anal pressure to a greater extent in women than in men and the maximal squeeze pressure is reduced with ageing in women only. They found no effect of childbearing on anal canal pressures. They also noticed a consistent effect of tube diameter on resting anal pressures as well as maximal squeeze pressures. The effect of the diameter of the measuring probe has also been noted by other workers (Duthie and Watts 1965; Gutierrez et al. 1975). Another important source of error with these pressure systems is that anal canal irritation due to the infused fluid may produce an artefactual contraction. However, perfused tube systems allow simultaneous recording from multiple sites, both on the longitudinal as well as the radial axes.

Sleeve Catheters

Sleeve catheters are often used in conjunction with the perfused manometry system. A silastic membrane is glued over a silastic base and fluid is perfused through this sleeve (Dent 1976). Sleeve sensors are useful in assessing the overall function of sphincters. The main drawback of sleeve catheters is that they measure pressure along a length of bowel rather than from a specific point along that segment. Also, sleeve assemblies cannot distinguish differences between the internal and the external anal sphincter activity.

Effect of Bowel Preparation

Studying a clean and empty colon is generally regarded as unphysiological since its motor action may be different from normal, although if the colonoscopic route is chosen for study then it is almost essential to prepare the bowel for adequate positioning of the tube. The agent chosen for bowel preparation may also modify the motor response of the colon. A tap water enema 3 hours prior to the commencement of study has been shown not to alter motility indices (Dinoso et al. 1983). However, it could be argued that the stimulating effect of an enema may mask the hypomotility in patients who had colonic distension prior to the administration of the enema (Reynolds 1988). Another important consideration must be that the response to cathartics is not uniform. It must not therefore be assumed that since all the subjects have received bowel preparation, the state of cleanliness of their colons will be the same, and more importantly, that colonic movements will be comparable. More work is needed before we can conclude that there are not important motor differences between the prepared and the unprepared bowel.

Ambulant Recordings

Ambulant recordings from the human gastrointestinal tract were first made by a radiotelemetric system (Connell et al. 1963). This system employs a radiotelemetry capsule which operates at a fixed frequency. The capsule is swallowed and then allowed free transit in the gut. The signal is collected with the help of an aerial belt, amplified and recorded on audiotape in a portable tape recorder. Since the system utilizes radiofrequency modulation, signal loss is a major problem. The other major drawback is the lack of knowledge of the position of the telemetry capsule in the gastrointestinal tract at any given time. Thus, the recorded activity cannot be assigned to a specific region of the gut. Several technological advances have been made in the design of telemetry capsules (Browning et al. 1981). The improved capsules have a pressure sensitive microtransducer embedded at one end. The output from this microtransducer is converted into a fixed frequency radiosignal. Signal loss with the new type of capsule is claimed to be minimal.

The obvious advantage of such studies is that the subjects can carry out their normal activities, thus providing more physiological data. Womack et al. (1985) have utilized this principle in monitoring rectal motor activity during defaecating proctograms. Also, the stress effects of some of the more invasive techniques can be avoided (Welgan et al. 1988).

Anorectal manometry for short periods of time provides some understanding of the function of the anorectum during controlled voluntary activities such as cough, change in posture and anal squeeze. However, physiological functions such as defaecation, micturition and passage of flatus are private and are therefore difficult to study in this manner. For the complete description and understanding of anorectal physiology and pathophysio-

logy, a technique that allows acquisition of physiological data, and at the same time preserves the mobility and freedom of the subject, must be a desirable aim.

We have developed a method for the continuous measurement of anorectal pressure under ambulatory conditions for a prolonged period of time (Kumar et al. 1990). Recently, Miller et al. (1988) described a technique for the ambulant recording of anorectal pressure. This was for a short period of time (3 h) and, more importantly, did not include recording during normal sleep. We believe sleep recordings are important because during sleep local reflex events are dissociated from the central nervous system dominance.

The recording system consists of a probe carrying the pressure-sensitive sensors (Fig. 3.1), a battery powered interface unit containing three amplifiers and a portable cassette recorder (Medilog 4–24, Oxford Medical Systems, Abingdon, UK). The tape recorder is capable of recording continuously for 24 hours on a single C120 cassette.

With the subject in the left lateral position, the probe is introduced and advanced until the proximal sensor is positioned in the rectum and the distal sensor in the midanal canal. The probe is then firmly taped as close to the anal verge as possible. This avoids displacement of sensors during the study. Once in position, the probe is connected to the interface box and the tape recorder. Using this technique we have studied 14 healthy subjects: in addition to measurements of resting and squeeze activity, it enabled us to study physiological events like micturition, passage of flatus and the sampling reflex during sleep.

Rectal Manometry

Based on conventional short recordings, the rectum has been shown to have contractions with a frequency of 5–10 cycles/min and slow contractions with a frequency of 3 cyles/min (Whitehead et al. 1980). The use of such techniques does not allow the study of periodic activity in the anorectum. In a prolonged manometric study of 12 healthy subjects, we have demonstrated the presence of periodic motor activity (rectal motor complexes) recurring at an interval of 92 ± 1.9 minutes (mean$\pm$SEM) during the day and 56 ± 1.7 minutes at night (Fig. 3.2) (Kumar et al. 1989). The detection of rectal motor complexes may prove useful in the assessment of anorectal neural integrity in patients with anorectal dysfunction.

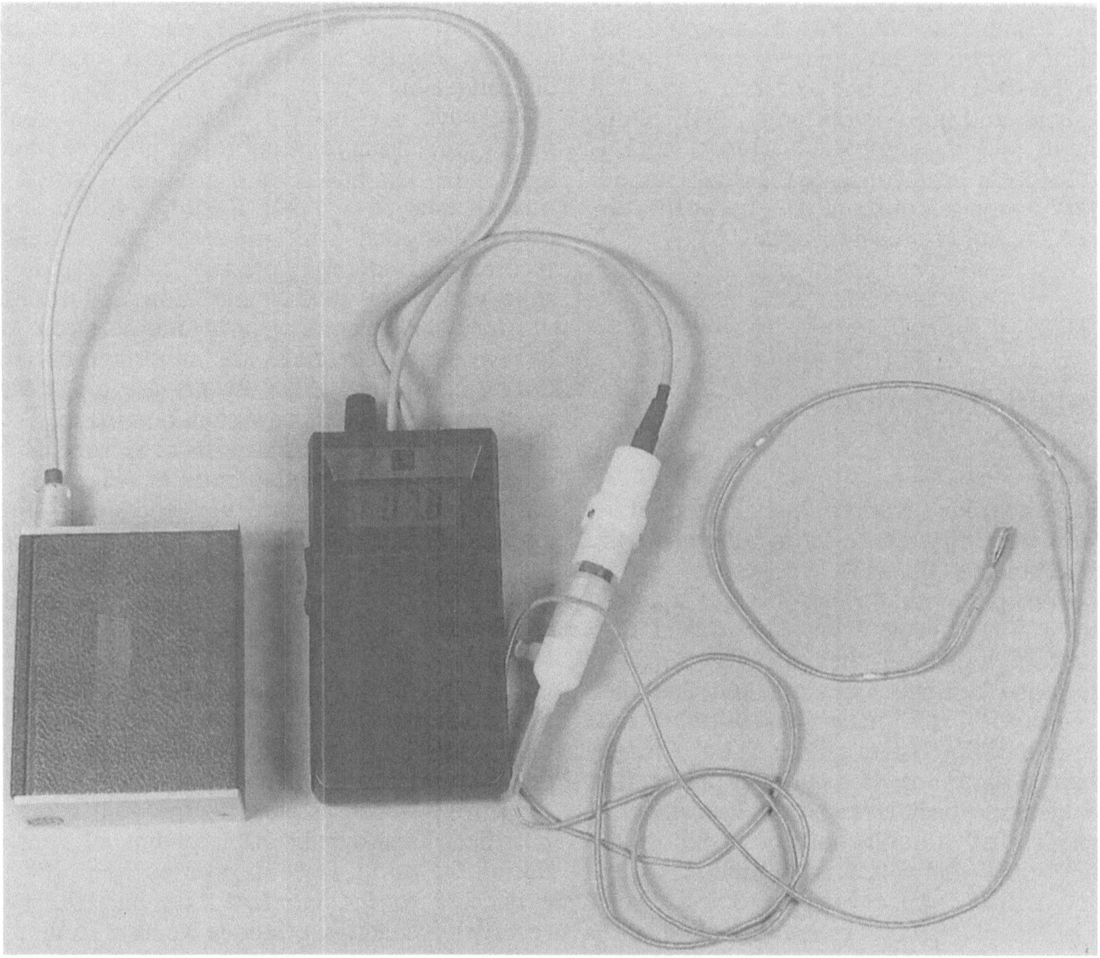

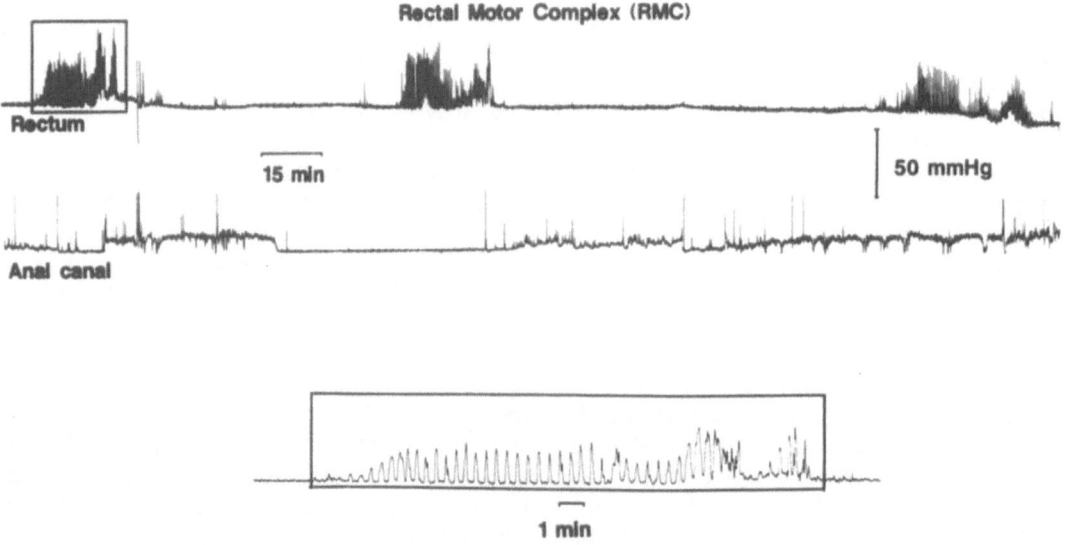

Fig. 3.1. The anorectal recording probe, the encoding box and the portable tape recorder.

Rectal Motor Complex (RMC)

Rectum

15 min   50 mmHg

Anal canal

1 min

Fig. 3.2. Example of rectal motor complexes in a healthy volunteer. The inset shows an RMC at a faster speed. Note the regular and sustained nature of contractions.

Anal Canal Manometry

Three main motility indices – resting pressure, squeeze pressure and reflex activity – have been studied using short recordings. Thus far it has not been possible to study variations in these indices over a period of 24 hours under physiological conditions. We have performed anal manometry for 24 hours under ambulant conditions. The anal canal shows considerable variation in motor activity during wakefulness and sleep (Fig. 3.3). The predominant pattern of anal activity during sleep is motor quiescence. Slow waves and ultra-slow waves are seen with a frequency of 1–2/min on waking and prior to defaecation.

We believe these observations may allow better understanding of mechanisms of defaecation and continence. Prolonged ambulant manometry, therefore, not only allows for evaluation of var-iations in contractile patterns of anorectal motility but also enables assessment of the role of various reflex mechanisms that are considered important in maintaining continence.

Interpretation of Records

Too much attention has been paid to the description of various methods and their relative merits and too little to the interpretation of records. The interpretation of manometric data requires a clear understanding of the validity of the recording method and its signal source. Manometric data is usually interpreted for: (a) contractile patterns and (b) quantification of contractions. Contractile patterns by themselves do not provide much infor-

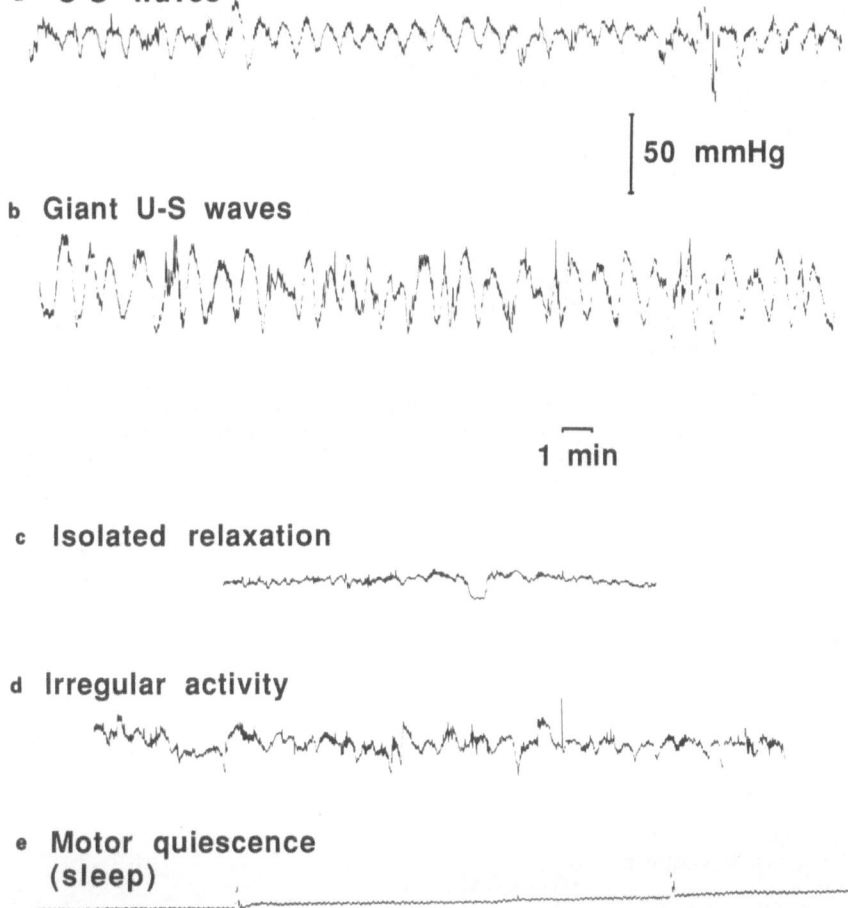

Fig. 3.3. Example of different types of motor activity in the anal canal of a healthy volunteer. **a** Ultra slow waves at a frequency of approximately 2/min. **b** Giant ultra-slow waves at a frequency of 1/min. Note the greater amplitude in comparison to the ultra-slow waves. **c** Isolated relaxation of the anal canal. **d** Irregular contractile activity with multiple relaxation responses. **e** Motor quiescence during sleep.

mation other than to suggest contractions of the muscular walls of the colon. Therefore, researchers have only used quantitative measurement of the amplitude or number (or both) of contractions per unit time. Whatever the method of analysis, interpretation of manometric data must take into account factors like emotional state of the subject, diurnal variations, nature of luminal contents and stimuli such as meals.

Normal Values of Anorectal Manometry

Although most laboratories have data on control subjects, few have control values for sex or for age. It has been reported that men have increased rectal compliance and a shorter duration of the recto-anal inhibitory reflex than women. Men also have higher maximal resting and squeeze anal canal pressures than women. Advancing age, on the other hand, produces a fall in maximal resting and squeeze anal pressures, especially in women. The wide variation in control values makes comparison between patients and healthy subjects difficult. Also, difficulties in recruitment of healthy subjects may introduce a bias in the selection of control subjects and data thus obtained. Although it is desirable to have one's own control data, due to low intra-observer error and a high interobserver correlation, it is in my view acceptable to refer to normal values from other laboratories, provided standard methodologies are used.

References

Browning C, Valori R, Wingate DL, MacLachlan D (1981) A new pressure sensitive ingestible radiotelemetric capsule. Lancet ii:504–505

Connell AM, McCall J, Misiewicz J, Rowlands EN (1963) Observations on the clinical use of radiopills. Br Med J ii:771–774

Dent J (1976) A new technique for continuous sphincter pressure measurement. Gastroenterology 71:263–267

Dinoso VP, Murthy SNS, Goldstein J, Rosner B (1983) Basal motor activity of the distal colon. A reappraisal. Gastroenterology 85:637–642

Duthie HL, Watts JM (1965) Contribution of the external anal sphincter to the pressure zone in the anal canal. Gut 6:64–68

Frenckner B, Von Euler C (1975) Influence of pudendal block on the function of the anal sphincters. Gut 16:482–489

Gutierrez JG, Oliai A, Chey WY (1975) Manometric profile of the internal anal sphincter in man. Gastroenterology 68:907

Ihre T (1974) Studies on anal function in continent and incontinent patients. Scand J Gastroenterology 9: supp 25

Kielmann J, Bonnesen T (1985) Anal profilometry, a method of investigating the physiology of the anal canal and the pelvic floor. Dan Med Bull 35:61–63

Kumar D, Williams NS, Waldron D, Wingate DL (1989) Prolonged manometric recording of anorectal motor activity in ambulant human subjects; evidence of periodic activity. Gut 30:1007–1011

Kumar D, Waldron D, Williams NS, Browning C, Hutton MRE, Wingate DL (1990) Prolonged anorectal manometry and external anal sphincter electromyography in ambulant human subjects. Dig Dis Sci (in press)

Lubowski DZ, Nicholls RJ, Burleigh DE, Swash M (1988) Internal anal sphincter in neurogenic fecal incontinence. Gastroenterology 95:997–1102

McHugh SM, Diamant NE (1987a) Effect of age, gender and parity on anal canal pressures. Dig Dis Sci 32:726–736

McHugh SM, Diamant NE (1987b) Anal canal pressure profile: a reappraisal as determined by rapid pull through technique. Gut 28:1234–1241

Miller R, Lewis GT, Bartolo DCC, Cervero F, Mortensen NJ (1988) Sensory discrimination and dynamic activity in the anorectum: evidence using a new ambulatory technique. Br J Surg 75:1003–1007

Rao SSC, Real NW, Davison PA, Bannister JJ, Holdsworth CD (1987) Anorectal sensitivity and responses to rectal distension in patients with ulcerative colitis. Gastroenterology 93:1270–1275

Reynolds JR (1988) The application of radiotelemetric techniques in the investigation of gastrointestinal function in health and disease. MD Thesis, University of Nottingham

Taylor BM, Beart RW, Phillips SF (1984) Longitudinal and radial variations of pressure in the human anal sphincter. Gastroenterology 86:693–697

Welgan P, Meshkinpour H, Beeler M (1988) Effect of anger on colon motor and myoelectric activity in irritable bowel syndrome. Gastroenterology 94:1105–1106

Whitehead WE, Engel BT, Schuster MM (1980) Irritable bowel syndrome: physiological and psychological differences between diarrhoea predominant and constipation predominant patients. Dig Dis Sci 25:404–413

Womack NR, Williams NS, Holmfield JHM, Morrison JFB, Simpkins KC (1985) New method for the dynamic assessment of anorectal function in constipation. Br J Surg 72:994–998

Electromyography
R. I. Hallan

Introduction

Since the studies of such early pioneers of electromyography (EMG) as Lord Adrian (Adrian 1925), the techniques of EMG have gradually improved as a result of developments in electronics: firstly valves, than transistors and now computer technology. The basic principles of routine EMG have been well established since the 1950s, when the work of Buchthal and his colleagues (Buchthal et al. 1954), with careful quantitative analysis, laid the foundations for modern electromyography. Since then the changes seen in health and disease have been progressively defined.

Gowers was the first physiologist to display scientfic interest in anal sphincter function and described the recto-anal inhibitory reflex (Gowers, 1877). Reflex responses affecting the (smooth) internal anal sphincter were later studied in detail by Denny-Brown and Robertson (1935) using manometric techniques. The first studies utilizing EMG to investigate (striated) external anal sphincter function were reported by Beck (1930) and Floyd and Walls (1953). Investigation of anal sphincter function by conventional EMG techniques quickly established that these muscles were tonically active even at rest and during sleep (Floyd and Walls 1953) and that contraction was reflexly evoked by coughing, sneezing or lifting heavy weights (Taverner and Smiddy 1959). This activity is facilitated by a spinal reflex arc which is maintained in paraplegics if the level of cord section is above S2 (Parks et al. 1962).

Physiology

The motor unit is the physiological unit of muscle function and is formed by a single alpha motor neurone in the anterior horn of the spinal cord, its nerve and the muscle fibres it supplies. When the unit fires its muscle fibres depolarize at the neuromuscular junctions, and action potentials are conducted along the muscle fibre cell membranes. The muscle fibre electrical activity conduction velocity is approximately 4 m/s, and can be recorded from individual fibres with needle electrodes or from many units with surface electrodes. The potentials are conducted along the muscle fibre membranes and spread through connecting tissues by volume conduction (Forster 1989). Concentric needles are usually used to pick up the resultant potentials as the EMG. Figure 3.4a shows the discharge recorded from a normal motor unit. In a myopathy the unit loses muscle fibres, in myasthenia some fibres are not activated, and in these disorders the recorded potentials are

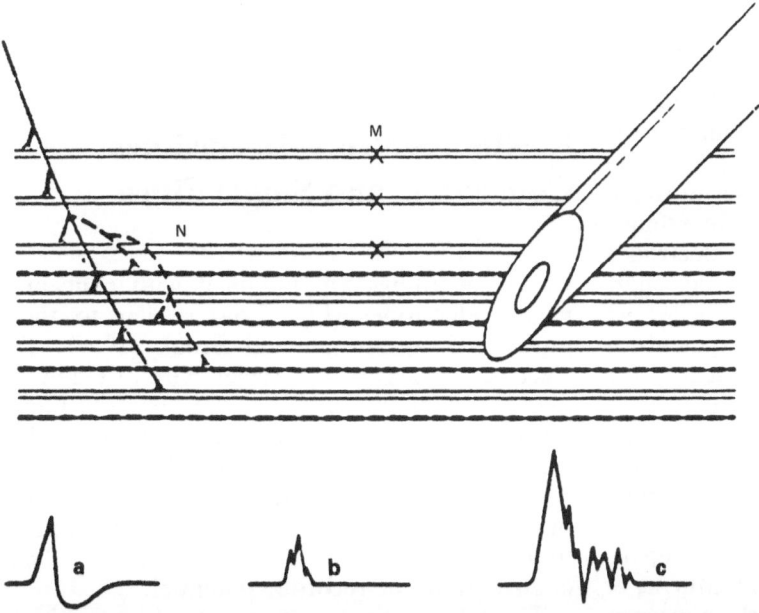

Fig. 3.4. Diagrammatic representation of a motor unit and changes in disease. The nerve fibre is on the left, normally supplying the muscle fibres shown with continuous lines. A concentric needle electrode is on the right. **a** Normal unit, all fibres contributing. **b** Myopathic change. Several fibres of original unit lost at damaged sites M: fewer fibres contribute to the recorded potential, and the EMG amplitude is reduced. **c** Neurogenic change with reinnervation. Nearby fibres (*dashed*) that have lost their nerve supply taken over by axon sprouting (at N) – more fibres contribute to the recorded potential, which is prolonged and of increased amplitude.

smaller (Fig. 3.4b). In a neuropathy, when axons are lost the surviving axons sprout and take over nearby denervated muscle fibres. These additions to the motor unit result in larger, longer units on EMG (Fig. 3.4c). The new axons usually conduct more slowly and less reliably, giving rise to variation in the shape of some of the components on repeated firing.

Patient Position and Electrode Sterilization for Anal Sphincter Electromyography

The left lateral position, as traditionally used for clinical and manometric anorectal physiological assessment, also serves well for most EMG studies of the anal sphincter muscles. It is important the patient is confident and relaxed, in a warm purpose-designed laboratory with all the necessary equipment available within easy reach of one of the investigator's hands, so that he can insert and manipulate EMG needles in the perineum at the same time with the other hand. The skin is adequately cleansed with an antiseptic solution and EMG needles are inserted quickly to the hilt (or as far as necessary) and then withdrawn for recording at several sites during a single needle insertion. This is because needle insertions are more uncomfortable than withdrawals. Inserting a blunt EMG needle is painful; the electrodes should therefore be well maintained and sharpened or replaced when indicated.

There is an ever present risk of patient-to-patient transmission of infectious disease, for example hepatitis and HIV, and it is nowadays essential to use high-pressure autoclave or ethylene dioxide sterilization of needle electrodes in a central sterilization department, rather than simple boiling water. The risk of infection of health care workers from patients carrying hepatitis or HIV is low (McEvoy et al. 1987). Murray et al. (1986) have set out guidelines for the appropriate precautions for dealing with these patients, including the sterilization of electrodes. However not all carriers of infectious diseases are recognized and it would be prudent to conform to these guidelines routinely.

Technique of EMG Recording

EMG apparatus is readily available commercially. A recording electrode, pre-amplifier, amplifier and loudspeaker, and an oscilloscope for the display of electrical activity are required. Modern EMG equipment provides variable amplitude and time-based duration controls within a range suitable for EMG recording, together with low and high pass filter options suitable for the various recording techniques in common use. Storage oscilloscopes with triggering facilities are required for some investigations.

Surface Electrodes

The recording of surface electrical activity is of limited value, but integrated anal sphincter EMG has been useful in long-term ambulatory recordings (Kumar et al. 1988). They are particularly good for recording sphincter EMG in normal subjects, but in neuropathic sphincters the EMG activity is too low to be of use. Surface electrodes are also useful for recording evoked potentials in stimulation techniques.

Needle Electrode Recordings, Concentric and Single Fibre

EMG recordings are obtained with concentric needle electrodes (Fig. 3.5a) similar to those introduced by Adrian and Bronk (1929). The electrode consists of a steel wire 0.1 mm in diameter contained within a thin-pointed cannula resembling a hypodermic needle. The wire electrode is separated from the cannula by insulating resin. The area of the recording surface is 0.07 mm^2, large enough to record the activity of many fibres within a motor unit. Fibres within 1 mm contribute to the recorded potential.

The other main type of needle electrode is the "single fibre" electrode (Fig. 3.5b), which has a very small recording surface of 0.0005 mm^2 (25 μm in diameter). This was first developed by Stålberg and Trontelj (1979) to examine the electrical activity of individual muscle fibres.

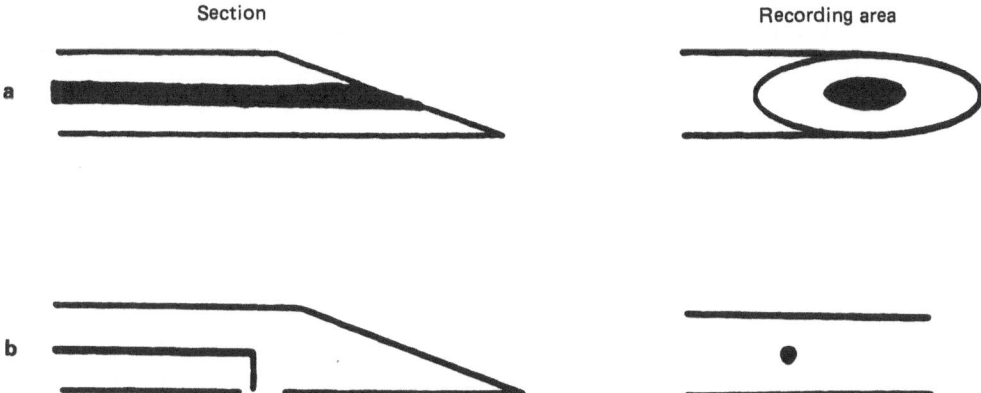

Fig. 3.5. Electrodes used in anal sphincter electromyography. **a** Concentric needle electrode. **b** Single fibre electrode.

Analysis of Concentric Needle Motor Unit Potentials

The potentials recorded from concentric needle electrodes can be subjected to quantitative analysis. The important parameters in analysis of motor units are amplitude, duration, number of phases and firing rate. As the uptake area of the concentric electrode is limited, it is essential that the recording electrode is in close proximity to the individual motor units. Volume conduction effects will modify these parameters when recordings are made at a distance. The major criteria for the proximity of a recording electrode to an active muscle fibre are a fast rise time of the action potential and an adequate amplitude (>150 μV) (Rosenfalck 1969).

The shape of the motor unit action potential during concentric needle EMG is dependent on the filtering characteristics of the amplifier. For most purposes it is conventional to set the low pass filter at 100 Hz and the high pass at 10 kHz, with sweep speeds from 2 to 20 ms.

A potential of more than four phases is termed a polyphasic motor unit potential. Buchthal (1977) defined a phase as those parts of the EMG which lie between two crossings of the base line. The parts of the EMG before the first and after the last crossing of the base line are also considered separate phases. Normal human skeletal muscle recordings contain up to 12% polyphasic motor unit action potentials (Caruso and Buchthal 1965), and this proportion is increased in neuropathic muscle. It is usual to assess the number of phases in individual motor unit action potentials, not during the free-running visualization of the oscilloscope trace during voluntary contraction, but with a trigger delay line. This is an electronic circuit which enables the isolation of individual potentials by triggering on a potential at a preset amplitude window and displaying the potential after a short delay, so that the earliest parts of the triggered potential can also be displayed. Examples of motor unit action potentials in a control subject and an incontinent patient are shown in Fig. 3.6.

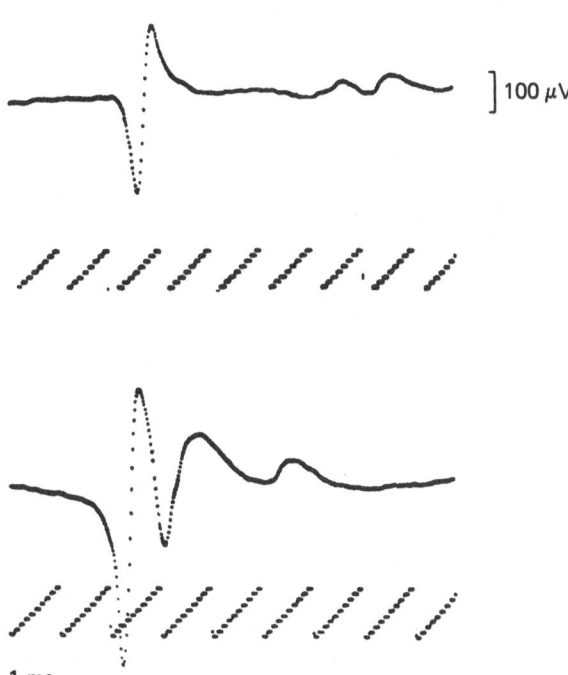

Fig. 3.6. Concentric needle EMG of external anal sphincter. *Upper trace*: normal subject with a biphasic motor unit potential of short duration (<2 ms). *Lower trace*: incontinent patient with a complex, four-phase, motor unit potential of longer duration (4 ms). In both traces the trigger delay line has been used to display the potential in the middle of the oscilloscope screen.

Analysis of Single Fibre Motor Unit Potentials

With concentric needle electrodes, individual muscle fibre action potentials cannot usually be recognized. The small leading-off surface of a single fibre electrode needle, with a 500 Hz low-pass filter and trigger delay line, allows single fibre action potentials to be recorded. When more than one single fibre action potential is recorded within the uptake radius of the electrode (270 μm; Stålberg et al. 1976) the variability in the time interval between the triggering potential and the other potential or potentials belonging to the same motor unit recorded in the uptake area can be measured and is called the neuromuscular jitter (Ekstedt 1964). The jitter is due to variation in the time of onset of the action potential generated by the end-plate potential and tends to be abnormal in myasthenia gravis, where the time course of the end-plate potential is abnormal. In normal subjects each component of the motor unit action potential recorded during single fibre EMG appears with each discharge; there is no impulse blocking. Impulse blocking is a feature of neuropathic muscle damage. Twenty different motor unit action potentials are usually studied. The mean duration of motor unit action potentials, consisting of more than one component recorded by single fibre EMG, is <8 ms. In the extensor digitorum communis muscle the duration did not exceed 4 ms in 95% of recordings in normal subjects (Stålberg and Trontelj 1979).

Fibre Density

The fibre density in single fibre EMG recordings is the mean number of single muscle fibre action potentials recorded within the uptake area of a single fibre EMG electrode in 20 different positions within the muscle (Stålberg and Thiele 1975). This implies four needle insertions into a muscle such as the external anal sphincter, with the recording of five potentials at each site. By convention the components of pelvic muscle motor unit potentials used for triggering must be greater than 100 microvolts. During the process of denervation and reinnervation, there is increased compaction of muscle fibres from an individual motor unit within the uptake area of a single fibre

electrode; i.e. the fibre density increases. It is important to recognize that the investigator must be scrupulous in his technique. There is a tendency to only include potentials with multiple components, but all potentials in which a component is greater than 100 μV must be included in the calculation of the mean derived from the 20 recordings. This avoids bias, which would tend to increase the fibre density.

In normal subjects the fibre density in most muscles is less than 2.0 (Stålberg and Trontelj 1979). It tends to rise slightly after 60 years of age. The fibre density of the external anal sphincter in normal subjects is 1.5 (SD 0.16) (Swash 1985). The fibre density is the most useful quantitative measure obtained from single fibre EMG and repeated investigations can be used for follow-up studies.

Fine Wire Electrodes

Needle EMG electrodes are uncomfortable for the patient, at times painful and are not suitable for recording sphincter EMG long term or during physiological acts such as defaecation. Fine wire electrodes, however, are painfree once inserted and do not appear to interfere with normal function. Their use for recording integrated sphincter EMG activity is an essential part of the technique of dynamic proctography, which is a useful investigation for patients with defaecatory disorders (Womack et al. 1985a).

Stimulation Techniques

The EMG tests described so far are able to determine whether there is evidence of denervation of the pelvic floor muscles, but do not define the site of any abnormality in their innervation. Several stimulation techniques have been developed to assess the conduction of the motor nerves supplying the pelvic floor muscles. The innervation of the external anal sphincter and external urethral sphincter can be assessed by stimulating the pudendal nerves transrectally. The more proximal innervation, including the pelvic sacral innervation of the puborectalis muscle, can be assessed by transcutaneous stimulation of the sacral motor roots at the L1 and L4 levels, allowing the investigation of proximal disorders such as spinal canal stenosis, lumbosacral spondylosis and cauda equina neoplasms, as well as the more common distal, nerve stretch lesions initiated by childbirth or abnormal bowel habit.

Pudendal and Perineal Nerve Terminal Motor Latencies

The pudendal nerve terminal motor latency (PNTML) is measured using a special stimulating and recording electrode combination devised by Kiff and Swash (1984) (Fig. 3.7). The device consists of a rubber finger-stall, which contains two stimulating electrodes at its tips and two recording electrodes at its base. The pudendal nerve is stimulated by digitally guiding the stimulating electrodes to the ischial spine during a rectal examination. Stimulation is by square wave pulses of 0.1 ms duration and 50 V at 1 s intervals. The evoked external anal sphincter (EAS) potential detected by the recording electrodes is displayed on an oscillosope screen, and the stimulating

electrode moved until an optimal response is obtained. The procedure is carried out on both sides of the pelvis so that both pudendal nerves can be examined. The latency of the EAS response is defined as the period from the beginning of the stimulus to the beginning of the response, and represents the terminal motor latency of the pudendal nerves to the external anal sphincter (PNTML).

The perineal nerve terminal motor latency is recorded using the same stimulating device and stimulation parameters. The latency of the evoked response of the periurethral striated sphincter muscle is measured by recording its EMG with an intra-urethral ring electrode mounted on a Foley catheter (Snooks and Swash 1984).

The values of pudendal and perineal nerve terminal motor latencies in control subjects and patients with faecal incontinence are shown in Table 3.1.

The original stimulation and recording device was reusable and required sterilization between patients. A disposable stimulating and recording electrode which can be mounted on an ordinary surgical glove is now available and has simplified the technique (Rogers et al. 1988) (Fig. 3.7).

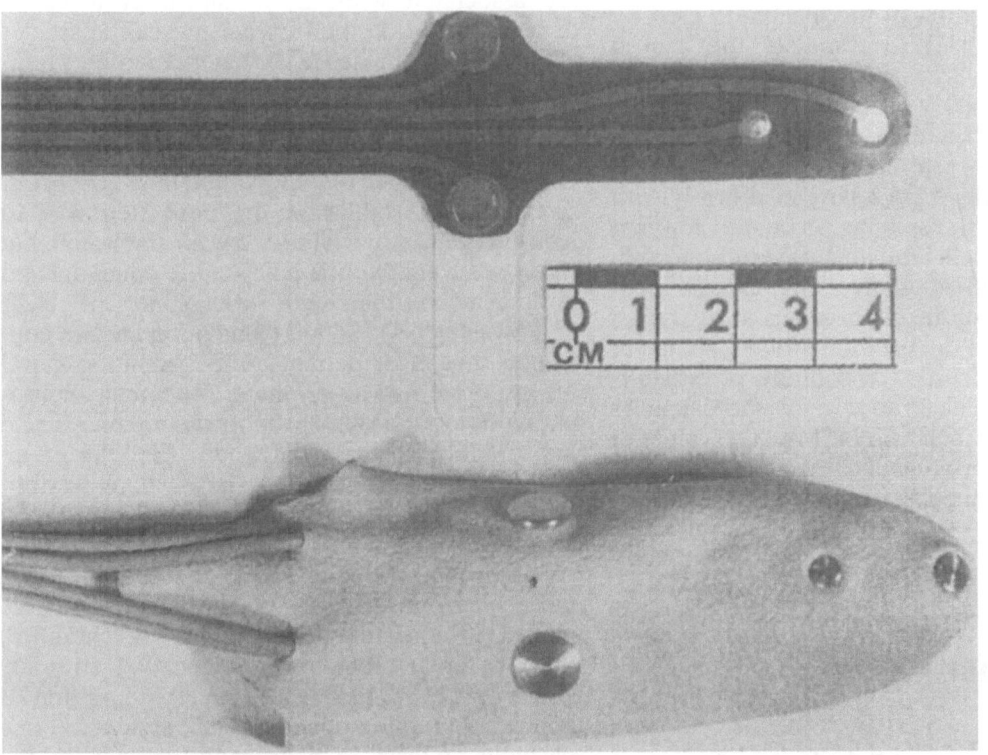

Fig. 3.7. *Above*: the disposable pudendal nerve terminal motor latency measurement device.
Below: the reusable digitally directed pudendal nerve terminal motor latency measurement device. The distance from the cathode to the recording surfaces at the base of the finger is 3 cm.

Table 3.1. The results of electrophysiological tests in control subjects and patients with faecal incontinence

	Normal subjects (n=20)	Faecal incontinence (n=20)
Single fibre EMG: fibre density of EAS	1.5 (0.16)	1.9 (0.2)
Pudendal nerve terminal motor latency PNTML (ms)	1.9 (0.2)	2.6 (0.8)
Spinal latency (ms)		
to EAS L1	5.5 (0.4)	6.0 (0.9)
L4	4.4 (0.4)	4.5 (0.7)
to PR L1	4.8 (0.4)	6.2 (1.4)
L4	3.7 (0.5)	3.5 (0.9)
Spinal latency ratio L1/L4 to PR	1.3 (0.1)	1.8 (0.2)

From Swash (1985).
Standard deviation in parentheses. EAS, external anal sphincter; PR, puborectalis.

Spinal Motor Latencies

Supramaximal transcutaneous stimulation at the L1 and L4 levels evokes compound action potentials in the three pelvic sphincter muscles with reproducible latencies (Swash 1985). The technique is a modification of the technique used by Merton et al. (1982) to stimulate the central nervous system transcutaneously. A single impulse of 800–1500 V, stimulus duration of 0.5 ms, decaying with a time constant of 50 μs, is delivered through two 1 cm diameter saline-soaked gauze pads, 5 cm apart, held firmly with the cathode over the spinous process of the first lumbar (L1) or fourth lumbar (L4) vertebrae, with the anode placed cranially. The evoked contraction response of the puborectalis, the external anal sphincter and the urethral striated sphincter musculature are recorded by digitally- or catheter-mounted surface electrodes, and the latencies calculated as described for PNTML. The values of spinal latencies for control subjects and patients with faecal incontinence are shown in Table 3.1.

Spinal Latency Ratio

The spinal latency ratio (SLR) is given by:

$$SLR = \frac{\text{latency to puborectalis after stimulation at L1}}{\text{latency to puborectalis after stimulation at L4}}$$

and is thus a comparison between the two latencies from different vertebral levels of spinal stimulation. With distal motor conduction delay, both L1 and L4 latencies increase similarly, and the SLR will remain approximately unchanged. However in the presence of proximal motor conduction delay, the L1 latency will be more increased than the L4 latency, and the SLR will be increased. Stimulation at two sites can thus be used to determine whether the conduction delay is within the lumbar canal or distal to the cauda equina, without the necessity for introducing unknown correction factors for the distance between the stimulating and recording electrodes (Swash 1985).

Contribution of Electromyography to Knowledge of Pelvic Floor Physiology and Pathophysiology

The early contribution of EMG to our understanding of pelvic floor physiology has been mentioned. Rectal prolapse and idiopathic faecal incontinence are associated with histochemical evidence of denervation of the pelvic floor muscles (Parks et al. 1977). The presence of denervation and reinnervation in these patients has been confirmed by both conventional (Bartolo et al. 1983) and single fibre (Neill and Swash 1980) electromyography. Once the presence of denervation in faecal incontinence was established the next step was to identify the anatomical site. It was established that there was a conduction delay in the pudendal and perineal nerves in patients with incontinence (Kiff and Swash 1984). Spinal stimulation studies confirmed that most patients with idiopathic faecal incontinence had a peripheral (pudendal) neuropathy, but that a small proportion of patients also had a more central component (Snooks et al. 1985a). Denervation of the pelvic floor has not only been identified in rectal prolapse and faecal incontinence, but may also be a factor in constipation (Snooks et al. 1985b) and solitary rectal ulcer syndrome (Snooks et al. 1985c). The role played in initiating this damage by childbirth (Snooks et al. 1984) and defaecation straining (Lubowski et al. 1988a) seems well established. It appears that idiopathic faecal incontinence is due partially at least to neurogenic damage to the striated sphincter muscles initiated by damage during childbirth and prolonged excessive defaecation straining.

Parks' original observation (Parks 1975) that patients with idiopathic faecal incontinence had poor internal anal sphincter function was largely ignored during the next decade as research workers concentrated on the striated pelvic floor muscles using histochemical and electrophysiological techniques. More recently the role of impaired internal anal sphincter function in the aetiology of idiopathic faecal incontinence has been rediscovered with EMG and ultrastructural evidence of smooth internal anal sphincter damage (Lubowski et al. 1988b; Swash et al. 1988). The name idiopathic, neurogenic, faecal incontinence appears to be inappropriate.

Relevance of Electromyography to the Practice of Coloproctology

It is clear that our understanding of the physiology of the maintenance of faecal continence and the pathophysiology of idiopathic faecal incontinence has paralleled the development of electrophysiological techniques for the investigation of the pelvic floor. The electromyographic and stimulatory techniques have been and still are unquestionably valuable research tools. What is their role in routine coloproctological practice?

In truth the role of EMG and stimulation tests is limited. The majority of coloproctologists practise, quite successfully, without access to these investigations. Felt-Bersma et al. (1989) found that anal sphincter EMG correlated with maximum anal canal pressure in a group of normal and incontinent patients. Indeed our group has found that the assessment of anal sphincter function digitally by an experienced investigator is as accurate as anal canal manometry in discriminating between continent and incontinent subjects (Hallan et al. 1989). There is a close correlation between the degree of denervation assessed by fibre density and the simple, and more acceptable, measurement of perineal position relative to the ischial tuberosities (Womack et al. 1985b).

Concentric needle EMG is particularly valuable in "sphincter mapping" to assess the extent of any remaining external anal sphincter in faecal incontinence due to sphincter disruption, in order to determine whether a sphincter repair is feasible. This applies both to anterior defects due to obstetric injuries or injuries to other segments of the sphincter caused by non-iatrogenic trauma, or iatrogenic trauma during injudicious fistula surgery. More sophisticated EMG investigations such as fibre density determination and stimulation techniques are valuable research tools. If anal canal pressures are low it is likely that the sphincters have been damaged by neuropathy, and the results of EMG and stimulation tests would merely confirm this. Their actual documentation would not usually contribute to clinical decision making. There are perhaps exceptions to this generalization. It may be advisable for women with EMG evidence of neuropathy to have a caesarian section in a future pregnancy rather than another vaginal delivery (Bartolo 1988). Patients with a severe neuropathy who undergo a sphincter repair for an obstetric tear have a worse outcome, and Laurberg et al. (1988) have suggested that these patients should also have a postanal repair. EMG and stimulation techniques are, however, useful for the assessment of the complicated patient.

The real benefit of an anorectal physiology laboratory, including sophisticated EMG techniques, to patients with difficult or rare coloproctological disorders is that with the technology comes the expertise of clinical neurophysiologists and surgeons with a particular interest in their disorders. The results of treating these patients by such a team must surely be better than if these patients are treated by surgeons who only see these disorders rarely. Studying these patients will lead to continuing progress in the understanding of normal physiology of the pelvic floor and its derangement in pelvic floor disorders. Greater understanding of these mechanisms in the long term could lead to improved treatment.

References

Adrian ED (1925) Interpretation of the electromyogram. Lancet i:1229–1233

Adrian ED, Bronk DW (1929) The discharge of impulses in motor nerve fibres. Part II. The frequency of discharge in reflex and voluntary contractions. J Physiol (Lond) 67:119–151

Bartolo DCC (1988) Pelvic floor disorders: incontinence, constipation, and obstructed defaecation. Perspect Colon Rectal Surg 1:1–24

Bartolo DCC, Jarratt JA, Read NW (1983) The use of conventional electromyography to assess external sphincter neuropathy in man. J Neurol Neurosurg Psychiat 46:1115–1118

Beck A (1930) Elektromyographische Untersuchungen am Sphinkter ani. Arch Physiol 224:278–292

Buchthal F (1977) Diagnostic significance of myopathic EMG. In: Rowland EP (ed) Pathogenesis of human muscular dystrophies. Exerpta Medica, Amsterdam, pp 205–218 (Exerpta Medica International Congress Series 404)

Buchthal F, Guld C, Rosenfalck P (1954) Action potential parameters in normal human muscle and their dependence on physical variables. Act Physiol Scand 32: 200–218

Caruso C, Buchthal F (1965) Refractory period of muscle and EMG findings in relatives of patients with muscular dystrophy. Brain 88:29–50

Denny-Brown D, Robertson EG (1935) An investigation of the nervous control of defaecation. Brain 58:256–310

Ekstedt J (1964) Human single muscle fiber action potentials. Act Physiol Scand 61 (supp 226): 1–98

Felt-Bersma RJF, Strijers RLM, Janssen JJWM, Visser SL, Meuwissen SGM (1989) The external anal sphincter: relationship between anal manometry and anal electromyography and its clinical relevance. Dis Colon Rectum 32:112–116

Floyd WF, Walls EW (1953) Electromyography of the sphincter ani externus in man. J Physiol (Lond) 122:599–609

Forster A (1989) Modern neurophysiology – electromyography. Br J Hosp Med 41:38–49

Gowers WR (1877) The automatic action of the sphincter ani. Proc R Soc (Lond) 26:77–84

Hallan RI, Marzouk DEMM, Waldron DJ, Womack NR, Williams NS (1989) Comparison of digital and manometric assessment of anal sphincter function. Br J Surg 76:973–975

Kiff ES, Swash M (1984) Slowed conduction in the pudendal nerves in idiopathic (neurogenic) faecal incontinence. Br J Surg 71:614–616

Kumar D, Williams NS, Waldron D, Browning C, Hutton MRE, Hallan RI, Wingate D (1988) Prolonged anorectal mechanical and electrical activity in ambulant human subjects. Gut 29:A734

Laurberg S, Swash M, Henry MM (1988) Delayed external sphincter repair for obstetric tear. Br J Surg 75:786–788

Lubowski DZ, Swash M, Nicholls RJ, Henry MM (1988a) Increase in pudendal nerve terminal motor latency with defaecation straining. Br J Surg 75:1095–1097

Lubowski DZ, Nicholls RJ, Burleigh DR, Swash M (1988b) Internal anal sphincter in neurogenic fecal incontinence. Gastroenterology 95:997–1002

McEvoy M, Porter K, Mortimer P, Simmons N, Shanson D (1987) Prospective study of clinical, laboratory, and ancillary staff with accidental exposures to blood or body fluids from patients infected with HIV. Br Med J 294:1595–1597

Merton PA, Hill DK, Morton HB, Marsden CD (1982) Scope of a technique for electrical stimulation of the human brain, spinal cord and muscle. Lancet ii:597–600

Murray NMF, Kriss A, Evans B (1986) Aids, Hepatitis B and Creutzfeld-Jacob disease: guidelines for dealing with patients and electrodes in the clinical neurophysiology laboratory. J Electrophysiol Technol 12:53–59

Neill ME, Swash M (1980) Increased motor unit fibre density in the external sphincter in anorectal incontinence: a single fibre EMG study. J Neurol Neurosurg Psychiat 43:343–347

Parks AG (1975) Anorectal incontinence. Proc R Soc Med 68:681–690

Parks AG, Porter NH, Melzak J (1962) Experimental study of the reflex mechanism controlling the muscles of the pelvic floor. Dis Colon Rectum 5:407–414

Parks AG, Swash M, Urich H (1977) Sphincter denervation in ano-rectal incontinence and rectal prolapse. Gut 18:656–665

Rogers J, Henry MM, Misiewiscz JJ (1988) Disposable pudendal nerve stimulator: evaluation of standard instrument and new device. Gut 29:1131–1133

Rosenfalck P (1969) Intra and extra cellular potential fields of active nerve and muscle fibres. Act Physiol Scand (supp) 321:1–168

Snooks SJ, Swash M (1984) Perineal nerve and transcutaneous spinal stimulation: new methods for investigation of the urethral striated sphincter musculature. Br J Urol 56:406–409

Snooks SJ, Setchell M, Swash M, Henry MM (1984) Injury to the innervation of the pelvic floor sphincter musculature in childbirth. Lancet ii:546–550

Snooks SJ, Swash M, Henry MM (1985a) Abnormalities in central and peripheral nerve conduction in patients with anorectal incontinence. J R Soc Med 78:294–300

Snooks SJ, Barnes PRH, Swash M, Henry MM (1985b) Damage to the innervation of the pelvic floor musculature in chronic constipation. Gastroenterology 89:977–981

Snooks SJ, Nicholls RJ, Henry MM, Swash M (1985c) Electrophysiological and manometric assessment of the pelvic floor in the solitary rectal ulcer syndrome. Br J Surg 72:131–133

Stålberg E, Thiele B (1975) Motor unit fibre density in the extensor digitorum communis muscle. J Neurol Neurosurg Psychiat 38:874–800

Stålberg E, Trontelj JV (1979) Single fibre electromyography. Miravelle Press, Old Woking

Stålberg E, Trontelj JV, Schwartz MS (1976) Single muscle fibre recording of the jitter phenomenon in patients with myasthenia gravis and in members of their families. Ann NY Acad Sci 274:189–202

Swash M (1985) Anorectal incontinence: electrophysiological tests. Br J Surg (supp) 72: S14–S15

Swash M, Gray A, Lubowski DZ, Nicholls RJ (1988) Ultrastructural changes in internal anal sphincter in neurogenic faecal incontinence. Gut 29:1692–1698

Taverner D, Smiddy FG (1959) An electromyographic study of the normal function of the external anal sphincter and pelvic diaphragm. Dis Colon Rectum 2:153–160

Womack NR, Williams NS, Holmfield JHM, Morrison JFB, Simpkins KC (1985a) New method for the dynamic assessment of anorectal function in constipation. Br J Surg 72:994–998

Womack NR, Morrison IFB, Williams NS (1985b) Non-invasive assessment of idiopathic faecal incontinence. Br J Surg (supp) 72:S128

Dynamic Assessment of Anorectal Function

N. R. Womack and P. R. O'Connell

Introduction

The rectum acts as a reservoir for faecal matter until evacuation is socially convenient. The rectum must therefore empty efficiently and completely when required. Evacuation depends on complex interactions between the sphincteric and reservoir components of the continence mechanism. These interactions have recently been the subject of considerable physiological investigation. With greater understanding of the physiology of continence has come a developing interest in disorders of evacuation and continence. Interaction among the rectum, the pelvic floor and the anal sphincters is a dynamic process and considerably more information is obtained from studies conducted during defaecation rather than in static situations. This chapter will deal with recently developed techniques of dynamic assessment of anorectal physiology.

Proctography

Examination of the rectum is part of every contrast study of the large intestine. Lateral pelvic, prone and decubitus views provide detail of anatomy and mucosal integrity. Such information is useful in diagnosis of neoplastic, inflammatory and developmental conditions but little information is provided concerning anorectal function. Although Hertz (1908) reported a radiological study of defaecation in humans, it was not until development of cineradiology that radiological investigation of anorectal function became possible.

In the first major study of anorectal physiology using cineradiography, Phillips and Edwards (1965) studied healthy volunteers in whom faeces had been rendered radio-opaque by ingestion of methyl cellulose and barium sulphate powder for 3 days prior to the study. Broden and Snellman (1968) investigated rectal prolapse using liquid barium suspension instilled into the rectum in combination with a cystogram and oral barium to outline the bladder and small intestine. To study defaecation in constipated patients, Kerremans (1969) devised a radio-opaque synthetic mixture of plasticine and barium sulphate which more accurately reproduced the consistency of constipated stool. These and other studies (Hardcastle and Parks 1970; Rutter 1974) greatly contributed to understanding of anorectal physiology. Maintenance of an acute anorectal angle was shown to be important for preservation of continence whereas failure of the pelvic floor to relax during defaecation was shown to contribute to obstructed defaecation.

During the past 20 years proctography has been developed in several different centres. No single technique has achieved widespread acceptance. There is, however, general agreement on a number of important points. Proctography should generally be performed on unprepared bowel. The contrast medium used should reproduce the consistency of faecal matter, as the radiological findings may differ if a liquid barium preparation is used (Shorvon et al 1989). Contrast media that are used include commercially available barium paste (Turnbull et al. 1988), a mixture of barium and potato starch (Mahieu et al. 1984), oat porridge (Womack et al. 1985) or methyl cellulose (Kodner 1988). There is no consensus regarding the amount of contrast that should be infused into the rectum and this varies widely from 50 ml (Read et al. 1984) to 300 ml (Womack et al. 1985). The anal canal is usually outlined with barium paste inserted digitally; however Bartolo et al. (1983) used a beaded metal chain to outline the anal canal. Proctography should be performed with the patient seated on a radiolucent commode. The design of commode varies between institutions. Most are constructed of perspex or plastic but Mahieu et al. (1984) recommend use of water-filled rubber tubing. Following insertion of the contrast the patient should be afforded the maximum possible degree of privacy. Lateral pelvic radiographs are taken at rest and during maximum squeeze effort. These are followed by a cine or video recording during which the patient is asked to evacuate. The following parameters are routinely measured: anorectal angle at rest; during squeeze effort; during evacuation; pelvic floor descent during evacuation. Changes in configuration of the rectal wall during evacuation are observed and the presence of a rectocoele or intussusception recorded. An estimation of the efficiency of evacuation may also be made.

The anorectal angle is the angle between the luminal axis of the anal canal and a line drawn along the lower border of the distal rectum (Figs. 3.8 and 3.9). The conventional method of measuring the anorectal angle has been criticized because the posterior border of the rectum is difficult to define and is rarely a straight line. Nevertheless, proposed alternatives, a line from the rectal centroid to the anorectal junction (Yoshioka et al. 1988) or determination of the central rectal angle (Shorvon et al. 1989) are complex to determine and have not met with widespread acceptance (Keighley et al. 1989). Using conventional measurement of the anorectal angle, we have found in healthy control subjects that the mean anorectal angle at rest is 93° (range 86–108). During evacuation the mean anorectal angle increased to 132° (range 120–145) (Womack 1988). These results

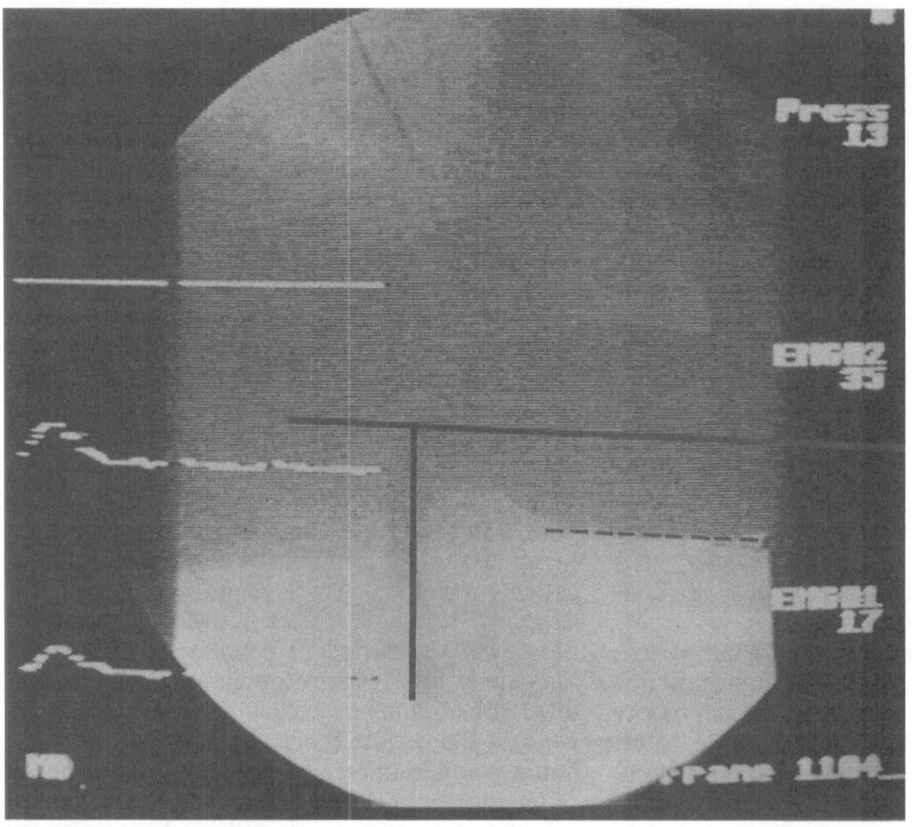

Fig. 3.8. Proctogram of a control subject at rest. The anorectal angle is measured between the axis of the anal canal and the axis of the rectum (a solid line parallel to the posterior wall of the rectum, indicated by the *hatched line*). Integrated pressure (*top white line*) and EMG recordings (*middle and lower white lines*) are superimposed on the proctogram (see Fig. 3.13).

are in close agreement with other reports (Mahieu et al. 1984; Ekberg et al. 1985; Skomorowska et al. 1987; Shorvon et al. 1989).

Pelvic floor descent is calculated from the proctogram by measuring the distance between the anorectal junction and the pubococcygeal line which joins the upper margin of the symphysis pubis and the tip of the coccyx. At rest this distance is normally less than 1.8 cm and on straining should not increase by more than 2 cm (Hardcastle and Parks 1970). The clinical importance of pelvic floor descent is controversial (Bartolo et al. 1983) and it has recently been shown that a considerable number of healthy control volunteers on straining demonstrate pelvic floor descent in excess of 2 cm (Shorvon et al. 1989).

Perineal descent may also be measured from the proctogram. It is taken as the distance between the pubococcygeal line and the anal margin. However significant, shortening of the anal canal occurs during straining. Thus measurement of perineal descent either radiologically or by use of a "perineometer" (Henry et al. 1982) results in an under-

estimate of pelvic floor movement during staining or defaecation (Oettle et al. 1985).

Changes in configuration in the rectal wall during defaecation are difficult to define and are open to observer variation. The most frequently seen changes are rectocoele and intussusception. A rectocoele results from inadequate support of the anterior rectal wall above the anal canal. During defaecation increased intra-abdominal and intrarectal pressure produce a bulge of the anterior rectal wall into the vagina (Fig. 3.10). Small rectocoeles are frequently asymptomatic and small outpocketing of the anterior rectal wall may even be observed in men (Bartram et al. 1987). The clinical importance of a proctographic rectocoele needs careful interpretation. Intrarectal intussusception varies greatly in degree and in clinical importance. A degree of anterior rectal wall prolapse is commonly seen even in healthy controls (Shorvon et al. 1989). Even intrarectal intussusception (Fig. 3.11) which results from a more prominent circumferential invagination of the rectal wall may be seen in asymptomatic

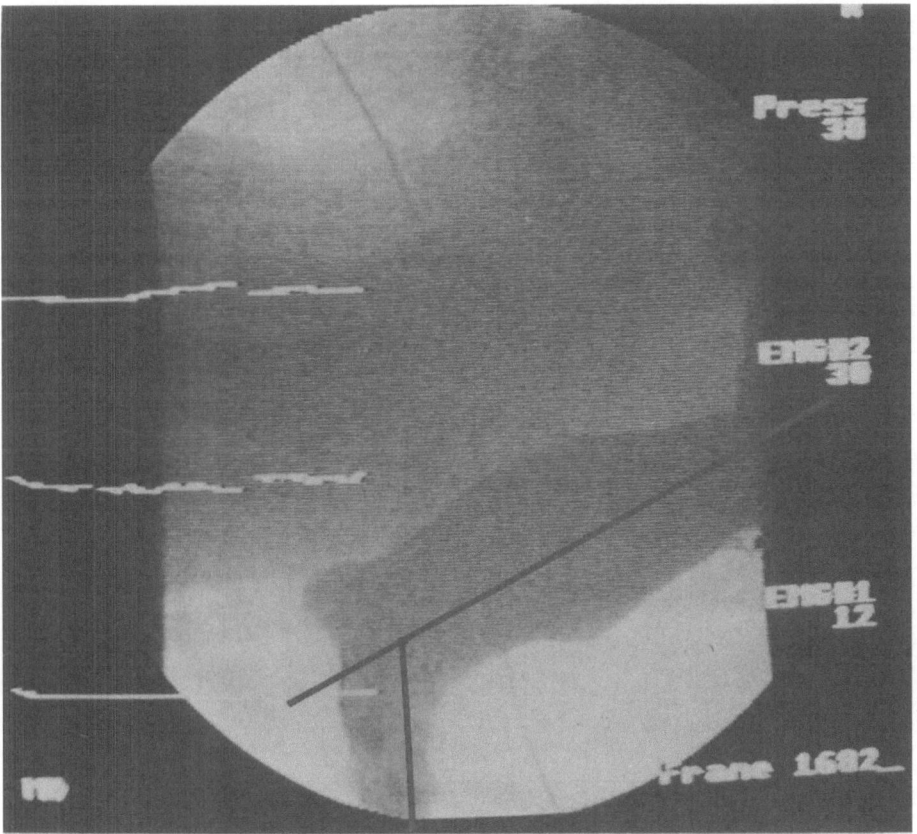

Fig. 3.9. Proctogram of a control subject during evacuation showing an obtuse anorectal angle. Intregrated pressure and EMG recordings are superimposed on the proctogram (see Fig. 3.13).

healthy controls (Womack 1988). Only when the intussusceptum reaches the anal canal, an intra-anal intussusception, is obstructed defaecation likely and further straining may produce a full thickness rectal prolapse (Fig. 3.12).

The advent of video radiography has reduced the radiation dose of proctography to about 25% of that of a conventional barium enema. This has allowed more widespread use of proctography as a research tool. Nevertheless the radiation dosage is significant and one of the considerable limitations of the technique at present is the relative paucity of data from healthy controls, particularly of women in the reproductive years. Only Skomorowska et al. (1987), Womack (1988) and Shorvon et al. (1989) have reported useful numbers of control studies, despite the world experience of proctography exceeding 4500 examinations (Finlay 1988). The control data available demonstrate "abnormalities" in over half the subjects studied (Shorvon et al. 1989) and illustrate that apparent abnormalities on proctography need to be correlated with the clinical picture and the results of other physiological investigations.

Balloon Proctography

The balloon proctogram was devised as a simple, quick and well tolerated technique which could provide much of the information available from standard proctography with a lower radiation dosage, without the need for preparation of special proctographic media (Preston et al. 1984). The test is performed by inserting a lubricated latex balloon mounted on a soft catheter into the rectum. The balloon is inflated with 100 ml of barium and water mixture. A lateral radiograph is taken with the patient seated on a radiolucent commode. A second radiograph is taken while the patient strains, simulating defaecation. The technique allows easy measurement of the anorectal angle and of pelvic floor descent.

Balloon sphincterography is an interesting variation of the balloon proctography technique (Lahr et al. 1988). The principle is similar except that the balloon is attached, outside the anal canal, by a hose to a bag of water-soluble x-ray contrast material. This bag of contrast material may be raised or lowered and the pressure within the

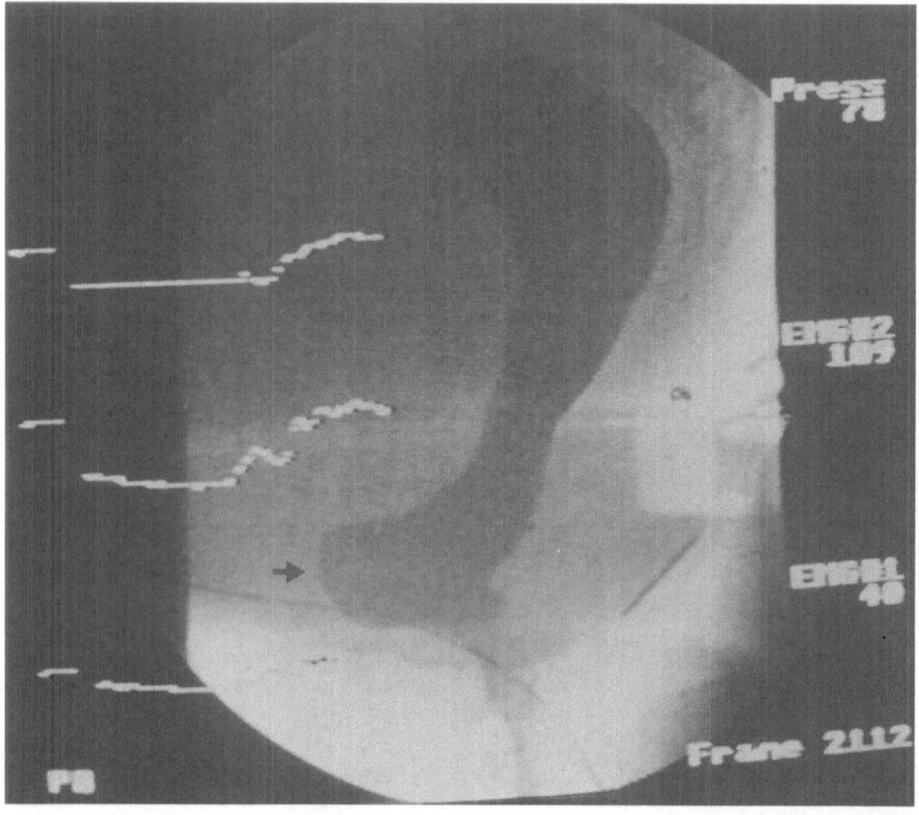

Fig. 3.10. Proctogram of a subject with a rectocoele (indicated by *arrow*). Intregrated pressure and EMG recordings are superimposed on the proctogram (see Fig. 3.13).

balloon is equal to the height of the bag. The pressure within the balloon at which the anal canal opens to allow flow of contrast into the intrarectal portion of the balloon correlates with resting pressure of the anal canal. The anorectal angle and pelvic floor measurements can be made in the standard fashion on lateral radiographs. The Lahr balloon, while ingenious, has been criticized as unreliable (Keighley et al. 1989) and is not widely used.

Balloon proctography has not achieved widespread application because measurement of the anorectal angle and pelvic floor descent alone are not considered to be of sufficient value to permit clinical decisions. As the technique does not provide dynamic imaging of the anterior and posterior rectal walls, abnormalities during defaecation such as rectal wall intussusception cannot be identified. It is clear that clinical decisions need to be based not on proctography alone, but in conjunction with other parameters of anorectal function.

Dynamic Synchronous Proctography

In response to the need for correlation between apparent abnormalities on proctography and other physiological investigations, we developed a technique capable of identifying both structural and functional anorectal abnormalities (Womack et al. 1985). The method, dynamic synchronous proctography, involves integration of proctographic, electromyographic and manometric data (Fig. 3.13). A semisolid contrast medium, made from oatmeal, barium sulphate and water, serves to simulate soft stool and allows the anorectum to be delineated by image intensification radiology. External anal sphincter EMG activity is recorded using fine wire electrodes inserted into the puborectalis and superficial components of the external anal sphincter. A pressure-sensitive radiotelemetry capsule is used to monitor changes in intrarectal pressure. The manometric and electromyographic changes during the proctogram are recorded and mixed with the video output of the image intensifier to produce a composite

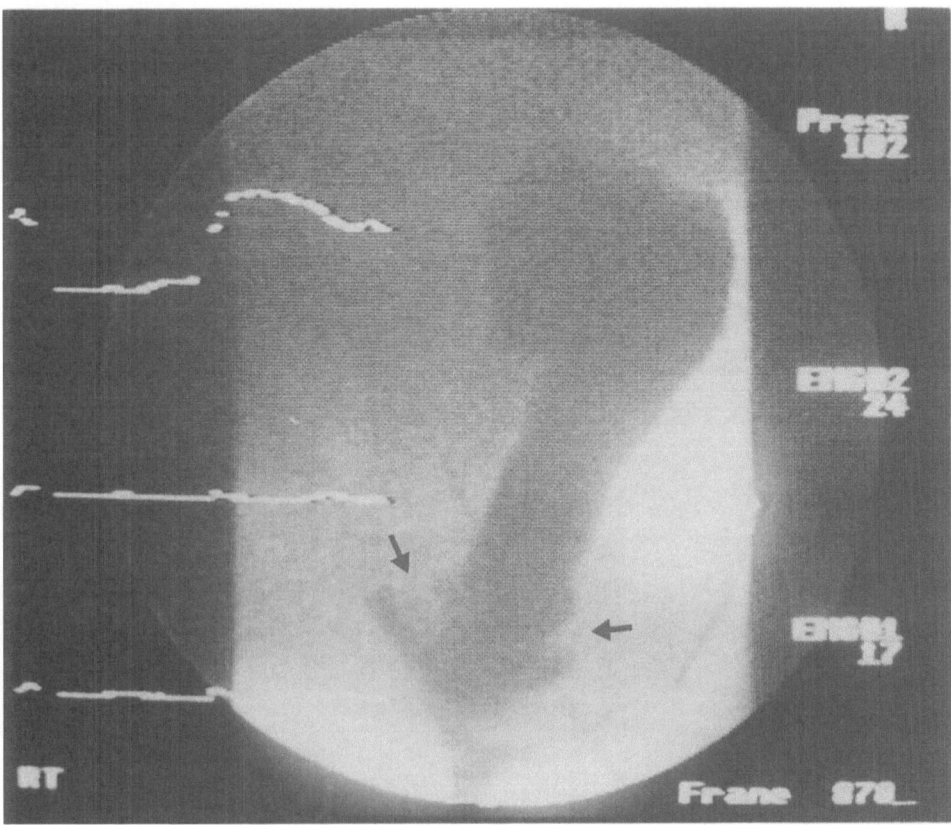

Fig. 3.11. Proctogram of a subject with rectal intussusception (*arrows* indicate the head of the intussusception). Intregrated pressure and EMG recordings are superimposed on the proctogram (see Fig. 3.13).

image which may be stored (Figs. 3.8–3.12). Alternatively the manometric and electromyographic data may be used to generate a graph of pressure and EMG changes against time (Fig. 3.14).

The technique has proved useful both as a research tool and in clinical practice as it allows correlation of EMG activity of the external anal sphincter and pelvic floor muscles with synchronous visualization of defaecation. It has proven of particular value in patients with symptoms of obstructed defaecation. In some, the puborectalis fails to relax during defaecation and the anorectal angle remains acute; this is termed anismus or spastic pelvic floor syndrome (Kuijpers and Bleijenberg 1985). In others, straining during evacuation produces anterior rectal wall prolapse. When this is associated with overactivity of the external anal sphincter, the combination of rectal prolapse and high pressure in the upper anal canal can produce mucosal ulceration. These abnormalities have been found in patients with the solitary rectal ulcer syndrome (Womack et al. 1987).

Scintigraphy

Conventional proctography provides clear definition of anorectal anatomy and function, particularly when combined with synchronous electromyographic recording. However, proctography is associated with substantial pelvic radiation. Furthermore, proctography does not permit the efficiency of emptying to be accurately measured. These problems tend to limit the use of standard proctography as a research tool, particularly in patients who have ileal pouch–anal anastomosis, many of whom will have had several preoperative barium radiographs. Quantification of ileal pouch emptying is important, as inefficient ileal pouch emptying has been shown, in certain situations, to contribute to postoperative problems (O'Connell et al. 1987). To overcome this, several investigators have used scintigraphic techniques to outline the "neorectum" and to measure the efficiency of evacuation (O'Connell et al. 1986a; Nasmyth et al. 1986; Heppell et al. 1987). Using scintigraphy it has been shown that the ileal pouch neorectum empties efficiently and

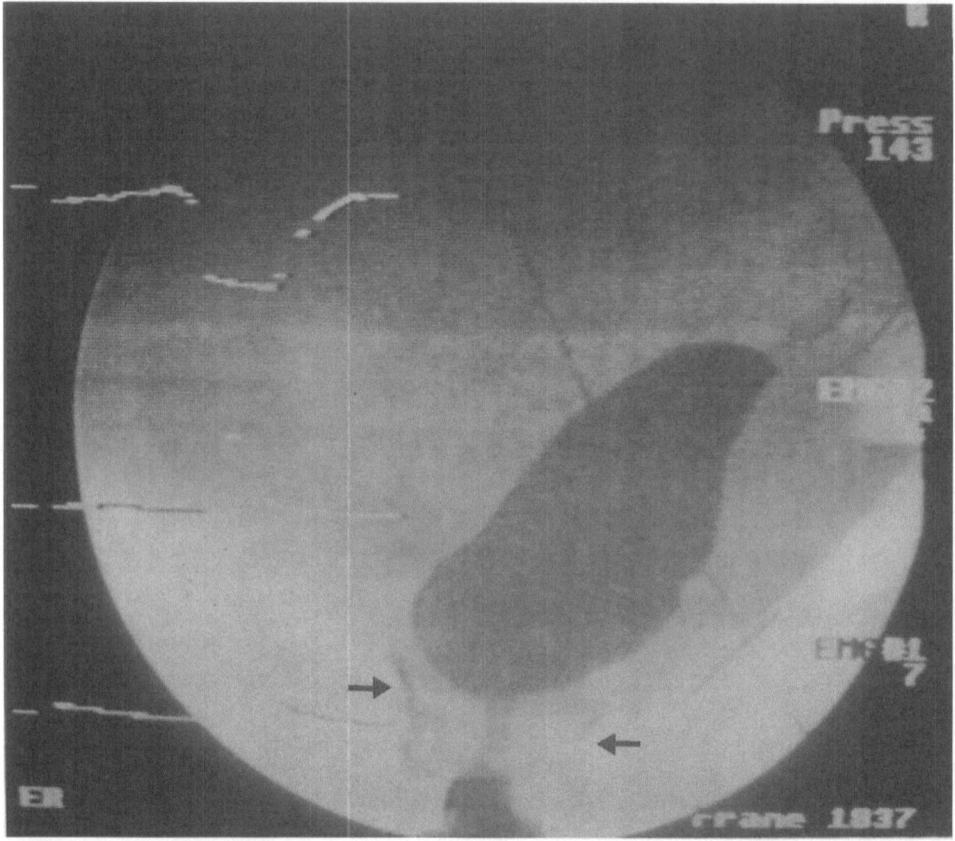

Fig. 3.12. Proctogram of a subject with full thickness rectal prolapse (*arrows* indicate the everted anorectal mucosa). Intregrated pressure and EMG recordings are superimposed on the proctogram (see Fig. 3.13).

that there is little difference in the emptying efficiency of the various reservoir designs in current use. Stasis within the ileal pouch has been shown not to underlie the condition of recurrent ileal pouch mucosal inflammation, termed "pouchitis" or "pouch ileitis" (O'Connell et al. 1986b; Heppell et al. 1987).

An interesting adaptation of scintigraphy and the balloon proctogram was described by Barkel et al. (1988). A balloon was inserted per anum into the rectum and it was filled with water containing technetium-99m. The scintigraphic technique using reference markers on the pubis and coccyx allowed measurement of the anorectal angle and pelvic floor descent. The radiation dosage to reproductive organs was approximately 7% of that required for an equivalent study in which barium sulphate with fluoroscopy and spot films was used. While useful in a research setting, balloon scintigraphy, like conventional balloon proctography, is unlikely to be a useful clinical tool.

Proctometrogram

In common with other physiological reservoirs, the rectum demonstrates receptive relaxation in response to distension. The ability of the rectum to accommodate a faecal bolus with minimal increase in intrarectal pressure is reflected in the compliance or distensibility of the rectal wall. The proctometrogram, a technique developed from the cystometrogram (Lipkin et al. 1962), provides information on rectal compliance, the volume at which there is first rectal sensation and the maximum tolerable capacity of the rectum. The most commonly used technique records intrarectal pressure response to progressive rectal distension using a water-filled balloon (Varma and Smith 1986a). Others have used air-filled systems (O'-Connell et al. 1987). More recently, Akervall et al. (1989) have suggested that rectal reservoir and sensory function may be best ·measured using graded isobaric distension.

Distensibility is an important property of the

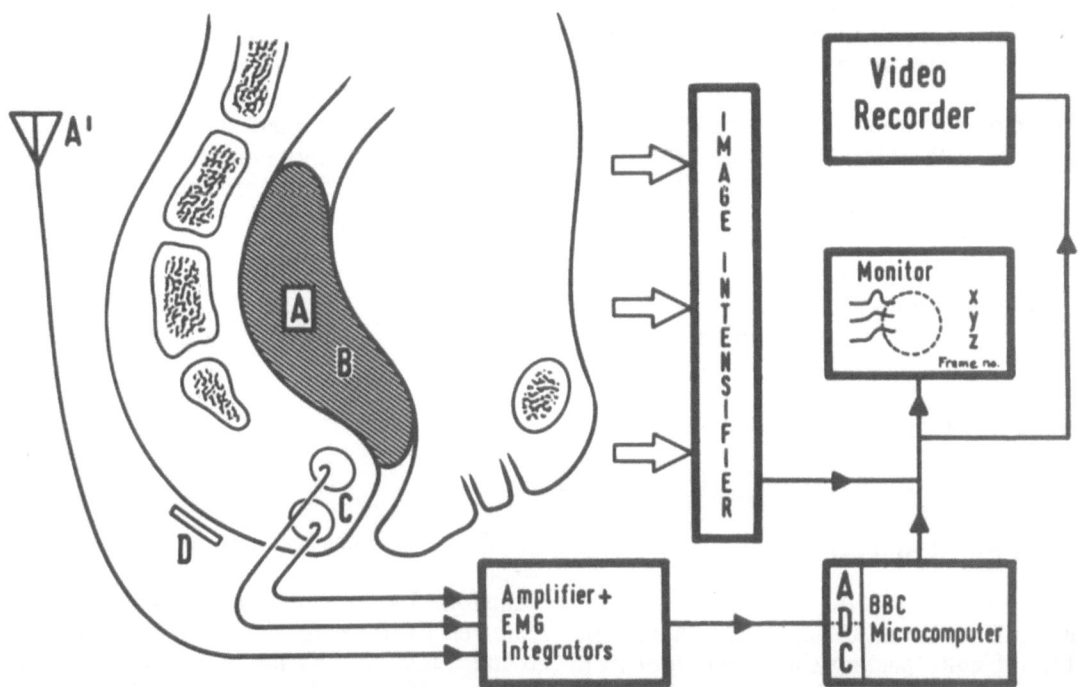

Fig. 3.13. Diagrammatic representation of data acquisition during dynamic synchronous proctography. A, pressure sensitive radiotelemetry capsule; A′, omnidirectional antenna strapped over sacrum; B, radio-opaque contrast medium in rectum; C, EMG electrodes in puborectalis and external anal sphincter; D, metal marker on perianal skin.

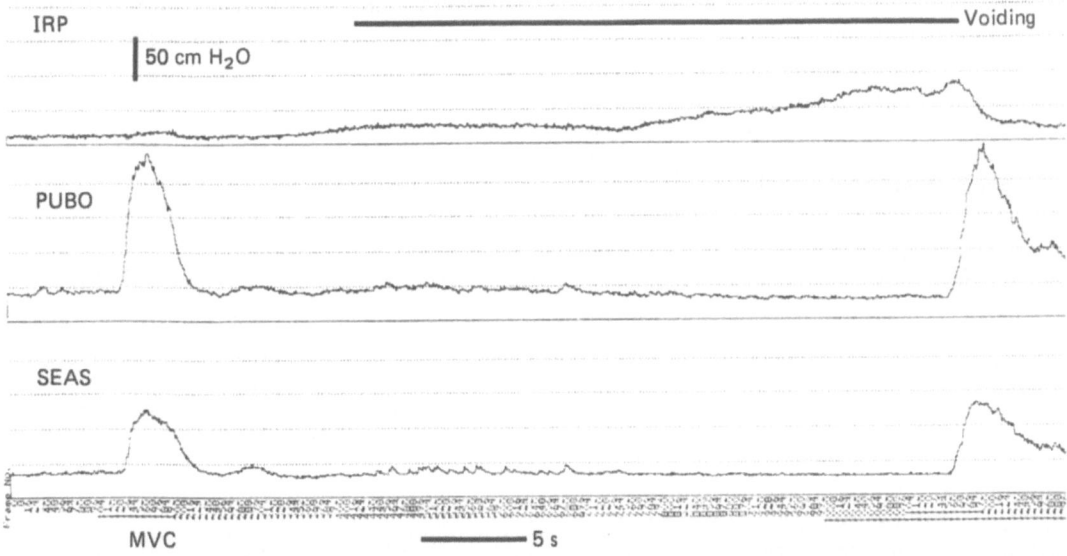

Fig. 3.14. Integrated intrarectal pressure (IRP, *top tracing*) and EMG recordings (puborectalis, *middle tracing*; superficial external anal sphincter, *lower tracing*), showing activity during maximal voluntary contraction (MVC) and voiding. Completion of voiding is associated with increased EMG activity, the "closing" reflex.

rectum. Using the proctometrogram it has been shown that loss of distensibility produces the urgency of defaecation experienced by patients with inflammatory (Denis et al. 1979), ischaemic (Devroede et al. 1982) or radiation proctitis (Varma and Smith 1986b). The unsatisfactory functional results experienced by patients after straight ileoanal anastomosis or coloanal anastomosis can be attributed to small reservoir capacity and reduced reservoir distensibility. Construction of an ileal pouch or colonic pouch "neorectum" overcomes these problems and greatly improves the clinical outcome (Beart et al. 1982; Nicholls et al. 1988).

The proctometrogram may be used to investigate patients with intractable constipation. In these patients, rectal distensibility is greatly increased. Large volumes are required to distend the rectum sufficiently to produce an intrarectal pressure sufficient to evoke a sensation of rectal filling and to induce an urge to evacuate. Soiling may occur in elderly patients in whom distension of the rectum produces inhibition of the internal anal sphincter, without perception, because of diminished rectal sensation (Read et al. 1985).

Balloon Expulsion Tests

Patients with intractable constipation have considerable difficulty passing simulated stool from the rectum. This may be demonstrated using a balloon expulsion test. A latex ballon filled with 50 ml water at 37 °C is inserted into the rectum. The patient is asked to expel the balloon and failure to do so is considered a positive test (Read et al. 1984). Recently, Lestar et al. (1989) have described an interesting new balloon expulsion test which provides information regarding rectal sensation as well as the ability to evacuate a simulated faecal bolus. The technique is simple to perform and provides similar information to the proctometrogram. It may find a clinical role.

Combined Urinary and Anorectal Assessment

The urinary bladder and the rectum have several common pathways of innervation. Damage to the spinal cord may produce both urinary and faecal incontinence or urinary retention and chronic constipation, depending on the level of injury. The pudendal nerve innervates both the external anal sphincter and the periurethral striated sphincter, via the perineal nerve. Damage may result in double incontinence (Snooks et al. 1984). Recent studies indicate that a high proportion of patients with idiopathic intractable constipation also give a history of urinary dysfunction (Bannis-

ter et al. 1988; Varma and Smith 1988). Combined urodynamic, proctometric and neurophysiological studies indicate that the common abnormality may lie in sacral segments of the spinal cord (Kerrigan et al. 1989). Prompted by these observations, research is currently being directed towards synchronous use of ambulatory anorectal and urological manometry to further elucidate the subtle abnormalities that may underlie "idiopathic" disorders of anorectal and urological function.

Conclusion

In the past decade there has been a virtual explosion of interest in disorders of anorectal function. Large numbers of patients are being referred for investigation. Dynamic tests of anorectal function provide clinically useful information. We have found that combined synchronous proctography adds little to performance of standard proctography and is as convenient as performing separate electomyographic and proctographic studies. At the London Hospital we recommend anal manometry, combined synchronous proctography and a proctometrogram as standard investigations for patients referred for assessment of anorectal function.

References

Akervall S, Fasth S, Nordgen S, Oresland T, Hulten L (1989) Rectal reservoir and sensory function studied by graded isobaric distension in normal man. Gut 30:496–502

Bannister JJ, Lawrence WT, Smith A, Thomas DG, Read NW (1988) Urological abnormalities in young women with severe constipation. Gut 29:17–20

Barkel DC, Pemberton JH, Pezim ME, Phillips SF, Kelly KA, Brown ML (1988) Scintigraphic assessment of the anorectal angle in health and after ileal pouch–anal anastomosis. Ann Surg 208:42–49

Bartolo DCC, Read NW, Jarratt JA, Read MG, Donnelly TC, Johnson AG (1983) Differences in anal sphincter function and clinical presentation in patients with pelvic floor descent. Gastroenterology 85:68–75

Bartram CI, Turnbull GK, Lennard-Jones JE (1987) Evacuation proctography: an investigation of rectal expulsion in 20 subjects without defecatory disturbance. Gastrointestinal Radiol 13:72–80

Beart RW, Dozois RR, Kelly KA (1982) Ileoanal anastomosis in the adult. Surg Gynecol Obstet 154:826–828

Broden B, Snellman B (1968) Procidentia of the rectum studied with cineradiography: a contribution to the discussion of causative mechanism. Dis Colon Rectum 11:330–347

Denis PH, Colin DR, Galmiche et al. (1979) Elastic properties of the rectal wall in normal adults and in patients with ulcerative colitis. Gastroenterology 77: 45–48

Devroede G, Vobecky S, Masse S et al. (1982) Ischaemic fecal incontinence and rectal angina. Gastroenterology 83:970–980

Ekberg O, Nylander G, Fork FT (1985) Defaecography. Radiology 155:45–48

Finlay IG (1988) Symposium on proctography. Int J Colorect Dis 3:67–89

Hardcastle JD, Parks AG (1970) A study of anal incontinence and some principles of surgical treatment. Proc R Soc Med 63 (supp): 116–118

Henry MM, Parks AG, Swash M (1982) The pelvic floor musculature in the descending perineum syndrome. Br J Surg 69:470–472

Heppell J, Belliveau P, Taillefer R, Dube S, Derbekyan V (1987) Quantitative assessment of pelvic ileal reservoir emptying with a semisolid radionuclide enema: a correlation with clinical outcome. Dis Colon Rectum 30:81–85

Hertz (1908) The passage of food through the human alimentry canal. Br Med J i:191–196

Keighley MRB, Henry MM, Bartolo DCC, Mortensen NJMcC (1989) Anorectal physiology measurement: report of a working party. Br J Surg 76:356–357

Kerremans RP (1969) Morphological and physiological aspects of anal continence and defaecation. Editions Arscia, Brussels

Kerrigan DD, Lucas MG, Sun WM, Donnelly TC, Read NW (1989) Ideopathic constipation associated with impaired urethrovesical and sacral reflex function. Br J Surg 76:748–751

Kodner I (1988) Proctography. In: Symposium on proctography. Int J Colorect Dis 3:67–89

Kuijpers HC, Bleijenberg (1985) The spastic pelvic floor syndrome. Dis Colon Rectum 28:669–672

Lahr CJ, Cherry DA, Jensen LL, Rothenberger DA (1988) Balloon sphincterography: clinical findings after 200 patients. Dis Colon Rectum 31:347–351

Lestar B, Penninckx FM, Kerremans RP (1989) Defecometry: a new method for determining the parameters of rectal evacuation. Dis Colon Rectum 32:197–201

Lipkin AT, Bell BM (1962) Pressure volume characteristics of the human colon. J Clin Invest 41:1831–1839

Mahieu P, Pringot J, Bodart P (1984) Defecography: I. Description of a new procedure and results in normal patients. Gastrointest Radiol 9:247–251

Nasmyth DG, Williams NS, Johnston D (1986) Comparison of the function of triplicated ileal reservoirs after mucosal proctectomy and ileoanal anastomosis for ulcerative colitis and polyposis coli. Br J Surg 73:361–366

Nicholls RJ, Lubowski DZ, Donaldson DR (1988) Comparison of colonic reservoir and straight colo-anal reconstruction after rectal excision. Br J Surg 75:318–320

O'Connell PR, Kelly KA, Brown ML (1986a) Scintigraphic assessment of neorectal motor function. J Nucl Med 27:460–464

O'Connell PR, Rankin DR, Weiland LH, Kelly KA (1986b) Enteric bacteriology, absorption, morphology and emptying after ileal pouch–anal anastomosis. Br J Surg 73:909–914

O'Connell PR, Pemberton JH, Kelly KA (1987) Determinants of stool frequency after ileal pouch–anal anastomosis. Am J Surg 153:157–164

Oettle GJ, Roe AM, Bartolo DCC, Mortensen NJMcC (1985) What is the best way of measuring perineal descent? A comparison of radiographic and clinical methods. Br J Surg 72:999–1001

Phillips SF, Edwards DAW (1965) Some aspects of anal continence and defaecation. Gut 6:396–405

Preston DM, Lennard-Jones JE, Thomas BM (1984) The balloon proctogram. Br J Surg 71:29–32

Read NW, Bartolo DCC, Read MG (1984) Differences in anal function in patients with incontinence to solids and in patients with incontinence to liquids. Br J Surg 71:39–42

Read NW, Abouzerkry L, Read MG, Howell P, Ottewell D, Donnelly TC (1985) Anorectal function in elderly patients with fecal impaction. Gastroenterology 89:959–966

Rutter KR (1974) Electromyographic changes in certain pelvic floor abnormalities. Proc R Soc Med 68:28–30

Shorvon PJ, McHugh S, Diamant NE, Somers S, Stevenson GW (1989) Defecography in normal volunteers: results and implications. Gut 30:1737–1749

Skomorowska E, Henrichsen S, Christiansen J, Hegedus V (1987) Videodefaecography combined with measurement of the anorectal angle and of perineal descent. Acta Radiol 28:559–562

Snooks SJ, Barnes RPH, Swash M (1984) Damage to the voluntary anal and urinary sphincter musculature in incontinence. J Neurol Neurosurg Psychiat 47:1269–1273

Turnbull GK, Bartram CI, Lennard-Jones JE (1988) Radiologic studies of rectal evacuation in adults with idiopathic constipation. Dis Colon Rectum 31:190–197

Varma JS, Smith AN (1986a) Reproducibility of the proctometrogram. Gut 1986:288–292

Varma JS, Smith AN (1986b) Anorectal function following colo-anal sleeve anastomosis for chronic radiation injury to the rectum. Br J Surg 73:285–289

Varma JS, Smith AN (1988) Neurophysiological dysfunction in young women with intractable constipation. Gut 29:963–968

Womack (1988) Proctography. In: Symposium on proctography. Int J Colorect Dis 3:67–89

Womack NR, Williams NS, Holmfield JHM, Morrison JFB, Simpkins KC (1985) New method for the dynamic assessment of anorectal function in constipation. Br J Surg 72:994–998

Womack NR, Williams NS, Holmfield JHM, Morrison JFB (1987) Pressure and prolapse – the cause of solitary rectal ulceration. Gut 28:1228–1233

Yoshioka K, Hyland G, Keighley MRB (1988) Physiological changes after postanal repair and parameters predicting outcome. Br J Surg 75:1220–1224

The Measurement of Anorectal Sensation

R. Miller

Sensory Endings in the Anorectum

The anorectum has a profuse sensory innervation, the nature and distribution of which reflects the embryology of the region. The rectum is supplied by autonomic fibres which terminate as free nerve endings in the muscularis propria, submucosa and mucosa (Sotolo 1954; Fan 1955). These fibres not only mediate local reflexes but also have extensive central connections and are more numerous in the lower rectum near the anal canal (Mei 1983).

The anal canal is supplied by somatic nerves as far as the junction with rectal type mucosa (Izumi 1955; Duthie and Gairns 1960). There are numerous encapsulated endings reaching as far as this level, together with nerve plexuses round hair follicles in the lower anal canal. The most striking feature, however, is the profusion of free nerve endings, particularly in the region of the anal valves. These endings are also to be found in large numbers throughout the anal transition zone above the valves (Duthie and Gairns 1960).

Methods of Measurement

The measurement of sensation in the rectum and anal canal is usually performed separately, although the two probably work together as a co-ordinated unit.

Rectal Sensation

The rectum is primarily sensitive to distension of its lumen and a feeling of rectal fullness is usually felt in the rectum itself or referred to the sacral area (Goligher and Hughes 1951). In health, the rectum is extremely sensitive and as little as 10 ml of air and 1 ml of water can be felt (Scharli and Kiesswetter 1970). Reduced rectal sensation has been described in patients with idiopathic con-

stipation (Baldi et al. 1982; De Medici et al. 1986; Loening-Baucke 1984) and also in some patients with incontinence (Ihre 1974).

As in many areas of anorectal physiology, there is no standard method for the assessment of rectal sensation. The simplest method is to insert a collapsed balloon connected to a catheter into the rectum, making sure the lower margin of the balloon is well clear of the anal canal, and then inflate it with progressively larger volumes of air from a hand-held syringe (Wald et al. 1986; Buchman et al. 1980; Latimer et al. 1984; Buser and Miner 1986; Wald 1983). This will allow the threshold to rectal distension to be assessed, but the rate of inflation and position of the balloon are variable and investigator-dependent. These factors probably have a considerable effect on the result and may account for the variation in the literature on the threshold to rectal distension. Similarly the material, size and shape of the balloon will also have an effect on the degree of rectal distension and to obtain reproducible results they must be kept constant.

As the volume of inflation increases, a point is reached when it becomes uncomfortable and this is usually termed the "maximum tolerated volume" (Read et al. 1985). This is used to provide an indication of rectal capacity and is not strictly a sensory parameter, although it could be interpreted as the pain threshold. Somewhere between these volumes the sensation of rectal fullness becomes constant rather than transient and this has also been used as an end point in some studies, although it is subject to considerable subjectivity.

An alternative to the incremental method of distending the rectum is to pump water or air into the balloon at a constant rate (Varma et al. 1985; Roe et al. 1986a). It is important, particularly if water is used, that it is at 37 °C, otherwise the subject records the feeling of temperature change rather than that of distension. The balloon is made of thin latex so that it offers minimal resistance to inflation. A condom is ideal for this purpose. It is inserted into the rectum at a set distance from the anal verge, the time noted and the pump started. The subject is requested to inform the investigator when the feeling of rectal distension is first noted and then when it becomes intolerable. As the infusion is held constant at a known rate the volume to threshold sensation and maximum tolerated volume can be determined. In patients with proctitis from whatever cause, both these volumes will be low. In contrast, some patients with megarectum have very high volumes for threshold sensation, with the point of maximum tolerated volume being beyond the capacity of the balloon.

A manometric device is usually also incorporated into the balloon so that pressure change can be determined (Fig. 3.15). The resulting trace of pressure against volume (proctometrogram) provides an estimation of the compliance of the rectum (dV/dP) (Fig. 3.16). This method has been shown to produce highly reproducible results (Varma and Smith 1986).

In addition to its diagnostic use, rectal sensation also has a therapeutic role. Using biofeedback

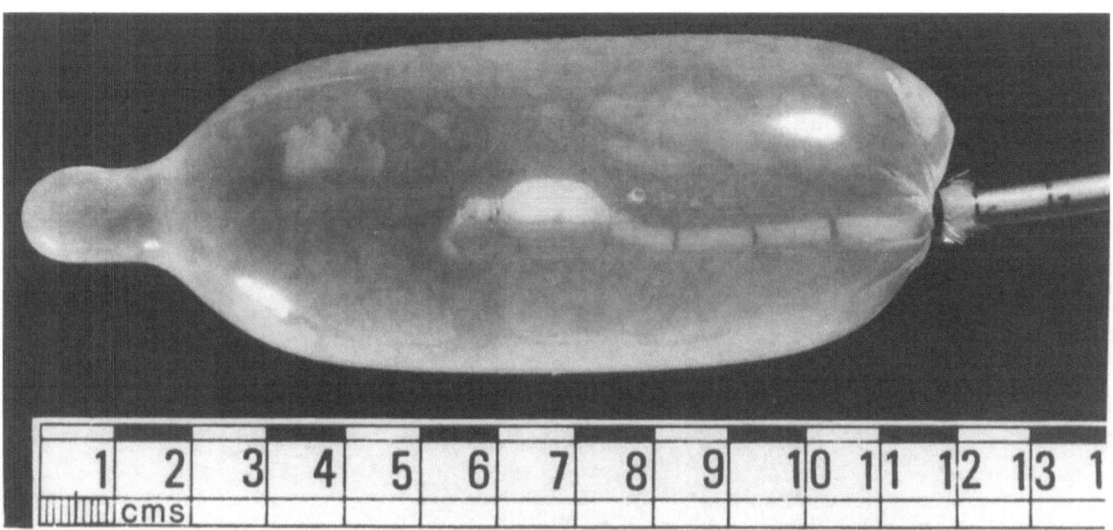

Fig. 3.15. Typical proctometrogram balloon used for assessment of rectal sensation and compliance studies.

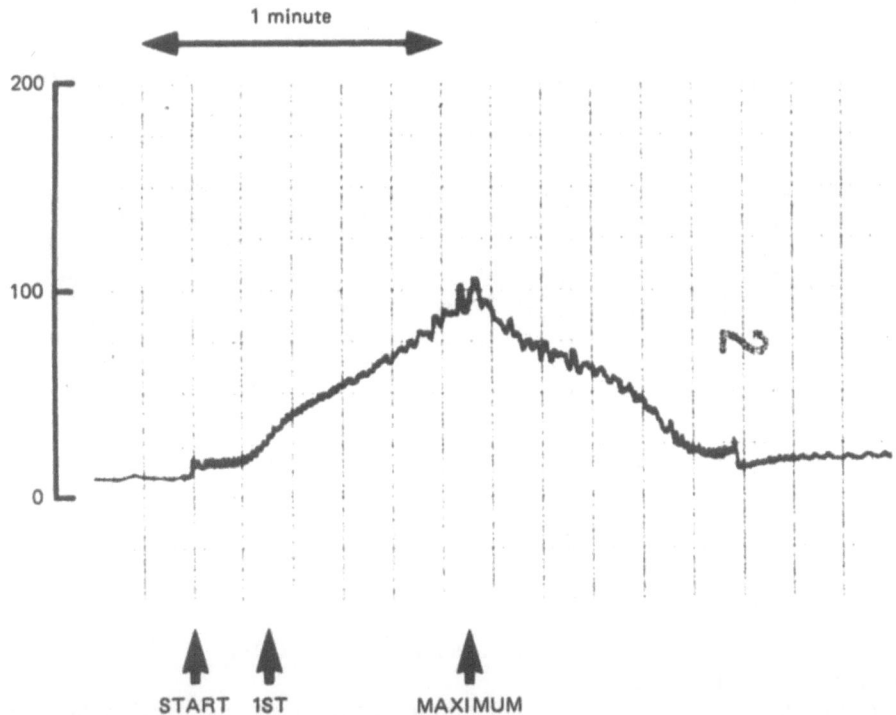

Fig. 3.16. Proctometrogram recording from a patient with proctitis. The threshold to rectal distension (*1st*) and point at which it became uncomfortable (*maximum*) are marked. The maximum tolerated volume and pressure can be measured from the trace at this point. The gradient of pressure versus volume infused gives a measure of compliance of the rectum. In this case the slope is steep, indicating low compliance.

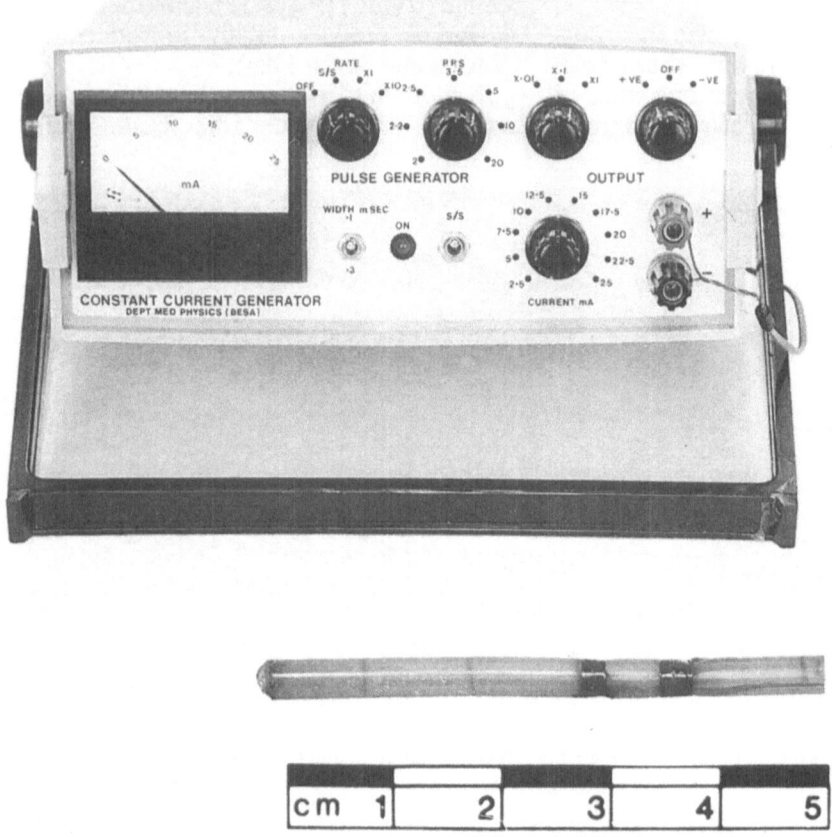

Fig. 3.17. The constant current generator and the probe used to measure mucosal electrosensitivity. (From R. Miller et al. (1988) *Dis Colon Rectum* 31:433–438, with permission of the publishers J. B. Lippincott.)

techniques, patients with incontinence can be trained to appreciate smaller and smaller volumes of rectal distension so that they are more aware of rectal contents. This is supplemented by contracting the external anal sphincter on feeling rectal distension and regular pelvic floor exercises (Buser and Miner 1986; MacLeod 1987; Whitehead et al. 1985; Cerulli et al. 1979). It would appear that rectal sensation is an important determinant of outcome (Latimer et al. 1984; Wald 1983).

Anal Sensation

While it has been recognized for many years that the anal canal is the seat of "a very acute special sense" (Andrews 1895; Stroud 1896), it has not been the subject of objective assessment until relatively recently. The histological studies of Duthie and Gairns indicate that the anal canal should be highly sensitive as far as the junction of

rectal type mucosa with the transitional zone (Duthie and Gairns 1960). These authors also assessed anal sensation using a von Frey hair, pinprick and metal plates at different temperatures. These techniques, however, can only give rough qualitative data and as the authors themselves comment, they are not suitable for quantitative measurement.

Two methods have been described to provide such a quantitative assessment of anal sensation, mucosal electrosensitivity and temperature sensation (Roe et al. 1986b; Miller et al. 1987). Both at present are primarily research tools.

Mucosal Electrosensitivity

The technique of cutaneous electrical stimulation has been used for many years. Sigel used a square wave electrical current with a fixed impulse duration and frequency to study cutaneous sensation as long ago as 1951 (Sigel 1951) and the same technique has been modified to investigate urethral sensory thresholds using a pair of electrodes on a urinary catheter (Kiesswetter 1977; Powell and Feneley 1980).

Roe was the first to apply the technique to study anal sensory thresholds (Roe et al. 1986b). The stimulating probe used consists of a 10 FG Dover catheter, which has two platinum wire electrodes exactly 1 cm apart near the tip (Department of Clinical Measurement, Royal Devon and Exeter Hospital, Devon, UK) (Fig. 3.17). This is connected to a battery-powered constant current generator which produces a square wave stimulus with a frequency of 5 Hz and 100 μs duration (Department of Medical Physics, Bristol Royal Infirmary, Bristol, UK) (Fig. 3.17). The functional sphincter length is first determined using station pull-through manometry and sensation is arbitrarily assessed in the upper, middle and lower thirds of the anal canal. The catheter is first lubricated with a conductive mixture of equal volumes of KY jelly (Johnson and Johnson) and normal saline and introduced into the anal canal so that the electrodes span the upper zone. The current across the electrodes is then increased in 1 mA increments until the subject feels the stimulus, which was often described as a tingling or prickling

sensation. The maximum stimulus is 25 mA. The average of three recordings is taken as the threshold value and the thresholds of the middle and lower zones assessed in the same way. The results from 44 normal subjects are shown in Fig. 3.18.

The technique provides a simple and rapid assessment of anal sensation. While it is not entirely clear which sensory fibres are being stimulated it is likely that the principal fibres are those subserving light touch (Vierck et al. 1986).

Temperature Sensation

The normal subject has the ability to distinguish solid stool from flatus. In the skin elsewhere in the body, temperature sensation plays an important role in this distinction as solids, liquids and gases have very different thermal conductivities and capacities (Hyndman and Wolkin 1943). To investigate whether temperature sensation could play a role in determining the presence and nature of rectal contents a technique has been developed to measure thermal thresholds in the anorectum for research purposes (Miller et al. 1987).

A hot and cold stimulus is provided by a

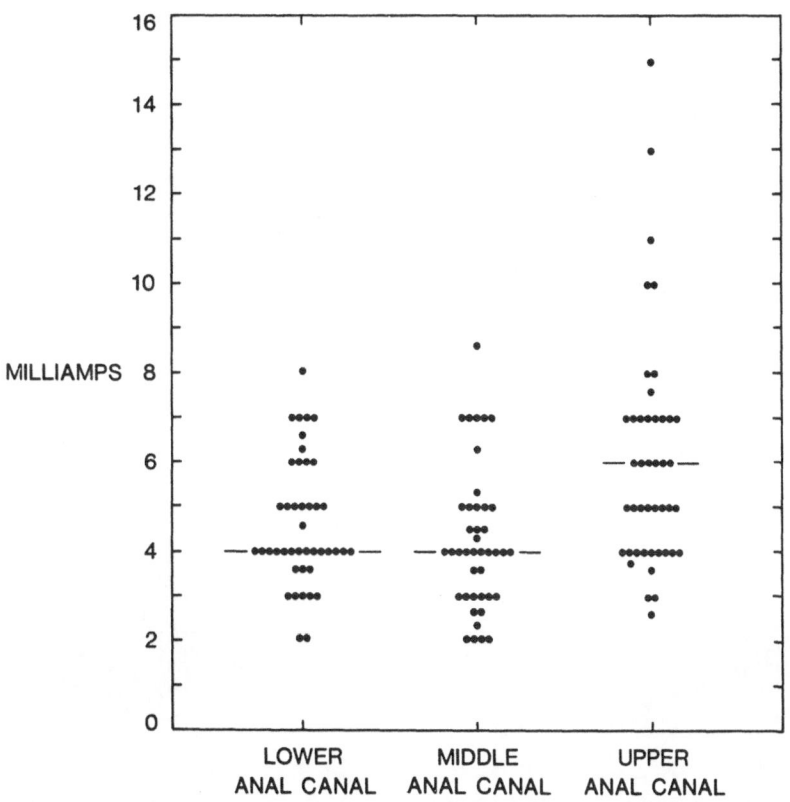

Fig. 3.18. Results of mucosal electrosensitivity in 44 control subjects.

specially constructed water-perfused thermode (Fig. 3.19). It consists of a hollow bullet-shaped probe, exactly 1 cm long, through which water of varying temperature can be pumped. The water is supplied from three thermostatically-controlled baths, the temperatures of which are set such that the thermode can be held at 37 °C and then rapidly increased or decreased by 4.5 °C (Fig. 3.20). The temperature at the thermode–mucosa interface is measured by a small thermocouple and conti-

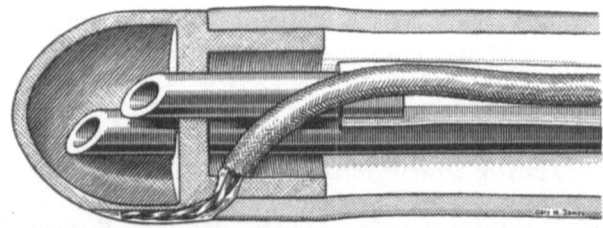

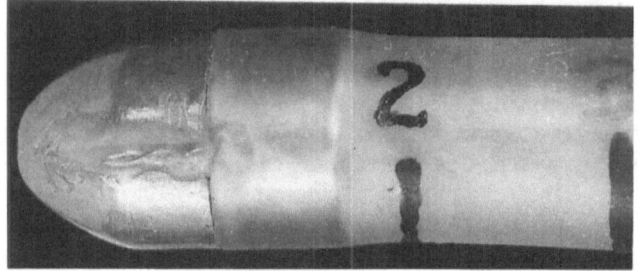

Fig. 3.19. Photograph of the thermode used to determine thermal thresholds in the anorectum, together with an illustration of its internal design. (From R. Miller et al. (1987) *Br J Surg* 74:511–515, with permission of the publishers Butterworth.)

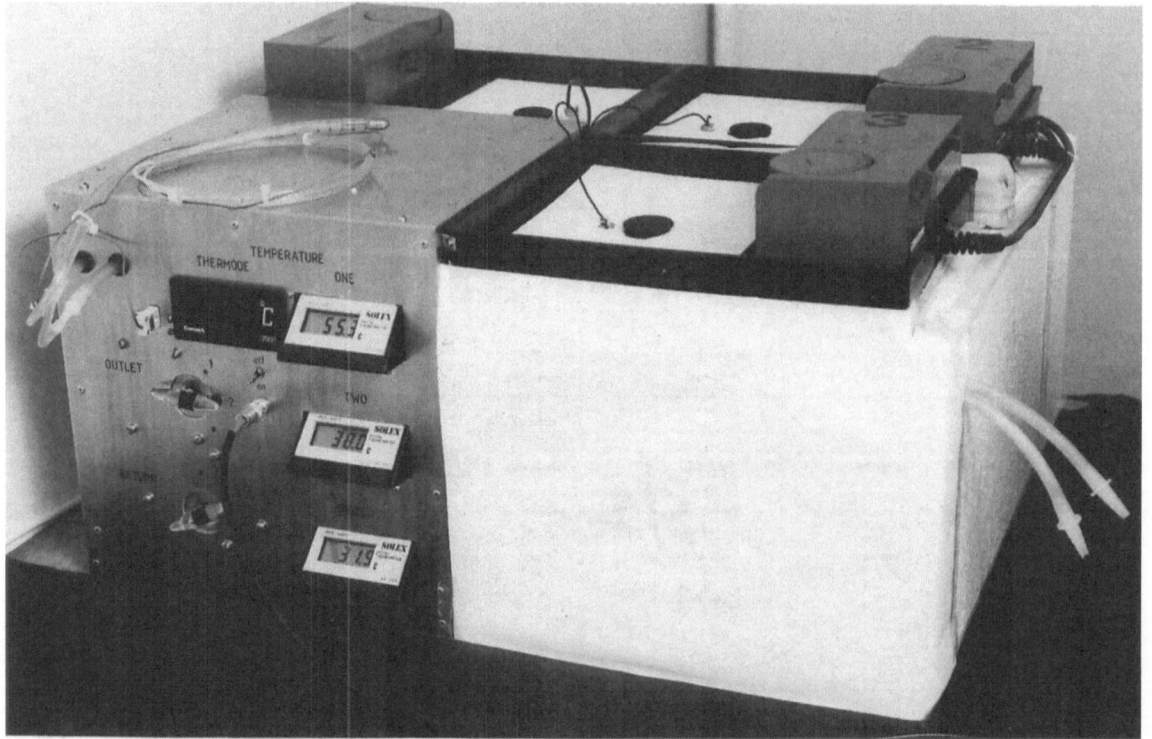

Fig. 3.20. The water baths and control box used to supply the thermode. Each bath temperature is thermostatically-controlled and the taps allowed water running through the thermode to be switched rapidly from one bath to another.

nuously recorded on a chart recorder. An example of the trace of temperature change is illustrated in Fig. 3.21.

The thermode is inserted into the lower zone of the functional sphincter and held at 37 °C. Its temperature is then either increased or decreased by switching the water flowing through it. The subject is requested to indicate immediately when any temperature change is felt and this point marked on the chart recorder. Using this mark the minimum detectable temperature change (MDTC) can be found for that particular shift in temperature. This thermal threshold is assessed for four temperature changes, normal to hot, hot to normal, normal to cold and cold to normal, in the same zones of the anal canal as tested for mucosal electrosensitivity. The median value of these four thresholds can then be used to obtain a single figure that represents temperature sensitivity for the zone, the median MDTC.

The results showed that the anal canal is extremely sensitive to thermal stimuli and that this is markedly diminished in patients with idiopathic faecal incontinence (Miller et al. 1987). There is a

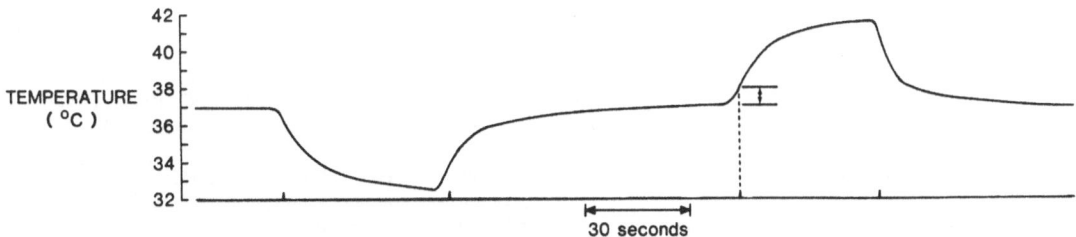

Fig. 3.21. Trace of temperature change induced by the thermode. The event marker trace is also shown with the measurement of the minimum detectable temperature change for normal to hot.

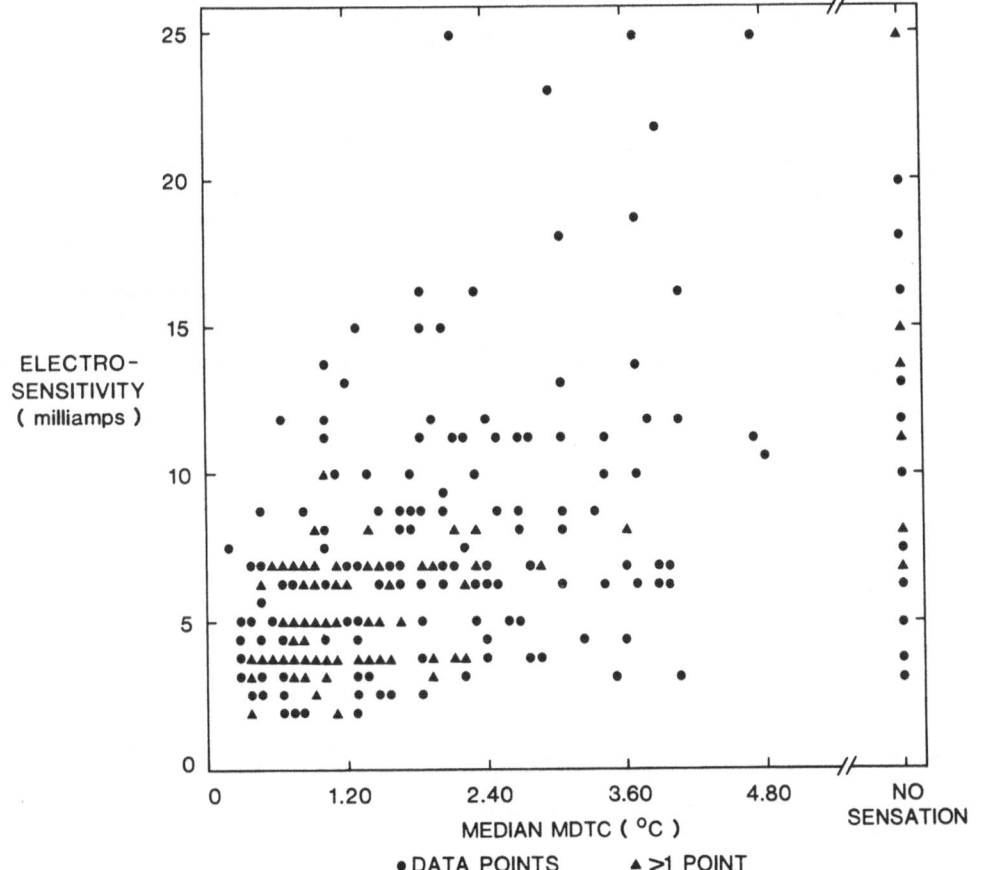

Fig. 3.22. Correlation between median minimum detectable temperature change (MDTC) and mucosal electrosensitivity, $r_s = 0.54$, $p < 0.001$.

degree of correlation between mucosal electrosensitivity and temperature sensation (Spearman ranked correlation coefficient 0.54, p<0.001), but a significant proportion of patients had high thresholds for one stimulus and not the other, as Fig. 3.22 illustrates. It follows that for a more complete assessment of anal sensation both tests should be performed, but if time is limited mucosal electrosensitivity provides a rapid measure of one sensory modality.

References

Andrews E (1895) Disastrous results following Whitehead's operation for piles and the so-called American operation. Mathews Med Quart (October): 303

Baldi F, Ferrarini R, Corinaldesi R et al. (1982) Function of the internal sphincter and rectal sensitivity in idiopathic constipation. Digestion 24:14–22

Buchman P, Mogg GAG, Alexander-Williams J, Allan RN, Keighley MRB (1980) Relationship of proctitis and rectal capacity in Crohns' disease. Gut 21:137–140

Buser WD, Miner PB (1986) Delayed rectal sensation with faecal incontinence: successful treatment with anorectal manometry. Gastroenterology 91:1186–1191

Cerulli MA, Nikoomanesh P, Schuster MM (1979) Progress in biofeedback conditioning for faecal incontinence. Gastroenterology 76:742–746

De Medici A, Badiali D, Anzini F, Corazziari E (1986) Rectal sensitivity varies with different types of constipation. Gastroenterology 90:1341

Duthie HL, Gairns FW (1960) Sensory nerves and sensation in the anal region of man. Br J Surg 47:585–595

Fan WW (1955) Histological studies of sensory nerves in the sigmoid and rectum. Arch Fur Jap Chir 24:567–574

Goligher JC, Hughes ESR (1951) Sensibility of the rectum and colon: its role in the mechanism of anal continence. Lancet i:543–548

Hyndman OR, Wolkin J (1943) Anterior chordotomy. Arch Neurol Psychiatry 50:129–148

Ihre T (1974) Studies in anal function in continent and incontinent patients. Scand J Gastroenterol 9: supp 25

Izumi I (1955) On the inervation, especially the sensory inervation, of anus in human adults. Arch Hist Jap 9:225–240

Kiesswetter H (1977) Mucosal sensory thresholds of urinary bladder and urethra measured electrically. Urol Int 32:437–448

Latimer PR, Campbell D, Kasperski J (1984) A component analysis of biofeedback in the treatment of faecal incontinence. Biofeedback Self Regul 9:311–324

Loening-Baucke VA (1984) Sensitivity of the sigmoid colon and rectum in children treated for chronic constipation. J Pediatr Gastroenterol Nutr 3:454–459

MacLeod JH (1987) Management of anal incontinence by biofeedback. Gastroenterology 93:291–294

Mei N (1983) Sensory structures in the viscera. Prog Sens Physiol 4:1–42

Miller R, Bartolo DCC, Cervero F, Mortensen NJMcC (1987) Anorectal temperature sensation: a comparison of normal and incontinent patients. Br J Surg 74:511–515

Powell PH, Feneley RCC (1980) The role of urethral sensation in clinical urology. Br J Urol 52:539–541

Read NW, Abouzekry L, Read MG, Howell P, Otterwell D, Donnelly CT (1985) Anorectal function in elderly patients with faecal impaction. Gastroenterology 89:959–966

Roe AM, Bartolo DCC, Mortensen NJMcC (1986a) Diagnosis and management of intractable constipation. Br J Surg 73:854–861

Roe AM, Bartolo DCC, Mortensen NJMcC (1986b) New method for assessment of anal sensation in various anorectal disorders. Br J Surg 73:310–312

Scharli A, Kiesswetter WB (1970) Defaecation and continence: some new concepts. Dis Colon Rectum 13:81–107

Sigel H (1951) Cutaneous sensory threshold stimulation with high frequency square wave current. J Invest Dermatol 18:441–445

Sotolo JR (1954) Nerve endings of the walls of the descendent colon and rectum. Z Zellforsch 41:S101–111

Stroud BB (1896) Of the anatomy of the anus. Ann Surg 24:1–15

Varma JS, Smith AN (1986) Reproducibility of the proctometrogram. Gut 27:288–292

Varma JS, Smith AN, Busuttil A (1985) Correlation of clinical and manometric abnormalities of rectal function following chronic radiation injury. Br J Surg 72:875–878

Vierck CJ, Greenspan JD, Ritz LA, Yeomans DC (1986) The spinal pathways contributing to the ascending conduction and descending modulations of pain sensation and reactions. In: Yaksh TL (ed) Spinal afferent processing. Plenum Press, New York, pp 275–329

Wald A (1983) Biofeedback for neurogenic faecal incontinence: rectal sensation is a determinant of outcome. J Pediatr Gastroenterol Nutr 2:302–306

Wald A, Chandra R, Chiponis D, Gabel S (1986) Anorectal function and continence mechanisms is childhood encopresis. J Pediatr Gastroenterol Nutr 5:346–351

Whitehead WE, Burgio KL, Engel BT (1985) Biofeedback treatment of faecal incontinence in geriatric patients. J Am Geriatr Soc 33:320–324

4 · Measurement of Absorptive and Secretory Function

D. S. Rampton

Introduction

The principal function of large intestinal mucosa is to absorb salt and water. This highly evolved and complexly regulated activity enables the daily ileal effluent of about 1000 ml fluid to be converted into a normally firm stool containing less than 200 ml water and 10 mmol each of sodium, potassium and chloride (Wrong et al. 1981). The aim of this chapter is to review the techniques available to study in man the colorectal mucosal fluxes which enable this modification of ileal output to occur; for reviews of large intestinal mucosal transport itself the reader is referred elsewhere (Powell 1979; Edmonds 1981; Schultz 1981; Wrong et al. 1981; Kerlin and Phillips 1983; Binder and Sandle 1987; Donowitz 1987; Powell 1987).

Allusion will be made to methods for investigating the transport not only of sodium and water, but also of other minerals, short-chain fatty acids, ammonia, bile salts and oxalate. How these have been applied to the study of regional variations in electrolyte transport, and the influences on it of luminal factors (such as bile salts and fatty acids), hormones (endocrine, paracrine and neurocrine), inflammatory mediators, drugs and disease will also be discussed. Techniques for evaluating the secretion of mucus will not be described (see instead Allen 1983; Bustos-Fernandez et al. 1983; Neutra and Forstner 1987). Discussion of methods for detecting, in exhaled breath, the colonic absorption of hydrogen and methane derived from nonabsorbable carbohydrates (Bond and Levitt 1972; Hofmann and Lauterburg 1977; Levitt et al. 1987), and of ^{14}C-glycine, measured after its hepatic conversion to $^{14}CO_2$, derived from bacterial deconjugation of exogenous radiolabelled glycocholate (James et al. 1973; Scarpello and Sladen 1977), will also be omitted from this review.

At the outset, it should be emphasized that the only role of conventional clinical investigations, such as barium enema, colonoscopy and histology, in the evaluation of colorectal absorption and secretion, lies in the identification and diagnosis of disease. The numerous techniques that have been adapted, mainly from animal work, for the study of human large intestinal mucosal transport can be broadly subdivided into in vivo and in vitro groups (Table 4.1), and have been applied to preparations ranging from the whole colon to cultured colonocyte monolayers (Table 4.2) (Parsons 1968; Shields 1972; Sladen 1975; Shields 1979; Wrong et al. 1981). Although their complexity has meant, as will be seen, that few of the available techniques have been incorporated into routine clinical practice, in experimental settings they have provided, as in the small bowel, an invaluable insight into large intestinal function in both health and disease.

It is hoped that by discussing the limitations and applications of individual techniques this chapter will help intending clinical investigators decide on the experimental method which most closely meets their needs. No single technique is sufficient for the characterization of all aspects of colorectal transport function, and the information derived

Table 4.1. Principal methods for investigating large intestinal mucosal transport in man

In vivo techniques
1. Input/output (balance):
   Direct and indirect faecal assays
   Assay of terminal ileal contents and flow rates (non-steady state)
2. Bolus infusions:
   Ligated colonic segments
   Balloon- and non-occluded colorectal segments
3. Mucosal dialysis
4. Transmucosal PD
5. Steady state perfusion:
   Whole large intestine
   Isolated colorectal segments

In vitro techniques
1. Short-circuit current:
   Mucosal sheets, cultured colonocyte monolayers
   Intracellular microelectrodes
2. Combined luminal and vascular perfusion of isolated colonic segments
3. Other:
   Everted sacs, epithelial rings or strips
   Colonocyte brush border vesicles (not yet in man)

Table 4.2. Large intestinal preparations used to study absorption and secretion in man

1. Whole colon
2. Isolated colorectal segments
3. Mucosal strips
4. Cultured colonic epithelial cell line monolayers
5. Isolated colonocyte brush border vesicles (not yet in man)

from different techniques is complementary rather than mutually exclusive. For any particular project the choice of method(s) will depend on the question to be asked, the advantages and disadvantages of the various techniques, the facilities available and the experience and expertise of the investigator. Lastly, it should be emphasized that, while in this review essential practical aspects of individual techniques will be outlined, investigators contemplating using any of them should consult the appropriate original articles for procedural and mathematical details.

In Vivo Techniques

General Remarks

The main theoretical advantage of the in vivo over the in vitro approach is that the tissue under investigation in situ is functioning under less physiologically abnormal conditions than when largely deprived, as in vitro, of its vascular and neurohumoral connections and of luminal influences such as bile salts, fatty acids and bacteria and their metabolic products. Nevertheless, in vivo studies have many limitations which must be borne in mind in their planning, execution and interpretation.

Before discussing the methods themselves, it is worth defining the most commonly used of the sometimes confusing nomenclature employed in the description of the results they provide (Code 1960; Fordtran and Dietschy 1966; Wrong et al. 1981). Net passage of a substance out of the bowel lumen is defined as absorption (denoted as +ve), and into the lumen as secretion (−ve). A substance moving in both directions is referred to as having a bidirectional flux, one from the mucosal to the serosal surface (+ve, J_{ms}, insorption), and the other in the reverse direction (−ve, J_{sm}, exsorption). Where the substance is not metabolized within the mucosa, the net flux (J_{net}) is the algebraic sum of the unidirectional fluxes.

Balance experiments (Table 4.1), in which caecal input and rectal output are compared, give information only about the overall effect of colorectal transport function; the large bowel is treated as a "black box" and no data about mucosal fluxes themselves is obtained. Experiments in which fluid of known composition is either instilled into or perfused through the whole or segments of the colon provide information about net or, when radio-isotopic tracers are used, bidirectional fluxes of water and solutes, but again cannot dissect out the nature of mucosal transport processes in the way that in vitro methods can (see p. 74). Further limitations of in vivo techniques will be discussed in detail where the relevant method is described.

Balance Studies

Faeces (Table 4.3)

Although theoretically simple, several factors hinder the analysis of faecal composition in practice. The usually solid and non-homogeneous state of faeces prevents the direct application of the assay methods commonly employed for the analysis of body fluids, and its colour interferes with colorimetric techniques. Much of its mineral content (e.g. calcium, phosphate, magnesium) is present in insoluble form. Faecal composition ex vivo, for example in relation to pH, osmolality, bicarbonate, short-chain fatty acid and ammonia content, changes with time as a result of ongoing bacterial metabolism (Gamble 1915; Tarlow and Thom 1974; Owens and Padovan 1976; Vince et al. 1976). Furthermore, data on daily output of faecal constituents is hampered by the necessity for prolonged stool collections using marker techniques to ensure representative figures for daily excretion (Branch and Cummings 1978).

Table 4.3. Methods used to assess faecal composition

1. Whole stool:
   Combustion
   Digestion with strong acid
2. Faecal water:
   In vivo faecal dialysis
   In vitro faecal dialysis
   High-speed centrifugation
   Ultrafiltration

Techniques. Despite these problems, extensive data for the faecal content of water, minerals and nitrogen have been obtained by *combustion* or *digestion* of stool with strong acids (Diem and Lentner 1970). However, because the exchangeable component of faeces is more likely than its total content to reflect colorectal absorption and secretion, several methods have been devised for the analysis of the composition of stool water.

Wrong and coworkers developed the ingenious technique of *in vivo faecal dialysis*, in which cellulose dialysis bags filled with dextran are swallowed and then collected after their passage in the stool (Wrong et al. 1961, 1965). Transit through the large intestine is usually slow enough to allow equilibration of the contents of the bag with those of the bowel lumen, at least for small molecules (Wrong et al. 1965; Tarlow and Thom 1974; Owens and Padovan 1976; Wrong et al. 1981).

Other workers have compared in vivo with in vitro faecal dialysis (Owens and Padovan 1976; Vernia et al. 1984), *high-speed centrifugation* (Findlay et al. 1973; Tarlow and Thom 1974; Owens and Padovan 1976) and *ultrafiltration* of homogenized stool (Mitchell et al. 1980; Vernia et al. 1984). While these three sometimes complex and time-consuming, as well as aesthetically unpleasant, techniques yield similar values for stool water electrolyte concentrations to those obtained by in vivo faecal dialysis, in some reports the values for pH and bicarbonate are lower and for osmolality, short-chain fatty acids, amino acids and ammonia higher (Tarlow and Thom 1974; Owens and Padovan 1976). As mentioned above, these differences probably result, at least in part, from continuing bacterial activity during the ex

vivo procedures of collection, storage, homogenization, freezing, thawing and separation of the water component of stool which precede its eventual analysis, and can be minimized by processing the stool anaerobically, at 4 °C and as quickly as possible (Owens and Padovan 1976; Vernia et al. 1984).

Applications. These techniques have been applied to the assessment of colorectal mucosal function in patients on differing diets (Metcalfe-Gibson et al. 1967), various drugs (Wilson et al. 1968a; Charron et al. 1969), and with renal failure (Wilson et al. 1968b), bowel resection (Cummings et al. 1973; Mitchell et al. 1980) and inflammatory bowel disease (Caprilli et al. 1978; Schilli et al. 1981; Roediger et al. 1982; Lauritsen et al. 1984; Vernia et al. 1988); they all suffer, however, from providing only an indirect and overall guide to mucosal transport in these situations.

Ileal Effluent

Techniques. In man, most of the earlier data about ileal effluent was achieved by collection of the excreta from *ileostomy* patients (Kanaghinis et al. 1963; Kramer 1966; Hill et al. 1975; Ladas et al. 1986). Unfortunately, however, the salt and water depletion common in such patients predisposes to reduced volume and sodium concentration and raised potassium concentration in ileostomy effluent (Kramer 1966; Clarke et al. 1967; Ladas et al. 1986). Furthermore, ileostomy output may well be modified by bacterial colonization of the distal ileum (Vince et al. 1973; Gorbach et al. 1973), residual disease (e.g. Crohn's) and postoperative small intestinal adaptation (Kanaghinis et al. 1963; Wright et al. 1969; Ladas et al. 1986).

Various groups have circumvented these difficulties by *intubation of the terminal ileum* perorally; its output is determined by a non-steady-state dye dilution technique in which ileal contents are repeatedly sampled during slow infusion of a nonabsorbable marker (Phillips and Giller 1973; Milton-Thompson et al. 1975; Cummings et al. 1976; Levitt and Bond 1977; Debongnie and Phillips 1978; Ladas et al. 1986). Although more likely to resemble physiological ileal flow rates than results obtained by studying ileostomists, values obtained by ileal intubation may be overestimates. Thus, small intestinal intubation may itself stimulate mucosal prostaglandin production, fluid secretion, motor activity and chyme flow velocity; in addition, high marker concentrations may inhibit small bowel fluid absorption (Davis et al. 1980). Other potential difficulties related to the use of nonabsorbable markers are discussed on page 73 (and see Table 4.4).

Applications. These methods have shown a rise in ileal flow rates after meals (Phillips and Giller 1973; Ladas et al. 1986) and, by simultaneous measurement of faecal volume, have quantified the ability of the colon to compensate, by enhanced absorption, for increased caecal input both acutely and over a 24-hour period (Debongnie and Phillips 1978; Palma et al. 1981).

Bolus Infusions

In experiments of this type, a bolus of fluid of known composition is infused into a segment of colon isolated proximally and distally by ligatures, balloons or, in studies of the rectum, the patient's posture. Information about mucosal transport and permeability is obtained by analysis of luminal contents, after a fixed time period, and, particularly when radio-isotopes are used, the rate of appearance of test substances in the blood.

Ligated Colonic Segments

Technique. For ethical and practical reasons, this simple technique, in which fluid is infused into a segment of colon ligated at both ends, but still connected, in vivo, to its vascular and neural supply, is difficult to apply in man.

Applications. Duthie and coworkers performed such studies intra-operatively, determining bi-directional water, sodium and potassium fluxes radio-isotopically, in patients undergoing colonic surgery for carcinoma (deemed controls), villous papilloma (Duthie and Atwell 1963) and ulcerative colitis (Duthie et al. 1964), but the application of this technique in human research is likely to remain limited.

Balloon- and Non-occluded Colorectal Segments

Technique. Although in principle more practicable in man, this kind of experiment is bedevilled in reality by failure satisfactorily to confine the infused solution to the supposedly isolated test segment. Thus, in studies of rectal absorption using balloons, both Levitan et al. (1963) and Devroede and Phillips (1970) were unable to occlude the sigmoid colon completely. Attempts to rely on the patient's posture alone to prevent proximal reflux of the test solution from the rectum were also ineffective (Levitan et al. 1963; Levitan and Brudno 1967); anal leakage has been an additional problem (Devroede et al. 1971). Consequent uncertainties about the area of mucosa in contact with the infusate makes quantitative interpretation of such investigations difficult.

As mentioned earlier, mucosal transport and permeability in isolated segment work has been assessed by measuring the rate of appearance in the blood of test substances, for example radio-isotopic tracers or drugs, placed in the gut lumen. Calculations of this type, however, may be compromised by failure to take into account the systemic distribution, metabolism and excretion of the test material. Other limitations of these techniques and perfusion studies are shown in Table 4.4 and discussed more fully on page 72–74.

Applications. Despite these problems, instillation methods have provided data about how mucosal transport and permeability vary in the rectum in health and ulcerative colitis (Levitan et al. 1963; Levitan and Brudno 1967; Devroede and Phillips 1970) and with site in the large intestine of normal subjects (Devroede et al. 1971).

Mucosal Dialysis

Technique. This method was originally adapted by Edmonds (1971) from the faecal dialysis technique of Wrong et al. (1961) (see p. 69) for the investigation of rectal mucosal absorption of sodium and water).

A cellulose dialysis tube, knotted at one end and containing about 2 ml fluid of known composition, is mounted on a cannula and inserted into the rectum (Fig. 4.1). After a defined period, usually 1 hour, during which exchange of water and solutes occurs between the dialysate and rectal mucosa, the tube is removed. Samples discoloured by faecal contamination are discarded. Changes in dialysate volume are determined by weighing, and of solute by appropriate biochemical techniques. Simple formulae allow calculation of rectal transport of water and solutes, making the assumptions that the rate of movement of the test substance

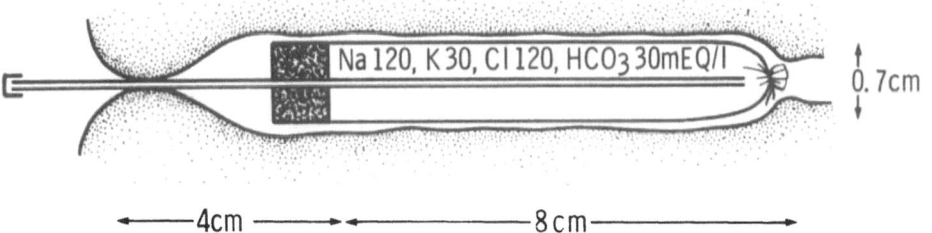

Fig. 4.1. In vivo rectal dialysis (Rampton et al. 1980a). Solutions of other composition can of course be used.

across the epithelium is slow compared to that across the dialysis membrane, and that the thin layer of fluid between the dialysis tube and the mucosal surface behaves as a compartment of small capacity (Edmonds 1971).

Although the theory of nonequilibrium dialysis depends on a number of suppositions that cannot be validated totally satisfactorily in intact man and cannot, in addition, detect net secretion of water in diarrhoeal states, the method has a number of advantages.

First, it is reproducible and sensitive, detecting, for example, rectal absorption of salt and water where perfusion techniques did not (Devroede and Phillips 1970; Edmonds 1971). Second, it leaves the physicochemical environment of the large bowel lumen relatively undisturbed, thereby permitting measurement of mucosal transport under conditions more physiological than is feasible with other methods. Furthermore, it is simple and cheap; it is also well tolerated by subject and researcher alike and therefore readily used repeatedly in appropriate individuals. Lastly, it can easily be adapted for simultaneous recording of transmucosal potential difference (see p. 71).

Applications. Since its initial description, in vivo rectal dialysis has been applied to the assessment of rectal mucosal water and electrolyte in patients with ulcerative colitis (Edmonds and Pilcher 1973; Rask-Madsen and Brix-Jensen 1973; Rampton and Sladen 1984) and after jejuno-ileal bypass (Rask-Madsen et al. 1974). It has also been used to investigate rectal mucosal absorption of short-chain fatty acids (McNeil et al. 1978) and its release of prostaglandins (Rampton et al. 1980a; Lauritsen et al. 1986), leucotrienes (Lauritsen et al. 1986) and histamine (Rampton et al. 1980b). Other applications include, in patients with appropriately sited colostomies, the investigation of regional differences in water and electrolyte transport (McNeil 1983).

Transmucosal Potential Difference (PD)

The PD across large intestinal mucosa is lumen-negative and reflects the activity of the sodium pump and the resistance of the tissue to the flow of ions: it can be used as a simple guide to mucosal integrity (Geall et al. 1969; Dalmark 1970; Edmonds 1975; Wrong et al. 1981).

Technique. Transmucosal PD can be conveniently recorded with electrodes incorporating a calomel cell or silver–silver chloride junction in a solution of normal saline in agar, and connected to a high impedance millivoltmeter (Fig. 4.2) (Edmonds 1975; Rampton et al. 1980a); the latter is necessary as the electrodes have a high resistance and it is essential that the meter draws little current. The probe electrode may be placed in the luminal fluid when the PD is measured during perfusion experiments, or alternatively directly in contact with the mucosa, for example via a dialysis bag (Fig. 4.2). The reference electrode is most easily placed in contact with an area of skin, the PD of which has been eradicated by an intradermal injection of saline; subcutaneous and intravenous electrodes are more cumbersome.

Measurement of PD is simple, quick, noninvasive, reproducible, safe and repeatable; it does not by itself, however, clarify mechanisms by which exogenous factors or disease affect mucosal transport processes. Methodological problems which may compromise the results include poor contact between the probe electrode and luminal fluid or mucosa, for example because of air bubbles in the electrode connections, and junction potentials due to contact in the circuitry between solutions of different ionic strengths (Edmonds 1975; Wrong et al. 1981).

Applications. The technique has been widely used in the in vivo assessment of the colorectal responses to, for example, changes in endoluminal composition (Archampong and Edmonds 1972),

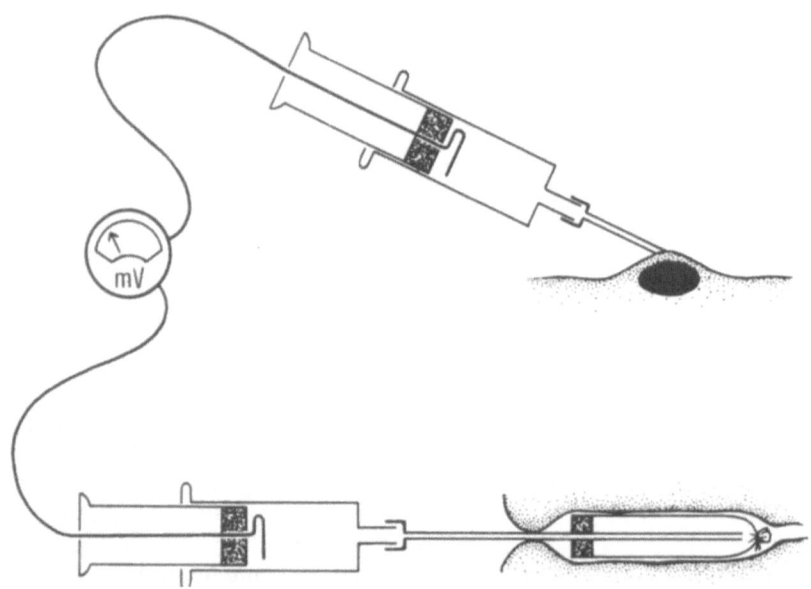

Fig. 4.2. Measurement of transmucosal rectal PD (Rampton et al. 1980a). In this system, contact with the mucosa is made through a dialysis bag, and the reference electrode is placed on the thigh in contact with an area of skin the PD of which has been abolished by an intradermal injection of saline.

drugs and hormones (Edmonds 1975; Wanitschke and Ewe 1983), and diseases such as ulcerative colitis (Edmonds and Pilcher 1973; Rask-Madsen and Brix-Jensen 1973; Rampton et al. 1980a) and cystic fibrosis (Orlando et al. 1989); regional variations in colonic PD have also been established (Rask-Madsen 1973a; Davis et al 1982; Schiller et al. 1988).

Perfusion Techniques

Whole Large Intestine

Since its introduction over 25 years ago (Levitan et al. 1962) and subsequent modification to take into account the passage of ileal effluent into the caecum (Devroede and Phillips 1969), the technique of perfusion of the whole colon in man has been widely and very profitably applied in the investigation of mucosal function.

In principle, all (or part) of the colon is perfused at a constant rate until achievement of a steady state, in which the flow rate and luminal solute concentrations at any single site are constant with respect to time. Net transport of water and solutes is estimated from changes in concentration of nonabsorbable markers such as polyethylene glycol 4000 (PEG 4000) or phenolsulphthalein (phenol red), using standard equations (Levitan et al. 1962; Whalen et al. 1966; Soergel 1968).

Technique. After fluoroscopically guided, usually peroral, intubation of the caecum with a tube containing at least two lumens, the colon is washed clean; it is then perfused with test solution via the caecal port for first equilibration, and subsequently steady state test periods, during which effluent is collected by a rectal tube. Additional lumens can be incorporated in the tube to facilitate aspiration of ileal contents proximal to the caecal infusion port (Fig. 4.3): this allows assessment of proximal reflux of perfusate and at least partial prevention of invalidation of the results by contamination from the ileum (Devroede and Phillips 1969). Other workers use a balloon in the terminal ileum to minimize ileocaecal fluid transfer and reflux (Wanitschke and Ewe 1983). Simultaneous measurements of PD and bidirectional ionic fluxes, using radio-isotopic tracers, facilitate evaluation of the intraluminal electrochemical forces and thus the active transport capabilities of the mucosa in vivo (Shields 1966; Rask-Madsen 1973a). Mucosal permeability has been assessed by measuring the rate of disappearance from the lumen of molecules of varying sizes, for example low molecular weight PEG (Chadwick et al. 1977).

A number of theoretical and practical problems are associated with this unpleasant, time-consuming, although nonetheless remarkably valuable procedure (Table 4.4) (Fordtran 1966; Soergel 1968, 1971).

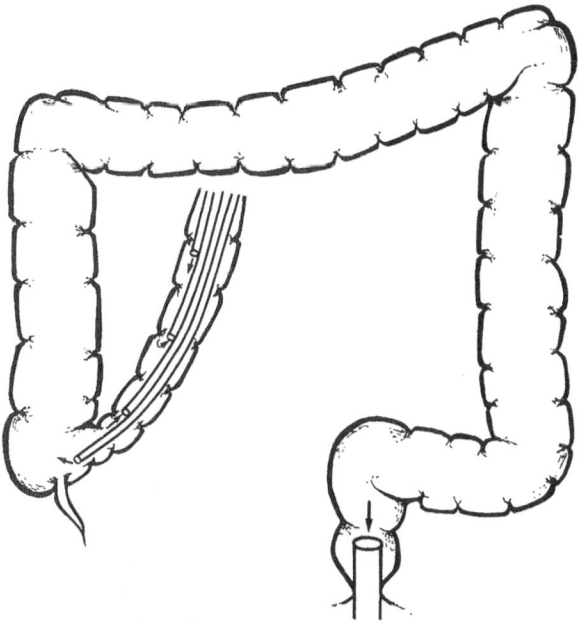

Fig. 4.3. Four-lumen tube for perfusion of whole colon in vivo.

Table 4.4. Limitations of in vivo perfusion techniques

1. Variable removal of luminal factors (bile salts, fatty acids, bacteria)
2. Variable mixing and dissipation of unstirred layer
3. Insufficient equilibration or too slow perfusion gives non-steady state
4. Rapid perfusion rate nonphysiological and inhibits detection of absorption
5. Altered bowel motility, transit, volume, distensibility and blood flow
6. Uncertain validity of nonabsorbable markers
7. Designation of mean solute concentration
8. Inappropriate composition of luminal solution
9. Contamination from lumen above test segment
10. Proximal reflux or distal leakage of infused/perfused solution
11. Uncertain length and surface area of test segment
12. Possible effect on transport of endoluminal tubes/balloons
13. Masking of regional differences in transport
14. Inability to control or analyse composition of serosal fluid
15. Cumbersome, unpleasant and time-consuming for subject

First, the perfusion rate is of critical importance (Devroede and Phillips 1969). Both the lavage and subsequent perfusion remove, to a variable and unpredictable extent, endogenous luminal factors, such as bile salts, fatty acids and the metabolic products of bacteria, which themselves may influence transport in vivo; the quantities of these factors present at the mucosal surface during the perfusion is uncertain. Slow perfusion predisposes to a relatively thick unstirred layer, together with

intracolonic fluid sequestration and a non-steady state, particularly when, as in human colon, the luminal diameter is large.

Unfortunately, while increasing the perfusion rate improves mixing, it may reduce the contact time between perfusate and mucosa to the extent that mucosal absorption, for instance, may not be detectable (Edmonds 1971). Furthermore, although colonic perfusion rates of 10–15 ml/min give reproducible results and a steady state after about 1 hour's equilibration, they are clearly nonphysiological when compared with resting ileal flow rates of <2 ml/min; secondary changes in colonic volume, motility, distensibility and blood flow, as well as transit time, may each affect the results.

Doubts have been raised about the validity of nonabsorbable markers. The necessary properties of these are several (Fordtran 1966; Soergel 1968, 1971). In diseased as well as healthy bowel, the marker must be completely nonabsorbable, non-adsorbable, uniformly miscible, chemically and biologically inert and totally recoverable from luminal contents; it should also be accurately and preferably easily measurable. While the commonly employed markers appear to fulfil most of these requirements satisfactorily, Davis et al. (1980) found that PEG produced a concentration-dependent reduction in absorption of water and electrolytes as measured by in vivo perfusion of human jejunum, perhaps by an osmotic effect; this observation calls into question results of studies in which high concentrations of PEG (>5 g/l) have been used.

Correct designation of the mean concentration of solute in the perfusate can be difficult. Thus, while for slowly absorbed test solutes the arithmetic mean of the infusate and effluent concentrations can be used, it is probably preferable to take the geometric mean in the case of rapidly absorbed substances (Soergel 1971; Shields 1972).

Other factors which require consideration in the interpretation of perfusion experiments (Table 4.4) include the composition of the perfusate, in particular its comparability to normal ileal effluent; measures taken to minimize contamination by ileal effluent and caeco-ileal reflux (Devroede and Phillips 1969; Wanitschke and Ewe 1983); uncertainties about the length and surface area of colon perfused; use of an equilibration period long enough to ensure steady state conditions before the test perfusion; the effects on transport of endoluminal tubes and/or balloons (see p. 69); the masking of regional differences in mucosal fluxes (e.g. ascending vs descending colon, surface vs crypt colonocytes); and an inability to control or determine the composition of the interstitial fluid at the contraluminal surface of the mucosa. Lastly, the possible effects of diurnal variation, the menstrual cycle and diet have rarely been taken into account (Wrong et al. 1981).

Applications. Notwithstanding this catalogue of potential pitfalls, the perfusion technique has proved extremely useful in the evaluation of human large intestinal water and electrolyte transport (see Wrong et al. 1981; Kerlin and Phillips 1983), and permeability (Billich and Levitan 1969; Rask-Madsen 1973a; Chadwick et al. 1977), as well as its handling of, for example, short-chain fatty acids (Ruppin et al. 1980), ammonia (Wolpert et al. 1970) and bile salts (Mekhjian et al. 1979). It has also provided important insights into the effects on the human colon of bile salts (Mekhjian et al. 1971), fatty acids (Ammon and Phillips 1973), hormones (see Kerlin and Phillips 1983), inflammatory mediators (Milton-Thompson et al. 1975), drugs (Wanitschke and Ewe 1983) and disease states (see Kerlin and Phillips 1983). In one study, simultaneous recording of intraluminal pressures has been undertaken (Chauve et al. 1974).

In the now extinct patients with colons surgically excluded for the treatment of chronic hepatic encephalopathy, whole colonic perfusion was relatively easy to perform. Transport data in such cases has been published about mucosal transport of water and electrolytes (Bown et al. 1972), ammonia (Castell and Moore 1971; Bown et al. 1975) and oxalate (Fairclough et al. 1977), but the confidence with which such results can be extrapolated to normal people is uncertain.

Isolated Colorectal Segments

Technique. The same principles as those employed for perfusion of the intact colon in vivo have been applied, to a limited extent, to the study of isolated segments of human large bowel. In these investigations many of the limitations listed in Table 4.4 pertain. Furthermore, as in infusion experiments (see p. 70), in man it is difficult to isolate satisfactorily and thereby accurately define the length and surface area of test segments. Moreover, when the test segment is short, it may be difficult to detect the small concentration changes which occur in the effluent during perfusion studies (Devroede and Phillips 1970; Edmonds 1971).

Applications. Despite these problems, the perfusion technique has been used in man to evaluate mucosal water and electrolyte transport and permeability in the normal (Devroede and Phillips 1970; Rask-Madsen 1973b) and inflamed rectum (Rask-Madsen et al. 1973), and to compare transport function in proximal and distal colon (Schiller et al. 1988).

In Vitro Techniques

General Remarks

The main advantage of in vitro over in vivo methods is the opportunity they provide to unravel mechanisms of ion transport by external control of experimental variables such as the transmucosal PD and the composition of the fluids in contact with the mucosal and serosal surfaces of the preparation. The short-circuit current technique (Ussing and Zerahn 1951), in particular, has proved extremely informative (Schültz 1981), even though the function of a small piece of mucosa deprived of its normal luminal environment, vasculature and neurohumoral connections is likely to be still less representative of its behaviour in situ than is that of mucosal preparations studied by the in vivo methods already reviewed (Tables 4.4 and 4.5).

Table 4.5. Limitations of short-circuit current techniques

1. Absence of vascular and neurohumoral connections
2. Variable removal of luminal factors (bile salts, fatty acids, bacteria)
3. Variable mixing and dissipation of unstirred layer
4. Limited availability of tissue
5. Edge damage
6. Small surface area may mask regional differences in transport
7. Inability to quantify movement of water
8. Uncertain effect of drugs, anaesthetics and disease in tissue host

Short-circuit Current Techniques

Technique. For human studies, samples of colon are obtained at surgery, for example, in the case of "controls", apparently normal areas adjacent to carcinoma or diverticulosis. The mucosa is dissected off the underlying tissue and mounted

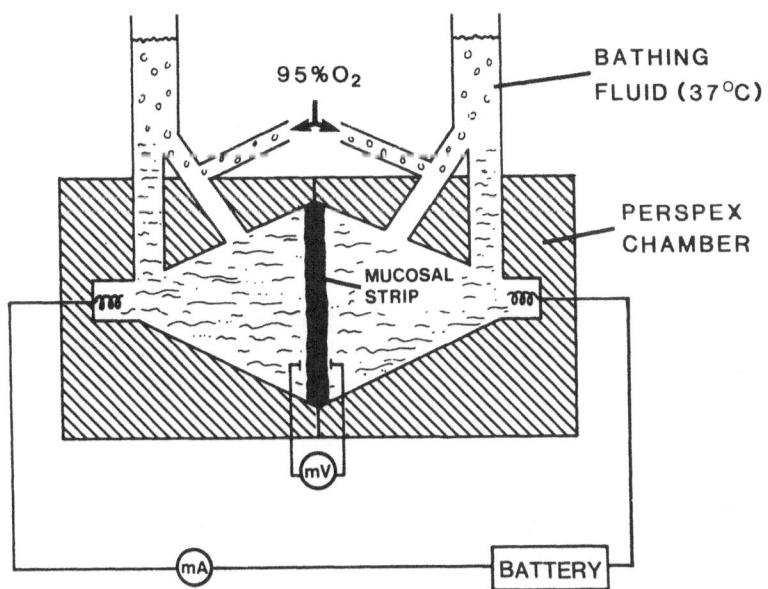

Fig. 4.4. Short-circuit current preparation for studying mucosal ion transport in vitro.

between half-chambers in a perspex box (Fig. 4.4) (Ussing and Zerahn 1951). The mucosal sheet then separates mucosal from serosal bathing fluid, the chemical and osmotic composition of which can, as already mentioned, be altered independently; furthermore, radio-isotopic tracers to measure bidirectional fluxes (J_{ms} and J_{sm}), and metabolic inhibitors and stimulants of active transport can be applied. Most importantly, the transmucosal PD (ψ_{ms}) can be monitored continuously and negated by opposing it with a short-circuit current (I_{sc}). If the bathing fluids are of identical composition, abolition of the PD removes the electrochemical gradient across the tissue: under these circumstances any net movements are a consequence of coupling to a source of metabolic energy (i.e. active transport). In addition, I_{sc} equals the algebraic sum of the net transepithelial flows of those ions whose movements are not due to simple diffusion.

In a recent modification of the short-circuit technique, measurement of the PD across the apical and basolateral membranes of the human colonocyte has been achieved by impaling mucosa, mounted in Ussing chambers, with intracellular microelectrodes (Sandle et al. 1986).

Various other modifications have also been introduced. For example, the tissue studied need not be whole mucosal strips. Dharmsathaphorn et al. (1984a, b) and Grasset et al (1984a, b) have applied the method to monolayers of cultured human colonic epithelial cell lines derived originally from carcinomas; monolayers derived from normal colonocytes (Gibson et al. 1989) may soon

be studied in this way. Such preparations allow the study of a homologous cell population free from the influence of vascular or neurohumoral factors. Moreover, by providing equal accessibility of both apical and basolateral membranes, they make possible improved localization of transport processes, particularly when intracellular microelectrodes are used (Grasset et al. 1984a, b). How closely the function of such monolayers resembles that of adult colonic epithelial cells in vivo, of course, is uncertain: monolayers derived from Caco-2 cells, for example, exhibit characteristics, depending on the experimental conditions, more suggestive of human foetal colonocytes (Blais et al. 1987) and small intestinal villous cells (Hidalgo et al. 1989).

As with any of the other techniques available for the study of human colonic absorption and secretion, the short-circuit preparation has a number of limitations (Table 4.5) apart from those related to the absence of the normal surrounding tissues.

Like perfusion techniques, this method causes variable removal of endogenous luminal factors which may affect transport; in addition, there remains a substantial unstirred layer on both the mucosal and serosal surfaces which may interfere with interpretation of the results (Wrong et al. 1981).

Viability of such tissue is restricted even with meticulous oxygenation before and during the study. Furthermore, damage inevitably sustained by the edges of the dissected mucosa can compromise results (Dobson and Kidder 1968). Because only small pieces of tissue (surface area <2 cm^2)

are used, possible regional differences in function may be missed. Lastly, this technique does not permit quantification of transmucosal water fluxes, and the effects are unclear of disease (e.g. carcinoma), drugs and anaesthetics given to patients prior to the colonic surgery at which the specimens for studies of supposedly normal mucosa are obtained.

Applications. The short-circuit technique, in its various modifications, has proved very valuable in the elucidation of ion transport across epithelia in general, and mammalian colon in particular (Schultz 1981). Grady et al. (1970), Archampong et al. (1972), Rask-Madsen and Hjelt (1977), Hawker et al. (1978) and Wills et al. (1984) have reported (sometimes conflicting) results in normal descending or sigmoid colon, while, more recently, Sandle et al. (1986), Hubel et al. (1987) and Sellin and de Soignie (1987) have used the method to investigate regional differences in human colonic transport function; Hubel et al. also tested the effects of electrical stimulation of intrinsic nerves. Electrolyte transport in vitro in inflamed colon has been studied by Archampong et al. (1972) and Hawker et al. (1980).

More recently, short-circuit experiments using cultured human colonic carcinoma-derived mono-layers have explored responses to ricinoleic acid, VIP and PGE_1 (Dharmsathaphorn et al. 1984a,b; Grasset et al. 1984b; Weymer et al. 1985).

Other In Vitro Techniques

A variety of other in vitro methods has been employed in the investigation of intestinal muco-sal transport in animals (see Parsons 1968), but few have found widespread application in man (Table 4.1).

It is worth mentioning, however, Roediger and Moore's (1981) study of the inter-relationships between sodium absorption, PD and short-chain fatty acids using an elegant but technically difficult technique in which the lumen and vascular bed of a human colonic segment are simultaneously per-fused in vitro (Parsons and Powis 1971).

More recently, it has become possible to isolate brush border vesicles by differential centrifugation and sucrose density gradient centrifugation of epithelial cells separated from colonic mucosa by chelation and mechanical dissociation. Although already used to study sodium–hydrogen exchange across the membrane of brush border vesicles derived from animal large intestine (Binder et al.

1986; Foster et al. 1986), this technique does not appear to have yet been applied to the study of human colonic function.

Conclusions

The ingenuity and imagination of their inventors is well illustrated by the wide variety of methods that has been devised and adapted for the investigation of human colorectal absorption and secretion. Unfortunately, however, no single technique has proved, as yet, capable of elucidating more than a narrow spectrum of mucosal functional proper-ties. More importantly, the majority of techniques presently available impose environmental con-ditions far removed from those pertaining in the normal or diseased bowel in situ. For the foresee-able future, therefore, caution must be exercised in the extrapolation of results obtained experi-mentally to intact man.

References

Allen A (1983) The structure of colonic mucus. In: Bustos-Fernandez L (ed) Colon: structure and function. Plenum Medical, New York, pp 45–64

Ammon HV, Phillips SF (1973) Inhibition of colonic water and electrolyte absorption by fatty acids in man. Gastroentero-logy 65:744–749

Archampong EQ, Edmonds CJ (1972) Effect of luminal ions on the transepithelial electrical potential difference of human rectum. Gut 13:559–565

Archampong EQ, Harris J, Clark CG (1972) The absorption and secretion of water and electrolytes across the healthy and the diseased human colonic mucosa measured in vitro. Gut 13:880–886

Billich CO, Levitan R (1969) Effects of sodium concentration and osmolality on water and electrolyte absorption from the intact human colon. J Clin Invest 48:1336–1347

Binder H, Sandle G (1987) Absorption and secretion in mammalian colon. In: Johnson LR (ed) Physiology of the gastrointestinal tract. Raven Press, New York, pp 1389–1418

Binder H, Stange G, Murer H, Stieger B, Harri H-P (1986) Sodium–proton exchange in colon brush-border mem-branes. Am J Physiol 251:G382–390

Blais P, Bissonette P, Berteloot A (1987) Common characteris-tics for sodium-dependent sugar transport in Caco-2 cells and human fetal colon. J Membr Biol 99:113–25

Bond JH, Levitt MD (1972) Use of pulmonary hydrogen measurements to quantitate carbohydrate absorption. J Clin Invest 51:1219–1225

Bown RL, Sladen GE, Rousseau B, Gibson JA, Clark ML, Dawson AM (1972) A study of water and electrolyte transport by excluded human colon. Clin Sci 43:893–902

Bown RL, Gibson JA, Fenton JCB, Snedden W, Clark ML, Sladen GE (1975) Ammonia and urea transport by excluded human colon. Clin Sci Mol Med 48:279–287

Branch WJ, Cummings JH (1978) Comparison of radio-opaque pellets and chromium sesquioxide as inert markers in studies requiring accurate faecal collections. Gut 19:371–376

Bustos-Fernandez L, Ledesma-Paolo MI, Kofoed JA et al (1983) The physiology of colonic mucus secretion. In: Bustos-Fernandez L (ed) Colon: structure and function. Plenum Medical, New York, pp. 65–78

Caprilli R, Sopranzi N, Colaneri O, Levi Della Vida M, De Magistris L (1978) Salt losing diarrhoea in idiopathic procto-colitis. Scand J Gastroenterol 13:331–334

Castell DO, Moore EW (1971) Ammonia absorption from the human colon. Gastroenterology 60:33–42

Chadwick VS, Phillips SF, Hofmann AF (1977) Measurements of intestinal permeability using low molecular weight poly-ethylene glycols (PEG 400). II. Application to normal and abnormal permeability states in man and animals. Gastroen-terology 73:247–251

Charron RC, Leme CE, Wilson DR, Ing TS, Wrong OM (1969) The effect of adrenal steroids on stool composition as revealed by in vivo faecal dialysis. Clin Sci 37:151–167

Chauve M, Devroede GJ, Sasseville J-L (1974) Continuous recording of multiple parameters during perfusion of human colon. J Appl Physiol 37:241–246

Clarke AM, Hill GL, MacBeth WAAG (1967) Intestinal adaptation to salt depletion in a patient with an ileostomy. Gastroenterology 53:444–449

Code CF (1960) The semantics of the process of absorption. Perpect Biol Med 3:560–562

Cummings JH, James WPT, Wiggins HS (1973) Role of the colon in ileal resection diarrhoea. Lancet i:344–347

Cummings JH, Milton-Thompson GJ, Billings JA, Misiewicz JJ (1976) The flow rate and composition of ileal contents during fasting and in response to a liquid meal in man. Gut 17:817–818

Dalmark M (1970) The transmucosal electrical potential differ-ence across human rectum in vivo following perfusion of different electrolyte solutions. Scand J Gastroenterol 5:421–426

Davis GR, Santa Ana CA, Morawski SG, Fordtran JS (1980) Inhibition of water and electrolyte absorption by polyethy-lene glycol (PEG). Gastroenterology 79:35–39

Davis GR, Santa Ana C, Morawski SG, Fordtran JS (1982) Permeability characteristics of human jejunum, ileum, proximal colon and distal colon: results of potential differ-ence measurements and unidirectional fluxes. Gastroentero-logy 83:844–850

Debongnie JC, Phillips SF (1978) Capacity of the human colon to absorb fluid. Gastroenterology 74:698–703

Devroede GJ, Phillips SF (1969) Studies of the perfusion technique for colonic absorption. Gastroenterology 56:92–100

Devroede GJ, Phillips SF (1970) Failure of the human rectum to absorb electrolytes and water. Gut 11:438–442

Devroede GJ, Phillips SF, Code CF, Lind JF (1971) Regional differences in rates of insorption of sodium and water from the human intestine. Can J Physiol Pharmacol 49:1023–1029

Dharmsathaphorn K, Mandel KG, Masui H, McRoberts JA (1984a) VIP-induced chloride secretion by a colonic epithe-lial cell line. J Clin Invest 75:462–471

Dharmsathaphorn K, McRoberts JA, Mandel KG, Tisdale LD, Masui H (1984b) A human colonic tumour cell line that maintains vectorial electrolyte transport. Am J Physiol 246:G204–208

Diem K, Lentner C (1970) Scientific tables, 7th edn. Geigy, Basle

Dobson JG, Kidder GW (1968) Edge damage effect in in vitro frog skin preparations. Am J Physiol 214:719–724

Donowitz M (1987) Small intestinal and colonic linked sodium chloride absorption. New understanding of distribution and regulation. Gastroenterology 93:640–651

Duthie HL, Atwell JD (1963) The absorption of water, sodium and potassium in the large intestine with particular reference to the effects of villous papillomas. Gut 4:373–377

Duthie HL, Watts JM, De Dombal FT et al. (1964) Serum electrolytes and colonic transfer of water and electrolytes in chronic ulcerative colitis. Gastroenterology 47:525–530

Edmonds CJ (1971) Absorption of sodium and water by human rectum measured by a dialysis method. Gut 12:356–362

Edmonds CJ (1975) Electrical potential difference of colonic mucosa. Gut 16:315–329

Edmonds CJ (1981) Water and ionic transfer pathways of mammalian large intestine. Clin Sci 61:257–263

Edmonds CJ, Pilcher D (1973) Electrical potential difference and sodium and potassium fluxes across rectal mucosa in ulcerative colitis. Gut 14:784–789

Fairclough PD, Feest TG, Chadwick VS, Clark ML (1977) Effect of sodium chenodeoxycholate on oxalate absorption from the excluded human colon – a mechanism for enteric hyperoxaluria. Gut 18:240–244

Findlay JM, Eastwood MA, Mitchell WD (1973) The physical state of bile acids in the diarrhoeal stool of ileal dysfunction. Gut 14:319–323

Fordtran JS (1966) Marker perfusion techniques for measuring intestinal perfusion in man. Gastroenterology 51:1089–1093

Fordtran JS, Dietschy JM (1966) Water the electrolyte move-ment in the intestine. Gastroenterology 50:263–285

Foster ES, Dudeja PK, Brasitus TA (1986) Sodium–hydrogen exchange in rat colonic brush-border membrane vesicles. Am J Physiol 250:G781–787

Gamble JL (1915) The ammonia and urea content of infants' stool. Am J Dis Child 9:519–532

Geall MG, Spencer RJ, Phillips SF (1969) Transmural electri-cal potential difference of human colon. Gut 10:921–923

Gibson PR, Van de Pol E, Maxwell LE, Gabriel A, Doe WF (1989) Isolation of colonic crypts that maintain structural and metabolic viability in vitro. Gastroenterology 96:283–291

Gorbach SL, Nahas L, Weinstein L (1973) Studies of intestinal microflora. IV. The influence of ileostomy effluent – a unique microbial ecology. Gastroenterology 53:874–880

Grady GF, Duhamel RC, Moore EW (1970) Active transport of sodium by human colon in vitro. Gastroenterology 59:583–588

Grasset E, Pinto M, Dussaulx E, Zweibaum A, Desjeux J-F (1984a) Epithelial properties of human colonic carcinoma cell line Caco-2: electrical parameters. Am J Physiol 247:C260–266

Grasset E, Pinto M, Bernabeu J (1984b) Epithelial properties of human colonic carcinoma cell line Caco-2: effect of secretagogues. Am J Physiol 248:C410–418

Hawker PC, Mashiter KE, Turnberg LA (1978) Mechanisms of transport of Na, Cl, and K in the human colon. Gastroen-terology 74:1241–1247

Hawker PC, McKay JS, Turnberg LA (1980) Electrolyte transport across colonic mucosa from patients with inflam-matory bowel disease. Gastroenterology 79:508–511

Hidalgo IJ, Raub TJ, Borchardt RT (1989) Characterisation of the human colon carcinoma cell line (Caco-2) as a model system for intestinal epithelial permeability. Gastroentero-logy 96:736–749

Hill GL, Mair WSJ, Edwards JP, Morgan DB, Goligher JC (1975) Effect of a chemically defined liquid elemental diet on composition and volume of ileal fistula drainage. Gastroenterology 68:676–682

Hofmann AF, Lauterburg BH (1977) Breath tests with isotopes of carbon: progress and potential. J Lab Clin Med 90:405–411

Hubel KA, Renquist K, Shirazi S (1987) Ion transport in human cecum, transverse colon and sigmoid colon in vitro. Baseline and response to electrical stimulation of intrinsic nerves. Gastroenterology 92:501–507

James OFW, Agnew JT, Bouchier IAD (1973) Assessment of the ^{14}C-glycocholic acid breath test. Br Med J iii:191–195

Kanaghinis T, Lubran M, Coghill NF (1963) The composition of ileostomy fluid. Gut 4:322–338

Kerlin P, Phillips SF (1983) Absorption and secretion of electrolytes by the human colon. In: Bustos-Fernandez L (ed) Colon: structure and function. Plenum Medical, New York, pp 17–44

Kramer P (1966) The effect of varying sodium loads on the ileal excreta of human ileostomised subjects. J Clin Invest 45:1710–1718

Ladas SD, Isaacs PET, Murphy G, Sladen GE (1986) Fasting and post-prandial ileal function in adapted ileostomates and normal subjects. Gut 27:906–912

Lauritsen K, Hansen J, Bytzer P, Bukhave K, Rask-Madsen J (1984) Effects of sulphasalazine and disodium azodisalicylate on colonic PGE$_2$ concentrations determined by equilibrium dialysis of faeces in patients with ulcerative colitis and healthy controls. Gut 25:1271–1278

Lauritsen K, Laursen LS, Bukhave K, Rask-Madsen J (1986) Effects of topical 5-aminosalicylic acid and prednisolone on prostaglandin E$_2$ and leukotriene B4 levels determined by equilibrium in vivo dialysis of rectum in relapsing ulcerative colitis. Gastroenterology 91:837–844

Levitan R, Brudno S (1967) Permeability of the rectosigmoid mucosa to tritiated water in normal subjects and in patients with mild idiopathic ulcerative colitis. Gut 8:15–19

Levitan R, Fordtran JS, Burrows BA, Ingelfinger FJ (1962) Water and salt absorption in the human colon. J Clin Invest 41:1754–1759

Levitan R, Bikerman V, Burrows BA, Ingelfinger FJ (1963) Rectosigmoidal absorption of phenolsulfonphthalein (PSP), sulfisoxazole diethanolamine (Gantrisin) and radioiodine (I^{131}) in normal subjects and patients with idiopathic ulcerative colitis. J Lab Clin Med 62:639–645

Levitt MD, Bond J (1977) Use of the constant perfusion technique in the non-steady state. Gastroenterology 73:1450–1454

Levitt MD, Hirsch P, Fetzer CA, Sheaman M, Levine AS (1987) H$_2$ excretion after ingestion of complex carbohydrates. Gastroenterology 92:383–389

McNeil NI (1983) Differences in electrolyte handling through the human large intestine. In: Skadhauge K, Heintze K (eds) Intestinal absorption and secretion. MTP Press, Boston, pp 111–116

McNeil NI, Cummings JH, James WPT (1978) Short chain fatty acid absorption by the human large intestine. Gut 19:819–822

Mekhjian HS, Phillips SF, Hofmann AF (1971) Colonic secretion of water and electrolytes induced by bile acids: perfusion studies in man. J Clin Invest 50:1569–1577

Mekhjian HS, Phillips SF, Hofmann AF (1979) Colonic absorption of unconjugated bile acids. Perfusion studies in man. Dig Dis Sci 24:545–550

Metcalfe-Gibson A, Ing TS, Kuiper JJ, Richards P, Ward EE, Wrong OM (1967) In vivo dialysis of faeces as a method of stool analysis. II. The influence of diet. Clin Sci 33:89–100

Milton-Thompson GJ, Cummings JH, Newman A, Billings JA, Misiewicz JJ (1975) Colonic and small intestinal response to intravenous prostaglandin F$_{2alpha}$ and E$_2$ in man. Gut 16:42–49

Mitchell JE, Breuer RI, Zuckerman L, Berlin J, Schiller R (1980) The colon influences ileal resection diarrhoea. Dig Dis Sci 25:33–41

Neutra MR, Forstner JG (1987) Gastrointestinal mucus: synthesis, secretion and function. In: Johnson LR (ed) Physiology of the gastrointestinal tract. Raven Press, New York, pp 975–1010

Orlando RC, Powell DW, Croom RD, Berschneider HM, Boucher RC, Knowles MR (1989) Colonic and oesophageal transepithelial potential difference in cystic fibrosis. Gastroenterology 96:1041–1048

Owens CWI, Padovan W (1976) Limitations of ultracentrifugation and in vivo dialysis as methods of stool analysis. Gut 17:68–74

Palma R, Vidon N, Bernier JJ (1981) Maximal capacity for fluid absorption in human bowel. Dig Dis Sci 26:929–934

Parsons DS (1968) Methods for investigation of intestinal absorption. In: Code CF (ed) Handbook of physiology, section 6, Alimentary canal, vol III, Intestinal absorption. American Physiological Society, Washington, pp 1177–1216

Parsons DS, Powis G (1971) Some properties of a preparation of rat colon perfused in vitro through the vascular bed. J Physiol 217:641–663

Phillips SF, Giller J (1973) The contribution of the colon to electrolyte and water conservation in man. J Lab Clin Med 81:733–746

Powell DW (1979) Transport in the large intestine. In: Giebisch G, Tosteson DC, Ussing HH (eds) Membrane transport in biology. Springer, New York, pp 781–809

Powell DW (1987) Intestinal water and electrolyte transport. In: Johnson LR (ed) Physiology of the gastrointestinal tract. Raven Press, New York, pp 1267–1306

Rampton DS, Sladen GE (1984) Relationship between rectal mucosal prostaglandin production and water and electrolyte transport in ulcerative colitis. Digestion 30:13–22

Rampton DS, Sladen GE, Youlten LJF (1980a) Rectal mucosal prostaglandin E$_2$ release and its relation to disease activity, electrical potential difference and treatment in ulcerative colitis. Gut 21:591–596

Rampton DS, Murdoch RD, Sladen GE (1980b) Rectal mucosal histamine release in ulcerative colitis. Clin Sci 59:389–391

Rask-Madsen J (1973a) Simultaneous measurement of electrical polarisation and electrolyte transport by the entire normal and inflamed human colon during in vivo perfusion. Scand J Gastroenterol 8:327–336

Rask-Madsen J (1973b) The relationship between sodium fluxes and electrical potentials across the normal and inflamed human rectal wall in vivo. Acta Med Scand 194:311–317

Rask-Madsen J, Brix-Jensen P (1973) Electrolyte transport capacity and electrical potentials of the normal and the inflamed human rectum in vivo. Scand J Gastroenterol 8:169–175

Rask-Madsen J, Hjelt H (1977) Effect of amiloride on electrical activity and electrolyte transport in human colon. Scand J Gastroenterol 12:1–6

Rask-Madsen J, Hammersgaard EA, Knudsen E (1973) Rectal electrolyte transport and mucosal permeability in ulcerative colitis and Crohn's disease. J Lab Clin Med 81:342–353

Rask-Madsen J, Bruusgaard A, Munck O, Nielsen MD, Worning H (1974) The significance of bile acids and aldosterone for the electrical hyperpolarisation of human rectum in obese patients treated with intestinal bypass operation. Scand J Gastroenterol 9:417–422

Roediger WEW, Moore A (1981) The effect of short chain

fatty acid on sodium absorption in isolated human colon perfused through the vascular bed. Dig Dis Sci 26:100–1

Roediger WEW, Heyworth M, Willoughby P, Piris J, Moore A, Truelove SC (1982) Luminal ions and short chain fatty acids as markers of functional activity of the mucosa in ulcerative colitis. J Clin Pathol 35:323–326

Ruppin H, Bar-Meir S, Soergel KH et al (1980) Absorption of short chain fatty acids by the colon. Gastroenterology 78:1500–1507

Sandle GI, Wills NK, Alles W, Binder H (1986) Electrophysiology of the human colon: evidence of segmental heterogeneity. Gut 27:999–1005

Scarpello JH, Sladen GE (1977) Appraisal of the ^{14}C-glycocholic acid test with special reference to the measurement of faecal ^{14}C excretion. Gut 18:742–748

Schiller LR, Santa Ana CA, Morawski SG, Fordtran JS (1988) Effect of amiloride on sodium transport in the proximal, distal and entire human colon in vivo. Dig Dis Sci 33:969–976

Schilli R, Breuer RI, Klein F et al (1981) Comparison of the composition of faecal fluid in Crohn's disease and ulcerative colitis. Gut 23:326–332

Schultz SG (1981) Ion transport by mammalian large intestine. In: Johnson LR (ed) Physiology of the gastrointestinal tract. Raven Press, New York, pp 991–1002

Sellin JH, de Soignie R (1987) Ion transport in human colon in vitro. Gastroenterology 93:441–448

Shields R (1966) Absorption and secretion of electrolytes and water by the human colon with particular reference to benign adenoma and papilloma. Br J Surg 53:893–897

Shields R (1972) Absorption and secretion by human colon. In: Badenoch J, Brooke BN (eds) Recent advances in gastroenterology. Churchill Livingstone, Edinburgh, pp 215–249

Shields R (1979) Absorption from the human colon. In: Duthie HL, Wormsley KG (eds) Scientific basis of gastroenterology: Churchill Livingstone, Edinburgh, pp 398–415

Sladen GE (1975) Methods of studying intestinal absorption in man. In: McColl I, Sladen GE (eds) Intestinal absorption in man. Academic Press, New York, pp 1–49

Soergel KH (1968) Inert markers. Gastroenterology 54:449–452

Soergel KH (1971) Intestinal perfusion studies: values, pitfalls, limitations. Gastroenterology 61:261–263

Tarlow MJ, Thom H (1974) A comparison of stool fluid and stool dialysate obtained in vivo. Gut 15:608–613

Ussing HH, Zerahn K (1951) Active transport of sodium as the source of electric current in the short circuited isolated frog skin. Acta Physiol Scand 23:110–127

Vernia P, Breuer RI, Gnaedinger A, Latella G, Santoro ML (1984) Composition of fecal water. Comparison of in vitro dialysis with ultrafiltration. Gastroenterology 86:1557–1561

Vernia P, Gnaedinger A, Hauck W, Breuer RI (1988) Organic ions and the diarrhoea of inflammatory bowel disease. Dig Dis Sci 33:1353–1358

Vince A, O'Grady F, Dawson AM (1973) The development of the ileostomy flora. J Infect Dis 128:638–641

Vince A, Down PJ, Murison J, Twigg FJ, Wrong OM (1976) Generation of ammonia from non-urea sources in a faecal incubation system. Clin Sci Mol Med 51:313–322

Wanitschke R, Ewe K (1983) Drugs and the colon. In: Bustos-Fernandez L (ed) Colon: structure and function. Plenum Medical, New York, pp 275–292

Weymer A, Huott P, Liu W, McRoberts JA, Dharmsathaphorn K (1985) Chloride secretory mechanism induced by prostaglandin E_1 in a colonic epithelial cell line. J Clin Invest 76:1828–1836

Whalen GE, Harris JA, Geenen JE, Soergel KH (1966) Sodium and water absorption from the human small intestine; the accuracy of the perfusion method. Gastroenterology 51:975–984

Wills NK, Lewis SA, Eaton DC (1984) Active and passive properties of rabbit descending colon: a microelectrode and mystatin study. J Membr Biol 45:81–108

Wilson DR, Ing TS, Metcalfe-Gibson A, Wrong OM (1968a) In vivo dialysis of faeces as a method of stool analysis. III. The effect of intestinal antibiotics. Clin Sci 34:211–221

Wilson DR, Ing TS, Metcalfe-Gibson A, Wrong OM (1968b) The chemical composition of faeces in uraemia, as revealed by in vivo dialysis. Clin Sci 35:197–209

Wolpert E, Phillips SF, Summerskill WHJ (1970) Ammonia production in the human colon. Effects of cleansing, neomycin and acetohydroxamic acid. N Engl J Med 283:159–164

Wright HK, Cleveland JC, Tilson MD, Herskovic T (1969) Morphology and absorptive capacity of the ileum after ileostomy in man. Am J Surg 117:242–245

Wrong OM, Morrison RBI, Hurst PE (1961) A method of obtaining faecal fluid by in vivo dialysis. Lancet i:1208–1209

Wrong OM, Metcalfe-Gibson A, Morrison RBI, Ing TS, Howard AV (1965) In vivo dialysis of faeces as a method of stool analysis. I. Technique and results in normal subjects. Clin Sci 28:357–375

Wrong OM, Edmonds CJ, Chadwick VS (1981) The large intestine. MTP Press, Lancaster, pp 15–24, 33–58

5 · Histological Measurement in Coloproctology

M. Swash

Coloproctological disorders have been studied by a variety of different techniques. Limitations are imposed by the necessity to do no harm as a consequence of the investigation; thus, radiological and other imaging methodologies such as ultrasonography, functional estimates based on manometric and flow methodologies, and electrophysiological techniques have been used to investigate the function of the colon, anorectum, and its associated smooth and striated muscle both in normal subjects and in patients with colorectal disorders. These investigations address particular aspects of functions of the colorectum, anal canal, and its associated tissues but do not give direct information concerning the morphological and pathological basis of such disturbed function. The latter is the role of pathology and its associated measurement techniques.

The structural system that must be addressed consists of the anal canal, the rectum and the colon together with its associated structures, particularly the pelvic floor itself. The colorectum consists of the most caudal part of the gut. It is lined with villous mucosa, and consists of a muscular wall made up of longitudinal and circular components of smooth, non-striated muscle cells. Embedded in this muscular coat is the myenteric plexus of Auerbach and the submucosal plexus of Meissner, representing the enteric nervous system, itself a third component of the autonomic nervous system recognized by Langley (1921). The activity of the myenteric nervous system is itself modulated by CNS input from the parasympathetic outflow derived from the lumbosacral segments, and from sympathetic nerve fibres derived from the intermediolateral cell column in the thoracic spinal cord. Afferents from the gut provide feedback control mechanisms in relation to this extrinsic innervation. The anal canal itself marks a junction point between the caudal part of the gut and the skin of the perineum. Its lower part consists of squamous epithelium innervated by somatic afferent fibres that project through the pudendal nerves to the S2, S3 and S4 spinal segments. Receptors are found in this squamous epithelium that closely resemble those found in skin elsewhere in the body (Duthie and Gairns 1960).

The pelvic floor consists of a muscular diaphragm made up of the levator ani, puborectalis, pubococcygeus, puboanalis, together with the striated sphincter muscles of the urethra, i.e. the periurethral striated sphincter musculature, and of the anal canal, i.e. the external anal sphincter muscle. Anteriorly the pelvic floor is perforated in the female by the vagina and the urethra. In the male the anatomy of the small muscles of the anterior part of the pelvic floor is specialized to take account of the functions of ejaculation and erection. The pelvic floor diaphragm is innervated by direct pelvic branches derived from somatic nerve fibres that pass through the lumbosacral plexus; more caudally the external anal sphincter muscle is innervated by the inferior rectal branches of the pudendal nerves. The puborectalis, a muscle that histologically and functionally is closely related to the external anal sphincter, is innervated by branches from the lumbosacral plexus, an arrangement that illustrates the phylogenetic origin of this muscle (Percy et al. 1981; Snooks and Swash 1986). In this chapter the techniques and scope of morphometric methods in the assessment of these structures will be addressed.

Histometric Studies of Human Muscle Biopsies

Histopathological studies of the striated sphincter and pelvic floor musculature have been important in formulating current ideas on the pathogenesis of incontinence and other pelvic floor disorders. Human striated muscles consist of a mixture of muscle fibre types defined by their twitch and fatigue characteristics, and by their histochemical profiles (Dubowitz 1986; Swash and Schwartz 1988). Thus, the Type 1 muscle fibres consist of fibres with relatively slow twitch characteristics that are resistant to fatigue and the Type 2 fibres of fibres with relatively rapid twitch characteristics; they are subdivided into two types, Type 2a which are resistant to fatigue and Type 2b which fatigue relatively rapidly. A third variety of Type 2 fibres, Type 2c fibres, take up an intermediate position. The Type 1 muscle fibres, specialized for continued tonic activity, with slow twitch times, react strongly in the myosin ATPase reaction at acid pH, are strongly positive in mitochondrial oxidative enzyme stains such as NADH and SDH, and contain little glycogen or phosphorylase, but plentiful neutral lipid. Type 2 fibres, on the other hand, react strongly for myosin ATPase at alkaline pH, contain relatively low mitochondrial NADH and SDH enzyme activity, but plentiful glycogen and myophosphorylase activity, and relatively little neutral lipid. Thus Type 2 fibres are adapted to rapid maximal contractions of phasic type, but are not suited to tonic continuous low-level activity. Type 1 muscle fibres are activated before Type 2 fibres during gentle sustained contractions of a muscle, as in maintaining a limb against gravity. Thus fast twitch, phasic tasks, such as weightlifting and sprinting, can be thought of as predominantly the function of Type 2 fibres, and long-distance athletic events such as long-distance skiing as predominantly dependent on Type 1 fibre activity. The relative proportions of Type 1 and Type 2 fibres within a given muscle vary from muscle to muscle, and in relation to the genetic constitution of the individual.

Studies of the distribution of muscle fibre types in different muscles have largely been limited to muscles that are commonly subjected to biopsy for diagnostic purposes in patients with myopathies and neuromuscular diseases, such as biceps, triceps, deltoid and quadriceps muscles. Muscles that contain particularly large numbers of Type 1 fibres include the tibialis anterior muscle and the soleus muscle. Other limb muscles, for example the deltoid, triceps and vastus medialis contain more Type 2 fibres in their superficial than in their deep layers. The levator ani, external anal sphincter, puborectalis, and periurethral striated sphincter muscles contain a marked predominance of Type 1 muscle fibres (Beersiek et al. 1979) and this relative predominance of Type 1 fibres is increased in patients with anorectal incontinence (Fig. 5.1). The levator ani muscle more closely resembles striated limb girdle muscles than the puborectalis and external anal sphincter muscles in its fibre type proportions.

The diameter characteristics of muscle fibres in normal and abnormal skeletal muscles were investigated in some detail by Brooke and Engel (1969) in a series of studies of muscle biopsies taken from adults and children. In conducting such investigations it is important to standardize the methods of preparation of the biopsy and most studies currently reported utilize tissue that has been frozen and sectioned in a cryostat in the unfixed state (Polgar et al. 1973). Measurements are made either directly at the microscope or from measurements of photomicrographs, utilizing fibres whose histochemical profile has been recognized in the myofibrillar ATPase reaction. In cross sections of muscles the orientation of muscle fibres varies somewhat and it is usual to measure the lesser diameter of the muscle fibre in a plane through the centre of the fibre in such measurements. The normal adult diameter of muscle fibres is reached between the ages of 12 and 15 years. In men Type 2 fibres are usually larger than Type 1 but in women Type 1 fibres are slightly larger than Type 2. The mean diameters of both Type 1 and Type 2 fibres are larger in men than in women. The variation in mean fibre diameter in striated limb muscles can be expressed by the standard deviation, or the standard error of the mean of the group of fibres measured. Usually, 200 fibres of each fibre type are measured in constructing such statistical algorithms. Brooke (see Dubowitz 1986) suggested the use of a coefficient of variation based on the relation between the standard deviation and the mean fibre diameter. The formula, standard deviation divided by mean fibre diameter × 1000, represents this variability coefficient and

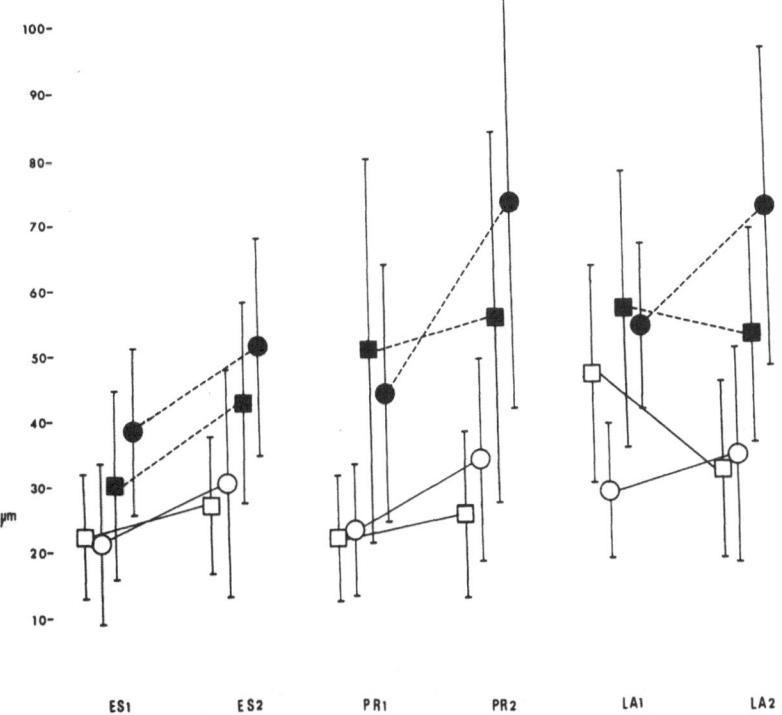

Fig. 5.1. Fibre size relationships in external anal sphincter, puborectalis and levator ani muscles in normal subjects and patients with incontinence. *Open symbols*, normal subjects; *filled symbols*, incontinent subjects; *round symbols*, male; *square symbols*, female. (From Beersiek et al. 1979.)

its value should be less than 250 in a normal muscle.

In constructing measurements of fibre type predominance it is important to sample representative areas of muscle. This is most easily achieved by counting muscle fibres of Type 1 or Type 2 histochemical type at the microscope using a ×16 objective, and simply counting the numbers of fibres of each histochemical type in five microscope fields. By this means at least 200 muscle fibres of each type will be counted. In very abnormal muscles, where there has been substantial destruction of muscle tissue, it may not be possible to achieve counts of 200 fibres of each histochemical type and, in this case, *all* the fibres of each type present in the biopsy should be counted. Similarly, in measurements of fibre diameter, using the criterion of the lesser diameter based on a line bisecting the centre of the muscle fibre, as described above, it is similarly important to sample representative areas of the muscle, and to measure at least 100 fibres of each fibre type. This is more accurately achieved using a ×25 objective than with lower power objectives. An eyepiece micrometer can be used and, with practice, data can be acquired relatively rapidly.

A number of automated techniques are available for measurement of fibre diameter and many of these, utilizing desktop computers, also provide the facility for measuring fibre area. Many laboratories have developed their own programmes for use with such systems, and commercially available equipment is now widely available. However, because of variations in the histochemical reaction for myosin ATPase in sections of muscle, it is not appropriate to rely on automatically collected data; all fibres used for diameter measurements and for calculations of fibre type predominance should be checked by hand with regard to their histochemical fibre type. Further, it is not appropriate to use mitochondrial enzyme reactions such as NADH to characterize fibre types because of the wide variation and intensity of this reaction, which does not conform exactly to the fibre type characterization achieved by the myosin ATPase reaction (Dubowitz 1986; Swash and Schwartz 1985, 1988).

Much emphasis has been placed in diagnostic histopathology of muscle on counts of the numbers of fibres containing central nuclei. Generally, less than 4% of muscle fibres in the biopsy contain centrally-located sarcolemmal nuclei, and a tendency for this number to increase is a characteristic principally of myopathic disease.

An important characteristic of the histopathology of muscle in neuromuscular disease is the fundamental division between *primary myopathic* and *primary neurogenic* disorders. In the former, the disease process falls upon the muscle fibre resulting in a characteristic series of pathological changes in individual muscle fibres, principally consisting of degeneration and regeneration, suggesting the presence of a primary disease of the muscle fibres themselves (see Dubowitz 1986; Engel and Banker 1986; Swash and Schwartz 1988). In neurogenic disease, however, the primary pathological process involves the nerve supply to the muscle and the changes seen in the muscle fibres are secondary to rearrangement of the distribution of Type 1 and Type 2 fibres consequent upon the relative predominance of the effects of denervation, or of compensatory reinnervation, largely due to regrowth of axons by sprouting into the denervated segment of the muscle. This process results in a tendency for muscle fibres to become grouped together in clusters of fibres of similar histochemical type. Normally, there is a mosaic of Type 1 and Type 2 muscle fibres distributed in a random or pseudorandom fashion in the fascicles of the muscle. Thus it is uncommon for more than three muscle fibres of similar histochemical type to be oriented so that they are in contact with each other and within the muscle, provided that there is no predominance of one fibre type over the other. When one muscle fibre type is predominant there is clearly an increased probability that muscle fibres of similar histochemical type will be in juxtaposition so that the definition of "fibre type grouping" depends not only on the presence of neurogenic disease, but also on the relative degree of fibre type predominance. In muscles without fibre type predominance, fibre type grouping is recognized when 12 or more muscle fibres of similar histochemical type are in contact with each other and, generally, neuropathologists recognize the presence of fibre type grouping only when both Type 1 and Type 2 fibres show grouping. Thus, in a muscle consisting largely of Type 1 muscle fibres, as in the external anal sphincter or puborectalis muscles, fibre type grouping can be recognized only when there is grouping of Type 2 fibres.

In muscle biopsies the tissue examined consists not only of muscle fibres, but of blood vessels, fibrous connective tissue, fat, and small nerve fascicles or even motor end-plates. All these structures can be quantified using measurement techniques but, generally, there is little to be gained by exact quantification of changes in these tissues since qualitative assessment by a skilled pathologist is not only reliable, but can provide exact diagnostic information. Motor end-plates are seen only when the biopsy is taken from the motor point, that is the zone in the muscle containing the band of innervation. Quantification of changes in motor end-plates generally requires electron microscopy in order to evaluate the numbers of vesicles and the relative areas of the primary and secondary postsynaptic folds. Such measurements are not relevant to coloproctology. For light microscopy motor end-plates may be readily visualized with silver and acetylcholinesterase techniques but they can also be seen in HE preparations.

Smooth Muscle

The non-striated, involuntary smooth muscle of the longitudinal and circular layers of the rectum and of the internal anal sphincter consists of muscle cells joined together into a densely packed tissue. Individual muscle cells vary in their electron density and contain dark, electron-dense zones, but changes in these variables are not of functional or diagnostic significance. Individual smooth muscle cells are in close contact with each other through specialized zones of cell adhesion that allow electrical contact between individual muscle fibres, and that form zones of strong physical interconnection, important in the transmission of force from cell to cell. These zones are generally well preserved even when the muscle tissue is abnormal. Individual muscle cells are similarly joined by strands of elastic tissue, and are separated by fibrils of collagen. The elastic tissue may be stretched and damaged, particularly in the internal anal sphincter in patients with incontinence (Swash et al. 1988), and there is often an increase in fibrous connective tissue with an increase in the numbers of collagen fibrils, together with a loss of smooth muscle cells in incontinent patients. Changes in the myenteric plexus are, so far, poorly understood, consisting largely of reduction in the numbers of myenteric ganglia and of changes in neuronal morphology consisting of enlargement of neurones, relative loss of neurones, or a change in their impregnability with silver, using the Smith (1972) technique. Although these neurones are known to contain neuropeptides VIP, somatostatin and neuropeptide Y, little is known as to the quantitative aspects of the presence of these neuropeptides in disease states. In Hirschsprung's disease there is an absence of myenteric plexus and myenteric ganglia in the atonic segment and similar changes are found in patients with megacolon secondary to hollow visceral neuropathy (Anuras and Shirazi 1984; Schuffler et al. 1985). Primary myopathic disorders of the longitudinal muscle coat of the colon have also been described, in which vacuolated smooth muscle cells are found in the "sick" longitudinal muscle coat, but the circular muscle is relatively spared (Schuffler et al. 1981). It is believed that smooth muscle cells can readily be repaired, and can respond by hypertrophy or by atrophy to increased or reduced demands placed upon them in the gut, as in other tissues. Documentation of this change in the colorectum, however, is incomplete. The rectum and colon contain free nerve endings, probably representing sensory fibres derived from the parasympathetic nervous system. In the internal anal sphincter there is a sympathetic innervation that is in a close, but non-synaptic, relationship to individual smooth muscle cells.

Other Tissues

Sensory receptors in the anal epithelium have not been studied in disease states, although it is likely that they would show morphological changes in patients with neuropathy, whether generalized or localized, as in pudendal neuropathy, resembling those found in the skin in patients with neuropathies of nerves innervating other parts of the cutaneous sensory system. Changes in the mucosal morphology of the colon can be investigated by quantitative techniques involving measurement of the length of the mucosal folds, their density and their complexity. Line bisection or point counting techniques are applicable to this end (see Engel and Banker 1986). Muscle spindles are present in the pelvic floor muscles, including the puborectalis and external anal sphincter (Swash 1985a) but morphological changes in these stretch receptors have not been systematically investigated in relation to coloproctological disorders. The morphological characteristics of muscle spindles in myopathic disorder and in motor and sensory neuropathies have, however, been extensively investigated by Swash and colleagues (see Swash 1985b for review).

Striated Sphincter and Pelvic Floor Musculature

The levator ani consists of muscle fibres of a diameter comparable with that found in limb skeletal muscles. However, unlike the puborectalis and external anal sphincter muscles, the diameter of Type 1 fibres in the female levator ani is quite strikingly larger than Type 2 fibres (mean difference 20 micrometres) in women. The diameters of Type 1 and Type 2 muscle fibres in the external anal sphincter and puborectalis muscles are less than those of the lowermost fibres of the levator ani (Fig. 5.2). In investigations of the changes found in these muscles in anorectal incontinence it was found that hypertrophy in the remaining muscle fibres was far more marked in the puborectalis than in the external anal sphincter or levator ani muscles, but that the tendency for Type 2 fibres to be larger than Type 1 in both men and women in external anal sphincter and puborectalis muscles was maintained, whereas in the levator ani the Type 1 fibres were slightly larger than Type 2 fibres in incontinent women (Beersiek et al. 1979). In addition, striking changes consistent with chronic partial denervation and compensatory reinnervation were found in these muscles (Parks et al. 1977).

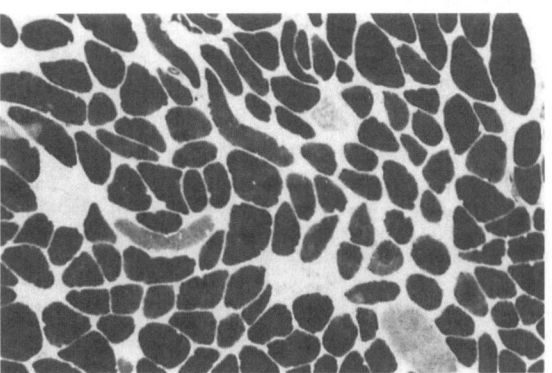

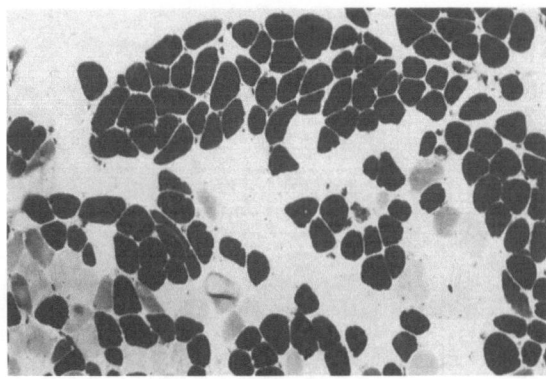

Fig. 5.2. a, b. External anal sphincter muscle. ATPase pH 4.6. Note the predominance of Type 1 muscle fibres, and the marked variations in fibre size.

Conclusions

Morphometric investigations of the tissues of the colon, rectum, anal canal and associated muscular and connective tissues can readily be carried out using established techniques. Investigations of changes in the innervation of the viscera, however, are in their infancy and relatively little is known about changes in the distribution of neurotransmitters in the neurones of the myenteric and submucosal plexuses. However, it is likely that changes in the state of the innervation of the colon and rectum are important in patients with slow transit constipation, Hirschsprung's disease, and in the primary visceral neuropathies and myopathies, with megarectum. The interaction of abnormalities in smooth muscle with the pelvic floor diaphragm and its voluntary sphincters remains incompletely understood, and detailed anatomical and pathological studies will be helpful in formulating appropriate questions.

References

Anuras S, Shirazi SS (1984) Colonic pseudo-obstruction. Am J Gastroenterol 79:525–532

Beersiek F, Parks AG, Swash M (1979) Pathogenesis of anorectal incontinence: a histometric study of the anal musculature. J Neurol Sci 42:111–127

Brooke MH, Engel WK (1969) The histographic analysis of human muscle biopsies with regard to fibre types. I. Adult male and female. Neurology 19:221–233

Dubowitz V (1986) Muscle biopsy: a practical approach, 2nd edn. Bailliere Tindall, London

Duthie HL, Gairns FW (1960) Sensory nerve endings in sensation in the anal region of man. Br J Surg 47:585–595

Engel AG, Banker BQ (1986) Basic reactions of muscle. In: Banker BQ, Engel AG (eds) Myology. McGraw-Hill, New York, pp 845–907

Langley JN (1921) In: The autonomic nervous system, part 1. Heffer, Cambridge

Parks AG, Swash M, Ulrich H (1977) Sphincter denervation in anorectal incontinence and rectal prolapse. Gut 18:656–665

Percy JP, Neill ME, Swash M, Parks AG (1981) Electrophysiological study of motor nerve supply of pelvic floor. Lancet i:16–17

Polgar J, Johnson MA, Weightman D, Appleton D (1973) Data on fibre size in 36 human muscles: an autopsy study. J Neurol Sci 19:307–318

Schuffler MD, Rohrmann CA, Schafee RG, Brand DL, Delaney JH, Young JH (1981) Chronic intestinal pseudo-obstruction: a report of 27 cases and review of the literature. Medicine (Baltimore) 60:173–196

Schuffler MD, Leon SH, Krishnamurthy S (1985) Intestinal psuedo-obstruction caused by a new form of visceral neuropathy: palliation by radical small bowel resection. Gastroenterology 89:1152–1156

Smith B (1972) In: Neuropathology of the alimentary tract. Edward Arnold, London

Snooks SJ, Swash M (1986) The innervation of the muscles of continence. Ann R Coll Surg Eng 68:45–49

Swash M (1985a) Histopathology of the pelvic floor muscles. In: Henry MM, Swash M (eds) Coloproctology and the pelvic floor: pathophysiology and management. Butterworth, London, pp 129–150

Swash M (1985b) Pathology of the muscle spindle. In: Mastaglia FM, Walton JN (eds) Skeletal muscle pathology. Churchill Livingstone, Edinburgh

Swash M, Schwartz MS (1985) In: Biopsy pathology of muscle. Chapman & Hall, London, p 206

Swash M, Schwartz MS (1988) In: Neuromuscular diseases: a practical approach to diagnosis and management, 2nd edn. Springer, Berlin Heidelberg New York

Swash M, Gray A, Lubowski DZ, Nicholls RJ (1988) Ultrastructural changes in internal anal sphincter in neurogenic faecal incontinence. Gut 29:1692–1698

COLOPROCTOLOGICAL DISORDERS

Before establishing the role of measuring functional parameters in abnormal states, it is important to understand fully the normal physiological functions of the large bowel, and how the structure of the organ itself allows these functions to be performed. There is no doubt that the physiology of the colon and anorectum are complex and probably not, as yet, completely understood. The first chapter in this section summarizes what is known in this area, to allow comparison with findings from investigation of the abnormal state, thus allowing the investigator to classify patients more accurately, and be better able to offer treatment options directed towards specific underlying aetiology.

Most clinicians with an interest in coloproctology, on scanning the list of disorders in the subsequent chapters, will recognize that the results of treatment of these conditions, whether medical or surgical, are unpredictable and, on the whole, generally poor. As it is likely that a complex series of events or physiological mechanisms contribute to these various abnormalities, it is essential to investigate these patients fully prior to commencing treatment. Improved detection of specific defects will allow better selection of patients for particular modes of therapy, and so should improve outcome in terms of relief of symptoms and duration of therapy. It must be emphasized that the following discussions relate to patients with relatively severe resistant problems with substantial implications for lifestyle, who are referred for specialist attention due to failure of conventional therapeutic approaches. An attempt is made in each chapter to relate the clinical usefulness of techniques already described to individual disorders and their influence on the clinical management of the patient.

6 · Physiological Mechanisms

D. Kumar

Introduction

The physiology of colonic function is less well understood than in other regions of the gastrointestinal tract. This is largely due to the relative inaccessibility of the colon in vivo, and the lack of a suitable animal model of the human colon. Colonic movements exhibit special features to serve a specific function. Firstly, the movements are organized to produce very slow flow which facilitates the extraction of water and electrolytes from the faecal mass. Secondly, the slow nature of colonic movements facilitates the growth of colonic microflora. In contrast, the contractions of the distal colon are designed to assist defaecation. It is now becoming increasingly clear that, although anatomically the colon is a single organ, in physiological terms the colon consists of three separate regions (right colon, left colon and the anorectum) which require precise coordination to produce normal function. Antiperistaltic contractions are predominant in the proximal colon, whereas slowly moving ring contractions directed aborally are more common in the distal colon.

Colonic Propulsive Activity

The colon shows two types of luminal flow patterns. The first is the movement of the contents of the single haustrum into the next and is known as individual haustral propulsion. The second is the coordinated contraction of multiple segments resulting in the spread of colonic contents over long distances. This is known as multihaustral propulsion (Richie 1971). A third type of colonic flow pattern has also been described (Holzknecht 1909; Hertz and Newton 1913). This comprises very fast moving and forceful contractions which propel colonic contents over long distances and is known as "mass movement" (Fig. 6.1). During a mass movement the colon loses its haustral pattern and is converted into a featureless tube. Colonic contents are then moved forward by a strong contraction wave. Mass movements are often accompanied by an urge to defaecate. This has now come to be recognized as one of the major propulsive forces in the colon (Holdstock et al. 1970).

During the passage of colonic contents from the right side to the left, water and electrolytes are absorbed, resulting in a firmer consistency of the contents as they arrive in the left colon. Due to the solid consistency of left colonic contents, individual haustral contractions are not very effective in propelling the contents forward. Moreover, there is no physiological need for gross movement of contents in this region unless there is a desire to defaecate. It is now believed that formed stool is stored in the left colon until there is an urge to defaecate.

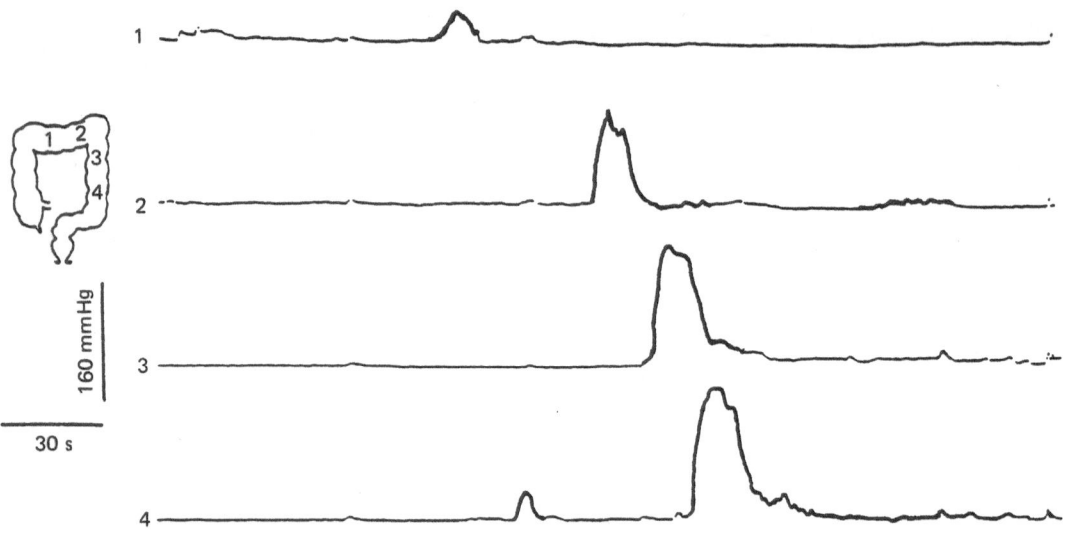

Fig. 6.1. Example of a high amplitude propagated contraction. It was associated with an urge to defaecate. (From Narducci et al. 1987, with permission.)

Control of Colonic Contractions

Myogenic Control

Smooth muscle of the colon generates two types of electrical signal: (a) the electrical slow wave and (b) the spike burst. The initiation of a contraction is thought to be accomplished by the spike bursts, whereas the slow waves are responsible for the integration of contractions (Christensen 1971). The slow waves occur at a constant frequency and contractions only occur in relationship to these slow waves. The spike bursts also occur at a fixed position in relationship to a slow wave producing an action potential. The slow waves appear to contain these action potentials to a fixed place in the muscular wall of the colon. The slow waves originate in the inner circular muscle layer of the colon (Caprilli and Onori 1972). In later studies it was noted that a spike burst was not a necessary electromyographic indication of contraction (Christensen et al. 1974). Another kind of spike burst was now identified, independent of slow waves and much more prolonged. This was called a long spike burst.

In humans, the slow waves show a much greater variation in frequency of slow waves ranging from 1–2/min to 10–20/min (Wankling et al. 1968). The pacemaker for the generation of electrical signals lies in the midcolon. Changes in slow wave frequency in man have been correlated with the diagnosis of irritable bowel syndrome (Snape et al. 1976; Sullivan et al. 1978).

Neurogenic Control

There are four different types of motor nerves in colonic muscle: excitatory nerves, which are cholinergic or non-cholinergic, and inhibitory nerves, which are adrenergic or non-adrenergic (Furness 1970). Most of the work on the regulation of colonic function has been done in experimental models, and due to the variability in colonic morphology among various species, the data have to be interpreted with caution, especially when extrapolating to the human colon. The parasympathetic outflow to the colon contains cholinergic excitatory neurones as well as non-cholinergic non-adrenergic inhibitory neurones (Jule 1975). The sympathetic flow to the proximal colon is via the splanchnic nerves, whereas the lumbar colonic nerves supply the distal colon (Jule and Gonella 1972). The spinal cord appears to be the source of tonic neural inhibition of the colon. This is evident in patients with lumber spinal cord lesions who have colonic hypermotility (Meshkinpour et al. 1983). There is also some evidence of a supraspinal centre having a facilitatory effect on the spinal inhibitory nerves. This is based on clinical observations that patients with a high spinal cord transection, with an intact cord below the lesion, have reduced colonic motility. As in other regions of the gut, the colonic nerves have been found to contain a variety of neurohormonal transmitters. In man the main colonic peptides of note include somatostatin, 5-hydroxytryptamine, substance P and vasoinhibitory peptide (Griffith and Burnstock 1983; Keast et al. 1984).

Colonic and Anorectal Reflexes

Peristaltic Reflex

Peristaltic reflex in the colon was first described by Bayliss and Starling in 1900. This was defined as excitation proximal to a pinch stimulus and inhibition distally. This work was later confirmed by Hukuhara and Miyaka (1959) and Jule in 1980 showed that distension of the rabbit proximal colon produces descending inhibition which was mediated by a serotonergic mechanism acting on the local cholinergic nerves. In clinical practice peristaltic reflex is seen in patients with intestinal obstruction. It is likely that the symptom of "absolute constipation" is due to the presence of this reflex.

Gastro-colic Reflex

Gastro-colic reflex signifies increased colonic activity following the ingestion of a meal. It is now recognized that this term is misleading because, firstly, the response is not specific to the presence of food in the stomach and, secondly, the response is not specific to the colon. The colon responds in a similar way to the presence of food in the small intestine and likewise the small intestine responds to the presence of food in the stomach. Moreover, it is not yet fully established that this response to food is solely mediated by extrinsic nerves (Christensen 1987).

Sampling Reflex

The term sampling reflex is used to describe relaxation of the anal canal in response to rises in rectal pressure. The concept was first put forward by Duthie and Bennett in 1963 when they plotted the distribution of the sensory area of the upper anal canal by pulling a pressure sensing unit through the sphincter. They found that the sensory zone was mainly confined to the high pressure zone, and with rises in intrarectal pressure there was shortening of the anal canal so that the sensory zone could come in direct contact with the rectal vault to facilitate sampling of rectal contents. These results were based on short-term recordings in the left lateral position; therefore only the effect of induced rectal distension on anal canal pressures could be monitored. Miller and colleagues in 1988 performed short-term ambulatory measurement of anorectal pressure and showed that sampling occurred spontaneously in 16 (89%) of their control patients. In nine of sixteen patients it occurred with no discernible increase in rectal pressure (Miller et al. 1988).

We have studied anorectal manometry continuously for 24 hours in 19 healthy ambulant subjects. Sampling reflex was observed in all subjects. There was a significant difference between the number of reflex episodes per hour during the day and during nocturnal sleep, as shown in Table 6.1. There was also a significant increase in the number of sampling reflex episodes after meals compared with the fasting state. These observations raised doubts about the possible explanation that relaxation in the upper anal canal is directly related to the sensory stimulus of rectal filling. It is likely that these transient relaxations in the upper anal canal (Fig. 6.2) are related to

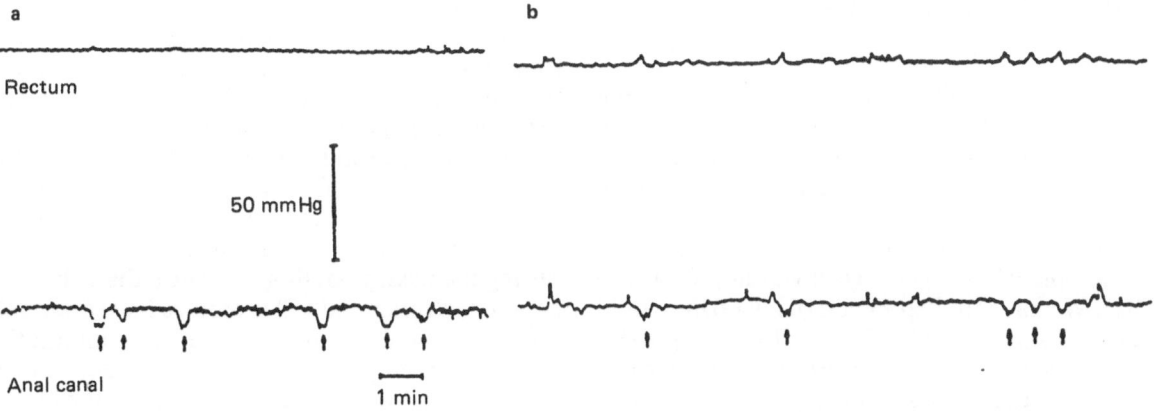

Fig. 6.2. Sampling reflex. **a** Spontaneous sampling (*arrows*) with no increase in rectal pressure. **b** Sampling associated with a rise in rectal pressure. (From Kumar et al. 1990, with permission.)

Table 6.1. Sampling reflex episodes (per hour)

Subjects	Awake (mean±SD)	Asleep (mean±SD)	Fasting (mean±SD)	Postprandial (mean±SD)
1	7.4±3.4	2.8±2.1	5.8±2.3	11.7±2.1
2	9.5±5.4	1.7±1.8	7.4±2.5	9.3±3.8
3	8.2±2.6	1.0±1.7	15.6±4.8	11.3±6.5
4	6.2±3.3	3.0±5.4	6.0±5.6	7.3±2.5
5	13.2±5.8	3.0±2.0	4.6±2.4	7.7±1.5
6	7.2±3.2	1.0±0.6	5.0±4.2	6.7±1.5
7	5.5±2.6	2.0±5.0	5.3±2.5	12.3±7.0
8	7.4±2.6	2.7±2.6	6.0±1.4	7.0±1.0
9	6.5±1.0	1.0±1.4	5.5±1.4	7.7±1.5
10	6.0±1.7	1.2±1.4	4.0±1.6	7.3±1.5
11	5.4±2.2	1.0±0.9		14.3±0.6
12	6.8±3.2	1.4±0.9	5.4±2.2	8.4±1.7
13	7.2±2.8	1.0±0.5	4.9±2.6	7.9±2.0
14	7.5±2.7	1.5±1.0	6.4±2.1	9.6±3.0
Mean±SEM	7.4±2.0	1.7±0.8[a]	6.3±2.9[b]	9.2±2.3[c]

[a] Asleep vs awake, $p<0.001$.
[b] Asleep vs fasting, $p<0.01$.
[c] Fasting vs postprandial, $p<0.01$.

contractile events in the rectosigmoid or proximal colon. This hypothesis is supported by the spontaneous occurrence of sampling in the absence of changes in rectal pressure (Miller et al. 1988). The decreased frequency of sampling episodes during sleep and an increase following meals suggests a central control.

Lubowski et al. (1987) studied the pathway of rectoanal reflex intra-operatively in three patients undergoing rectal excision and found that the reflex was present after presacral nerve blockade but was abolished by circumferential rectal myotomy. This suggests a local intramural pathway and supports the concept that in conditions like Hirschsprung's disease, the absence of this reflex is due to aganglionosis.

Vesicoanal Reflex

Urinary bladder filling in humans increases the EMG activity of the internal anal sphincter which returns to normal after voiding (Salducci et al. 1982). This reflex response is effectively mediated by the lumbar spinal cord via the hypogastric nerves, the inferior mesenteric ganglion and lumbar splanchnic nerves (Bouvier and Grimaud 1984). We have studied 21 acts of micturition in 14 subjects (Kumar et al. 1990). All these episodes were associated with an increase in anal canal pressure (range 10–23 mmHg) and increased EMG activity in the external anal sphincter (Fig. 6.3). This may simply reflect a continence mechan-

ism against raised intra-abdominal pressure during micturition. Alternatively this may be a protective rather than a reactive reflex response.

Passage of Flatus

Successful passage of flatus while maintaining continence is said to be achieved by a decrease in the anorectal angle, increases in the anal sphincter pressure and an increase in intrarectal pressure (Finlay et al. 1986). In an ambulant study of 14 healthy subjects we recorded 49 episodes of passage of flatus. In 35 of these episodes anal canal pressure increased (range 11–52 mmHg) in association with an action potential in the external anal sphincter (Fig. 6.4). In nine episodes there was transient relaxation in the anal canal pressure followed by contraction of the anal canal and external anal sphincter as shown in Table 6.2. In the remaining episodes the anal canal pressure and the external anal sphincter activity did not show any change. The inconsistency of this response perhaps represents a true physiological variation during the passage of flatus because the volume of gas passed varies and will therefore have a variable effect on anal canal pressure. An alternative explanation may be that the contractile event in the anal canal was a voluntary effort on the part of the subject; social circumstances may not have been appropriate for the release of flatus.

Rectum

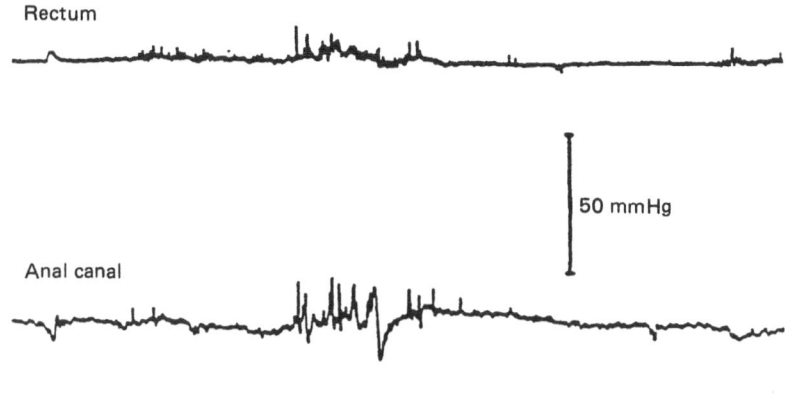

50 mmHg

Anal canal

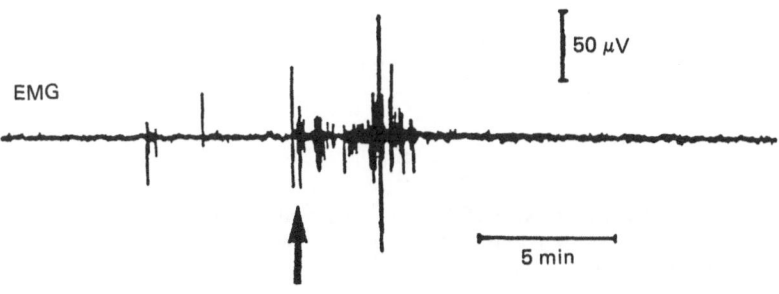

50 μV

EMG

5 min

Fig. 6.3. Pressure and EMG activity during micturition. Note the rise in anal canal pressure (*top trace*) and increased external sphincter activity (*lower trace*) during micturition. (From Kumar et al. 1990, with permission.)

Table 6.2. Changes in anorectal pressure and external sphincter EMG activity during passage of flatus

Number of episodes	Rectal pressure	Anal canal pressure	EMG
35	No change	Rise	Action potential
9	Rise	Relaxation followed by rise	Action potential
3	No change	No change	No change

Mechanism of Defaecation

Defaecation is a complex act under the influence of the central nervous system. The stimulus to the initiation of defaecation is rectal distension and excitation of anorectal mechanoreceptors (Garry 1933; Schuster et al. 1963; Scharli and Keisewetter 1970). There are two main components of the act of defaecation. The first is the rise in intra-abdominal pressure which is achieved by the contraction of the abdominal wall muscles, diaphragmatic descent, closure of the glottis and contraction of the pelvic floor muscles. The second component involves evacuation of the rectum which is achieved by relaxation of the anal sphincter complex, straightening of the anorectal angle and contraction of the rectal wall. The exact mechanism of integration of these complex movements is not known.

In addition to the central control, there is a spinal centre in the lumbosacral region of the spinal cord which can maintain reflex defaecation following transection of the spinal cord above this level.

Mechanism of Faecal Continence

Maintenance of faecal continence is a complex phenomenon which is mediated by local reflexes and is also subject to voluntary control. Certain factors such as anatomical integrity of the anal sphincter complex and the pelvic floor, coordination of the anal, rectal and pelvic floor musculature and the consistency of stool are important.

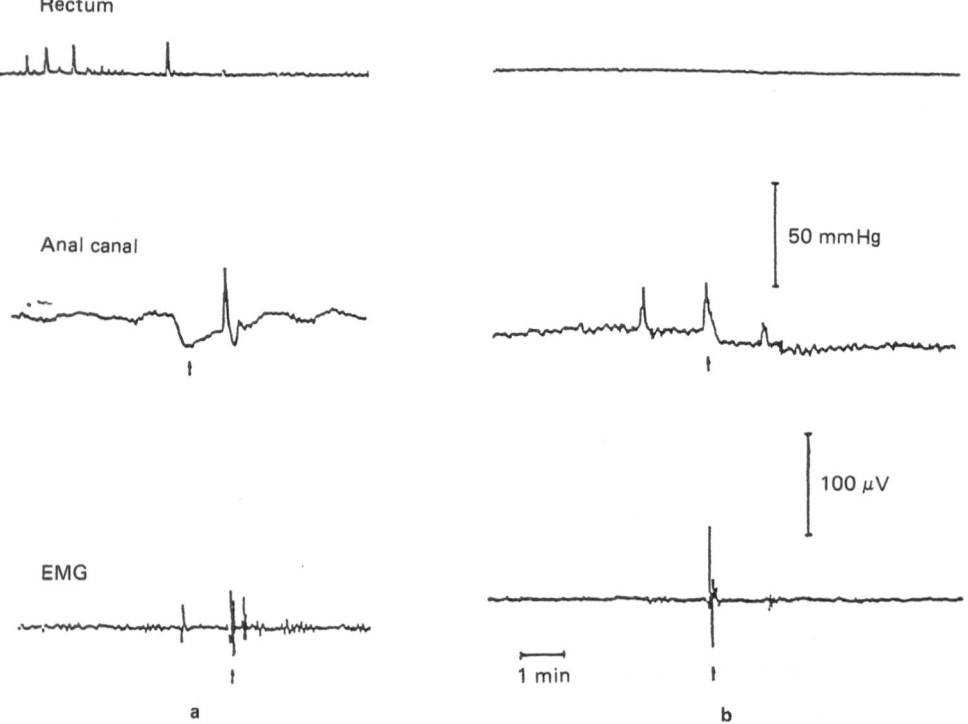

Fig. 6.4. Pressure and EMG activity during the passage of flatus. **a** Relaxation followed by contraction of the anal canal associated with an action potential in the external anal sphincter. **b** Contraction in the anal canal associated with action potential in the external sphincter. (From Kumar et al. 1990, with permission.)

Maintenance of faecal continence requires integration of internal and external sphincter function, maintenance of anorectal angle and an adequate sensory function. The internal anal sphincter contributes as much as 85% of the resting anal canal pressure (Bennett and Duthie 1964). The remaining 15% is due to activity of the external anal sphincter. These observations clearly suggest a role of the anal sphincter complex in the maintenance of continence. However it has been shown that division of the internal sphincter muscle alone only causes a minor functional abnormality (Bennett and Duthie 1964) and likewise division of the external anal sphincter causes minimal derangement of function (Milligan and Morgan 1934). The other contributory factor in maintaining faecal continence is the puborectalis muscle which is said to maintain the anorectal angle. In normal individuals this angle is in the order of 60–105° (Hardcastle and Parks 1970). It has been reported that whenever the anorectum becomes more obtuse it results in faecal incontinence. Phillips and Edwards (1965) put forward the theory of a flutter valve, postulating that intra-abdominal pressure was transmitted at the level of the levator ani to the lateral wall of the anal canal. The authors suggested that this mechanism keeps the two walls of the anal canal together whenever intra-abdominal pressure is raised.

However, this hypothesis does not take into account the activity of the puborectalis muscle. An alternative hypothesis of a flap valve was suggested by Parks et al. in 1966. This was based on a pressure differential between the intra-abdominal pressure and that of the anal canal. A rise in intra-abdominal pressure compresses the anterior rectal wall onto the upper anal canal thereby occluding its lumen.

Another contributor to the mechanism of faecal continence is anorectal sensation. The receptors responsible for the sensory function are probably located in the rectum and to some degree in the sigmoid colon (Gaston 1951; Schuster et al. 1963). Studies in normal humans have suggested that the reflex sensory pathways are mediated by the spinal cord.

References

Bayliss WM, Starling EH (1900) The movements and innervation of the large intestine. J Physiol (Lond) 26:107–118

Bennett RC, Duthie HL (1964) The functional importance of the internal sphincter. Br J Surg 51:355–357

Bouvier M, Grimaud JC (1984) Neuronally mediated interactions between urinary bladder and internal anal sphincter motility in the cat. J Physiol (Lond) 346:461–469

Caprilli R, Onori L (1972) Origin, transmission and ionic dependence of colonic electrical slow wave. Scand J Gastroenterol 7:65–74

Christensen J (1971) The controls of gastrointestinal movements: some old and new views. N Engl J Med 285:85–98

Christensen J (1987) Motility of the colon. In: Johnson LR (ed) Physiology of the gastrointestinal tract. Raven Press, New York, pp 665–693

Christensen J, Anuras S, Hauser RL (1974) Migrating spike bursts and electrical slow waves in the cat colon: effect of sectioning. Gastroenterology 66:240–247

Duthie HL, Bennett RC (1963) The relation of sensation in the anal canal to the functional anal sphincter. A possible factor in anal continence. Gut 4:179–182

Finlay IG, Carter K, McCleod I (1986) A comparison of intrarectal function of gas and mass on anorectal angle and anal canal pressure. Br J Surg 73:1025

Furness JB (1970) The origin and distribution of adrenergic nerve fibers in the guinea-pig colon. Histochemie 21:295–306

Garry RC (1933) The responses to stimulation of the caudal end of the large bowel in the cat. J Physiol (Lond) 78:208–224

Gaston EA (1951) Physiological basis for preservation of fecal continence after resection of rectum. JAMA 146:1486–1489

Griffith SG, Burnstock G (1983) Serotonergic neurons in human fetal intestines: an immuno-histochemical study. Gastroenterology 85:929–937

Hardcastle JD, Parks AG (1970) A study of anal incontinence and some principles of surgical treatment. Proc R Soc Med 63 (supp): 116–118

Hertz AF, Newton A (1913) The normal movements of the colon in man. J Physiol (Lond) 47:57–65

Holdstock DJ, Misiewicz JJ, Smith T, Rowlands EN (1970) Propulsion (mass movements) in the human colon and its relationship to meals and somatic activity. Gut 11:91–99

Holzknecht G (1909) Die normale Peristaltik des Kolon. Munch Med Wschr 56:2401–2403

Hukuhara T, Miyaka T (1959) The intrinsic reflexes in the colon. Jpn J Physiol 9:49–55

Jule Y (1975) Modification de l'activite electrique du colon proximal de lapin in vivo par stimulation des nerfs vagues et splanchniques. J Physiol (Paris) 70:5–26

Jule Y (1980) Nerve-mediated descending inhibition in the proximal colon of the rabbit. J Physiol (Lond) 309:487–498

Jule Y, Gonella J (1972) Modifications de l'activite electrique du colon terminal de lapin par stimulation des fibers nerveuses pel viennes et sympathiques. J Physiol (Paris) 64:599–621

Keast JR, Furness JB, Costa M (1984) Somatostatin in human enteric nerves. Distribution and characterization. Cell Tissue Res 237:299–308

Kumar D, Waldron D, Williams NS, Browning C, Hutton MRE, Wingate DL (1990) Prolonged anorectal manometry and external anal sphincter electromyography in ambulant human subjects. Dig Dis Sci 35:641–648

Lubowski DZ, Nicholls RJ, Swash M, Jordan MJ (1987) Neural control of internal anal sphincter function. Br J Surg 74:668–670

Meshkinpour H, Nowroozi F, Glick ME (1983) Colonic compliance in patients with spinal cord injury. Arch Phys Med Rehabil 64:111–112

Miller R, Bartolo DCC, Cervero F, Mortensen McC (1988) Anorectal sampling: a comparison of normal and incontinent patients. Br J Surg 75:44–47

Milligan ETC, Morgan CN (1934) Surgical anatomy of the anal canal with special reference to anorectal fistulae. Lancet ii:1150–1156

Narducci F, Bassotti G, Gaburri M, Mordli A (1987) Twenty four hour manometric recording of colonic motor activity in healthy man. Gut 28:17–25

Parks A, Porter NH, Hardcastle JD (1966) The syndrome of the descending perineum. Proc R Soc Med 59:477–482

Phillips SF, Edwards DAW (1965) Some aspects of anal continence and defaecation. Gut 6:396–405

Richie JA (1971) Movement of segmented constrictions in the human colon. Gut 12:350–355

Salducci J, Planche D, Nandy B (1982) Physiological role of the internal anal sphincter and the external anal sphincter during micturition. In: Wienbeck M (ed) Motility of the digestive tract. Raven Press, New York, pp 513–520

Scharli AF, Keisewetter WB (1970) Defaecation and continence: some new concepts. Dis Colon Rectum 13:81–107

Schuster MM, Hendrix TR, Mendeloff AI (1963) The internal anal sphincter response: manometric studies on its normal physiology, neural pathways and alteration in bowel disorders. J Clin Invest 42:196–207

Snape WJ Jr, Carlson GM, Cohen S (1976) Colonic myoelectric activity in the irritable bowel syndrome. Gastroenterology 70:326–330

Sullivan MA, Cohen S, Snap WJ Jr (1978) Colonic myoelectric activity in irritable-bowel syndrome. Effect of eating and anticholinergics. N Engl J Med 298:878–883

Wankling WJ, Brown BH, Collins CD, Duthie HL (1968) Basal electrical activity in the anal canal in man. Gut 9:457–460

7 · Constipation

D. J. Waldron

Introduction

Constipation can affect a significant percentage of the general population at any stage during life. In most sufferers a cause will be found (Table 7.1) and the vast majority will respond to dietary or specific therapy designed to correct the underlying cause. There is, however, a small group of patients who despite intensive investigations, often in multiple institutions over many years, continue to complain of severe constipation without any apparent cause. These patients, usually young to middle-aged females, are frequently tagged with the label of chronic idiopathic constipation (Pres-

Table 7.1. Causes of constipation

Physiological causes
Faulty diet
Pregnancy
Old age
Lack of exercise

Disorders of the large bowel
Anal fissure/stenosis
Colonic stricture (benign or malignant)
Aganglionosis (congenital or acquired)

Disorders outside the large bowel
Endocrine/metabolic (hypothyroid, hypercalcaemia, etc.)
Neurological (trauma to spinal cord and cauda equina, CNS disorders, sacral cord lesions)
Systemic sclerosis (connective tissue disorders)
Drug side effects (iron, aluminium antacids, anticholinergics, cough mixtures, purgative abuse, lead poisoning)
Psychological (depression, anorexia nervosa)

ton and Lennard-Jones 1986; Lancet Editorial 1986). They have been well categorized (Table 7.2) and as they pose most problems in management will be highlighted in this chapter. The tests used to investigate them have not all been proved to be of value. However, it is important that these patients are fully investigated, not only to exclude serious underlying conditions but also to select the mode of therapy most likely to be beneficial to them.

Table 7.2. Patient characteristics

History dating to childhood or adolescence
Bowel habit usually less than 1/week
Abdominal pain/distension prominent
Medications unhelpful (often worse with bran)
Symptoms dominate the patient's lifestyle
Association with pelvic operations
Barium enema usually normal

General Investigations

History and Physical Examination

A detailed history of duration of symptoms, degree and type of abdominal pain, associated abdominal bloating, consistency of stool, length of time spent straining at stool, frequency of bowel habit, episodes of faecal or mucus incontinence, necessity for digitation to achieve a bowel motion and a history of obstetric and pelvic operations are all necessary clues to the background of the patient's problem. Physical examination is generally unhelpful but obvious evidence of underlying disease must be sought. Patients with chronic severe constipation often have visible evidence of abdominal distension.

Dietary Assessment

In all patients a careful assessment of diet should be made preferably by a dietician. In particular, the dietary fibre content must be estimated.

Haematological and Biochemical Evaluation

Apart from the traditional baseline studies, glucose levels, thyroid function tests, serum calcium concentration and a urine test to exclude porphyria should be performed.

Radiological Assessment

A plain abdominal x-ray and barium enema should be performed in all patients. The degree of faecal loading and gaseous distension, with or without fluid levels, can best be assessed by simple erect and supine plain films. Underlying structural disease will commonly be seen on barium contrast studies although in functional disorders, barium studies are thought to be unhelpful (Varma et al. 1988; Patriquin et al. 1978).

Colonoscopy

Direct visualization of the large bowel by colonoscopy may be of greater value than barium contrast studies in the evaluation of patients with colonic disorders (Durdey et al. 1987).

EUA and Full Thickness Rectal Biopsy

In patients with chronic functional disorders an examination under anaesthesia allows a more thorough assessment of the anorectum than a physical examination in the clinic. A full thickness strip of rectal musculature and mucosa is necess-

ary to make a definitive histological diagnosis of Hirschsprung's disease and should be obtained in all difficult cases. In the less well-defined cases of aganglionosis or hypoganglionosis, immunohistochemical techniques are now available which can be diagnostic (Kluck et al. 1984).

Functional Assessment

Anorectal Manometry

Findings

In severe constipation, findings in different studies have been inconsistent (Table 7.3). In general, with occasional exceptions (Read et al. 1986), there is no evidence of weakness of either the internal or the external anal sphincters, as reflected in the maximum basal and maximum squeeze pressures. Some studies have demonstrated abnormalities in the recto-anal inhibitory response (Roe et al. 1988; Watier et al. 1983) but frequently control subjects can also have abnormal responses (Shouler and Keighley 1986). Increases in rectal compliance with associated inability to perceive small increases in rectal volume and pressure and to achieve a desire to defaecate at intrarectal volumes comparable to controls are more constant features in this group of patients (Table 7.4). Demonstration of the absence of a recto-anal inhibitory response has traditionally been considered diagnostic of Hirschsprung's disease but recent studies have cast doubt on its reliability (Yoshioka and Keighley 1987).

Clinical Implications

Anal hypertonia, either as a primary event or due to an absent recto-anal inhibitory response, could in theory account for difficulty in rectal evacuation. The results of various studies do not, however, support such an aetiology and while surgical division of the internal sphincter (lateral sphincterotomy or anorectal myectomy) has been performed with satisfactory short-term results (Martelli et al. 1978; Yoshioka and Keighley 1987), the overall impression is that this is of little therapeutic value. Lack of sensitivity in the rectum could be secondary to a chronically dilated flaccid rectum resulting from chronic faecal impaction. This,

Table 7.3. Anorectal manometry in chronic idiopathic constipation (1)

Author		Maximum basal pressure (cm H$_2$O)	Maximum squeeze pressure (cm H$_2$O)	Rectoanal inhibitory response
Read et al. (1986)	N	103±8	217±16	Normal
	C	74±10*	178±21	Normal
Shouler and Keighley (1986)	N	99±5.3	214±6	24% Abnormal
	C	99±5.7	196±12	36% Abnormal
Waldron et al. (1988)	N	109±13.8 (mmHg)		Normal
	C	111±32 (mmHg)		Normal
Roe et al. (1988)	N	85 (60–115)	158 (110–290)	Normal
	C	100 (55–135)	155 (90–270)	6% Abnormal
Varma and Smith (1988)	N	107±5.6	167±7	Normal
	C	101±4.6	159±8	Normal

N = controls; C = constipation.
* $p<0.05$.

Table 7.4. Anorectal manometry in chronic idiopathic constipation (2)

Author		Compliance	Initial rectal sensation (ml)	Defaecatory sensation (ml)
Shouler and Keighley (1986)	N	–	6.3±6.3	136±10.3
	C	–	5.6±5.9	269±21.2**
Waldron et al. (1988)	N	6.15±4.4	55±27.8	87.5±36.4
	C	7.19±4.4*	137±130*	180±162*
Roe et al. (1988)	N	5.1 (2.2–13.5)	68 (35–145)	–
	C	4.4 (1.8–19.5)	123 (35–325)	–
Varma and Smith (1988)	N	8.5±0.6	230±35	300±28
	C	14.4±1**	348±56	444±40**

N = controls; C = constipation.
* $p<0.05$; ** $p<0.01$.

however, is not borne out by the physiological tests discussed above. In a study of 355 patients undergoing rectal elasticity studies in Quebec, only 9.5% had manometric evidence of megarectum (Verburon et al. 1988). Similarly, chronically constipated patients generally do not have gross impaction of faeces in the rectum (Waldron et al. 1988). Patients with impaired rectal sensation would seem therefore to have an afferent neuropathy involving at least the rectum and possibly the more proximal colon.

Influence on Treatment

The demonstration of normal anal sphincter function in most of these patients highlights the importance of not dividing the sphincters in the hope of relieving an "outlet obstruction" due to a clinical impression of a failure of relaxation at this level. Such an operation is of even greater concern when the results of investigations of external sphincter function are reviewed (Table 7.3). There is a tendency towards lower squeeze pressures (reflecting deficient external sphincter function) in chronic constipation, possibly secondary to chronic straining. The internal sphincter

may thus be the important additional component in preventing mucus or faecal incontinence. Similarly, when colectomy is indicated in this group, patients should be warned that their sphincter muscle may be unable to cope with the inevitable loose bowel motions in the immediate postoperative period. Also, patients undergoing colonic resection for colonic inertia can be predicted to have a better outcome if their pre-operative rectal sensitivity is normal (Akervall et al. 1988).

Position of the Pelvic Floor

Findings

The position of the pelvic floor, which is related to the tone of the pelvic diaphragm and external sphincter muscles, can best be deduced by measurement of anorectal angles and the amount of perineal descent below the pubococcygeal line both at rest and during straining. The latter can be measured on a St Mark's perineometer (Henry et al. 1982) or on lateral x-ray visualization of the rectum during proctography (Skomorowska et al. 1988). Measurement of anorectal angles in con-

Table 7.5. Measurement of anorectal angles in chronic idiopathic constipation

Author		Anorectal angle (degrees) at rest	Anorectal angle (degrees) with sphincter contraction	Anorectal angle (degrees) during straining
Roe et al. (1988)	N	94 (78–102)	–	111 (80–130)
	C	95 (65–113)	–	108 (81–138)
Read et al. (1986)	N	88±3	–	115±7
	C	99±4*	–	110±6
Skomorowska et al. (1987)	N	108 (94–119)	–	–
	C	117 (100–134)	–	–
Shouler and Keighley (1986)	N	89±3.9	70±3.2	128±3.3
	C	90±2.7	78±2.9	111±4.4**

N = controls; C = constipation.
* $p<0.05$; ** $p<0.01$.

stipated patients have not shown any significant changes (Table 7.5) (Turnbull et al. 1988; Preston et al. 1984; Shouler and Keighley 1986) and similarly abnormal perineal descent has not been found to be a feature (Skomorowska et al. 1987). When these abnormalities are present they probably indicate the degree of straining employed by an individual patient over the course of many years. This leads to progressive weakening of the pelvic floor muscle secondary to the neuropathy associated with stretching of the pudendal nerve. It is therefore more likely a secondary effect of the symptoms rather than a primary cause.

Clinical Implications

An anorectal angle which remains closed during attempts at straining may indicate a non-relaxing puborectalis muscle (although ideally this should only be diagnosed on the basis of EMG recordings during defaecation). Marked descent of the pelvic floor during defaecation can be classified under the heading of the descending perineum syndrome, which is not an isolated syndrome but is associated with other related problems such as mucosal prolapse and rectal prolapse.

Influence on Treatment

An increased risk of incontinence following extensive colonic resection must be stressed to a patient in whom such surgery is contemplated in the presence of weak pelvic musculature. It is interesting to note that the prevention of pelvic floor displacement during defaecation does not necessarily result in therapeutic benefit to patients with difficulty in defaecation (Lesaffer 1989).

Dynamic Evacuation Studies

Findings

Patients with chronic constipation usually have difficulty in expelling rectal contents be they balloons (Preston et al. 1984), solid spheres (Bannister et al. 1986), fluid or simulated semisolid stool (Womack et al. 1985; Turnbull et al. 1988). The shape and size of an object can influence its evacuation; smaller objects are more difficult to defaecate. Some patients may have difficulty in emptying soft or liquid stool (Turnbull et al. 1986). The use of integrated dynamic proctography has demonstrated an inappropriate contraction of the puborectalis muscle at the point of maximum straining (Womack et al. 1985). This condition has been termed "anismus" due to its similarity to the spasm-induced vaginismus (Preston and Lennard-Jones 1985a). Internal prolapse or intussusception of the rectal wall during straining (Bartolo et al. 1985) and the presence of abnormally large rectocoeles (Turnbull et al. 1988; Womack et al. 1985) which may retain faeces have been demonstrated using these techniques.

Clinical Implications

The implications of anismus in chronic intractable constipation has received considerable attention in recent years. As the puborectalis muscle maintains the angulation between the anteriorly-projecting lower rectum and the posteriorly-directed anal canal, inappropriate contraction or lack of relaxation of this muscle prevents widening of the anorectal angle and so prevents spontaneous defaecation. Similarly, the presence of infolding of the rectal muscle walls, the head of such an indentation often progressing to the anorectal junction or anal canal, could act as an obstructing lesion during defaecation. A variation of this lesion – an anterior wall prolapse – can be compressed during defaecation and may be a factor in the development of the solitary rectal ulcer syndrome. A large rectocoele could allow misdirection of faeces anteriorly during defaecation and so prevent adequate pressure downwards. Whether these two conditions are of importance as a primary cause of constipation or are merely secondary features of chronic ineffectual straining at stool is unknown, but both can act as aggravating features and should be sought and perhaps treated in the absence of other pathology.

Influence on Treatment

In an effort to improve symptoms in a group of patients in whom management is often unsatisfactory, attempts have been directed towards reversing the effects of inappropriate puborectalis contraction during defaecation. Attempts surgically to divide the muscle, either posteriorly (Barnes et al. 1985) or laterally (Kamm et al. 1988a), have resulted in little improvement. However, a recent attempt to weaken the muscle by using a chemical toxin has produced more hopeful results on early follow-up (Hallan et al. 1988). The benefits obtained from surgical repair of rectal intussusceptions (Berman et al. 1985; Kuijpers and de Morree 1986) and of rectocoeles (Capps 1975; Sehapayak 1985) in chronic constipation do seem to have produced a significant level of success in relieving symptoms although this has not been a common experience (Roe et al. 1986).

Neurological Assessment of the Pelvic Floor

Findings

More detailed electromyographic studies, assessing the neurological reflexes which are necessary for the pelvic floor musculature to react to physiological stimuli, may provide some insight into chronic functional constipation. In this context Snooks et al. (1985) were able to demonstrate prolonged latency of the reflex produced by transcutaneous stimulation of the lower spine in more than 30% of patients with regard to conduction of

the stimulus to the external sphincter and in more than 50% to the puborectalis. The same authors demonstrated a prolonged pudendo-anal reflex in 43% of these patients, a finding later confirmed by Varma and Smith (1988). Varma and Smith's patients, however, did not show significant abnormality in the mean motor unit potential duration of the external anal sphincter, or in the sensory thresholds and stimulation strengths, suggesting a significant neurological abnormality situated centrally. From the same centre, elderly patients with chronic constipation were shown to have similar abnormalities, with 16% having an absent reflex (Varma et al. 1988).

Clinical Implications

The concept of chronic straining at stool with resultant traction injury to the pelvic floor nerves and subsequent deficits in neurological function (Kiff et al. 1984) is used by Snooks et al. (1985) to explain the prolonged latencies of the pudendo-anal reflex found in chronic constipation of young women, as most of their patients had evidence of abnormal perineal descent on straining. Not all these patients, however, had evidence of anal sphincter denervation. Varma and Smith's (1988) work strongly suggests a spinal cord origin for the neurological dysfunction in this group and it is of interest to note that 33% of their patients had an associated vertebral column dysraphism. The well-recognized associated urinary abnormalities in this group (Bannister et al. 1988) support a central rather than a peripheral neurological deficit.

Influence on Treatment

These findings may be the first indication of an underlying aetiology for this condition. It has been suspected for some time that the pelvic sacral outflow of nerves in these patients is compromised, so influencing the function of the pelvic floor muscles and, via the long colonic nerves, the motor function of the left colon (Devroede and Lamarche 1974). Investigation of the latter is obviously not practical in humans but their importance in colonic propulsion are well demonstrated in dogs. Perhaps further work in this area will provide definitive evidence of a localized spinal lesion which may be amenable to neurophysiological or stimulatory manipulation.

Large Bowel Transit Studies

Findings

The majority of colonic transit studies in constipation have been performed by using orally ingested inert markers or shapes with either a single radiograph at 4 days post ingestion or with daily x-rays. Approximately half of the patients with constipation will show evidence of slow colonic transit (Bannister et al. 1986; Roe et al. 1986). Those who have normal transit times may be shown to have pelvic outflow abnormalities or are eventually categorized as having irritable bowel syndrome (Preston and Lennard-Jones 1985b) or psychiatric overlay (Wald 1986). Occasionally it has been found that normal subjects also exhibit delayed transit times and delayed movement through the right side of the colon in the absence of any symptoms (Melkersson et al. 1983). While advancing age has been shown to have no effect on transit (Eastwood 1972; Varma et al. 1988), it has been demonstrated that elderly patients with constipation have predominantly distal rectosigmoid slowing (Varma et al. 1988); a feature also noted in patients with paraplegia with sacral nerve outflow damage who suffer from constipation (Menardo et al. 1987). Patients with pelvic floor dysfunction syndromes are frequently shown to have delay in colonic transit but this may be due to back pressure resulting from the distal obstruction, a feature supported by a study of segmental transit in these patients (Kuijpers et al. 1986). Constipation in childhood is also often associated with slow colonic transit, demonstrated by delayed passage of inert markers, but in contrast to adults with chronic constipation the problem can be frequently reversed by dietary and drug therapy (Cucchiara et al. 1984). More recently, intraluminal radio-isotopic markers have been used to monitor proximal colonic transit in response to surface acting stimulants demonstrating abnormalities in severe constipation (Kamm et al. 1988b). This study and others have also demonstrated delay in segmental transit in some patients who previously had normal studies using inert markers (Lanfranchi et al. 1984).

Clinical Implications

Accurate definition of slow colonic transit is desirable to categorize patients with constipation. Inert marker studies have generally proved satisfactory and the definition of slow transit provided by Hinton et al. (1969) is still generally accepted as the criterion of abnormally slow colonic transit. More recent attempts to define abnormalities of segmental colonic transit have had some success (Arhan et al. 1981) but in clinical practice it may be unacceptable due to the radiation exposure involved in daily x-rays. If a single x-ray exposure is used, segmental colonic transit measurements may not be reproducible (Waldron et al. 1989a) and therefore can be unreliable in selection of patients for surgical therapy directed towards an individual colonic segment. The more recently developed scintigraphic studies of colonic transit (Krevsky et al. 1986) seem more promising in defining segmental transit while avoiding excessive radiation exposure of the patient.

Influence on Treatment

Constipated patients with colonic inertia will probably not respond favourably to correction of distal pelvic floor abnormalities. Those patients with abnormalities of colonic transit respond poorly to traditional oral pharmaceutical preparations. However, some early reports suggest that newer prokinetic agents such as Cisapride may be of benefit (Krevsky et al. 1988). In the absence of a response to medical treatment subtotal colectomy is an option in patients with prolonged severe symptoms. This procedure should only be offered to patients with evidence of slow transit and while outcome in the short term is satisfactory, future attempts to define segmental defects may allow for less extensive surgery in selected cases.

Intraluminal Manometric Studies

Findings

Early studies using perfused tubes to measure rectosigmoid motility in constipation suggested that diminished transit in these patients may be associated with hypersegmentation and increased intraluminal pressure (Connell et al. 1965). Indeed, an aetiology based on a functional obstruction at the rectosigmoid level was advanced (Chowdhury et al. 1976). While subsequent studies have not upheld this theory it would seem to be present in some patients (Meunier 1986). More definite motor abnormalities have been seen in the rectosigmoid to external stimuli such as feeding (Schang and Devroede 1983) and stimulant drugs such as bisacodyl (Preston and

Lennard-Jones 1985b). Attempts to study the whole colon with intraluminal manometric assemblies are rarely reported due to problems with accessibility and accurate positioning of the pressure monitoring ports during the period of study. The best results have been obtained by the use of tubes passed orally which traverse the length of the intestine and are anchored at the anal canal (Kerlin et al. 1983). Such studies in normal subjects suggest that there is considerable individual variation from day to day. More recently it has been possible to measure intraluminal pressure activity in the distal large bowel of constipated subjects using a totally ambulant system of recording, so allowing recordings to be made over a prolonged period and in a more physiological, unstressed environment during the course of a 24-hour period (Kumar et al. 1989a). Abnormalities of rectal motor function have been identified in constipated patients using this technique (Waldron et al. 1990).

Clinical Implications

Abnormalities of motility are not as yet adequately understood to have direct clinical implications. However, the suggestion that hypersegmentation occurs in some patients may indicate that overactivity of mixing contractions of the colon rather than the commonly supposed inactivity may be a cause of constipation. This abnormality is thought to account for the symptomatology of patients with irritable bowel syndrome who suffer from constipation (Preston and Lennard-Jones 1985b). Studies showing diminished propulsive activity, however, are more likely to represent the real abnormality in chronic idiopathic constipation. This latter finding would suggest a role for the use of drugs which induce peristalsis, but most of these patients have had a poor response to such therapy. As peristaltic activity is thought to be dependent on an intact intramural nerve plexus, this lack of response may not be surprising in view of the fact that nerve plexus abnormalities have now been documented in tissue obtained at colectomy.

Influence of Treatment

Disordered motility in the colon may respond to drugs which correct such states in other areas of the gut. Cisapride is a new prokinetic drug which has shown some promise in chronic constipation (Muller-Lissner et al. 1987) and has been shown to reverse manometric abnormalities in the stomach and improve symptoms in some small bowel motility disturbances. However, the lack of response to a multiplicity of laxative agents, the demonstration of impaired propagative activity and histological evidence of damaged intramural nerve plexus suggest that drug therapy is unlikely to be effective in this condition. Therefore, when symptoms are severe and abnormalities are confined to the colon, surgical resection of the malfunctioning colon may be the only valid treatment option.

Colonic Electromyographic Studies

Findings

Extensive work has now been reported on EMG characteristics of the upper gastrointestinal tract and its relationship to normal and abnormal physiological events. These correlations become less obvious as one proceeds down the intestine. Abnormal excessive electrical activity in the small intestine is typically· seen in the presence of pseudo-obstruction syndromes (Sullivan et al. 1977). Investigation of EMG activity in the colon, however, is more difficult in man and most data have been obtained from animal experiments. Analysis of the complex recordings from the colon, as compared with the stomach, is also a problem. Initial work in humans demonstrated the presence of spiking and later slow wave activity in the sigmoid colon (Couturier et al. 1969). The spiking activity, associated with muscular contractions, has been further subdivided into short spike-bursts (SSB), which are not propagative and last for less than five seconds, and long spike-bursts (LSB) which have a duration longer than ten seconds, and are seen to propagate in an orad or aboral direction (Bueno et al. 1988). In constipated subjects with irritable bowel syndrome the former are seen to be much increased (Bueno et al. 1980a). In dogs with diet induced constipation, a similar increase in SSBs was also seen but in conjunction with a decrease in LSBs (Bueno et al. 1988). In contrast, patients with diarrhoea exhibit a reduction or complete absence of SSBs (Bueno et al. 1980b).

Clinical Implications

Short spike-bursts are most likely to be associated with the segmenting type movements of the colonic muscle wall particularly seen in the proximal colon. An increase in such activity, as has been previously documented by Connell et al. (1965), can be associated with constipation as it tends to cause excessive mixing as opposed to progression of content. Added to this, a decrease in the propagative type of contraction, probably represented by the LSB, would further lead to stagnation of content. Obviously further work needs to be done to define the role of motor abnormalities in the pathophysiology of chronic constipation.

Influence on Treatment

As yet this type of investigation plays little role in the management of patients with chronic constipation. Possibilities beckon in the area of selection for various methods of treatment such as specific laxative therapy in the presence of lack of propulsive activity or, failing this, surgical resection of specific areas of the colon showing this type of abnormality.

Upper Gastrointestinal Assessment

Findings

Chronic constipation is generally regarded as a disorder of the large bowel. Patients with the irritable bowel syndrome, while tending to have slightly prolonged total gut transit time, are not significantly different from controls (Cann et al. 1983). Oesophageal motor dysfunction has been reported in patients with chronic idiopathic constipation (Watier et al. 1983; Reynolds et al. 1987). Similarly, prolonged small intestinal transit has been documented in the majority of subjects with chronic idiopathic constipation (Howard et al. 1985; Bannister et al. 1986). While it is possible that slowing of small intestinal transit may be secondary to an impacted colon, reduced transit is not improved by disimpacting the colon by colonic irrigation (Bannister et al. 1986). Equally, while there are distinct abnormalities in small intestinal motor function in chronic idiopathic intestinal pseudo-obstruction (Stanghellini et al. 1987), where constipation can be part of the symptom complex, a recent review of motility disturbances of the gut in the pathogenesis of constipation suggested that "no typical motor alterations of the upper gut are associated with constipation" (Bueno et al. 1988). Recent work (Kumar et al.

1989b), however, shows that there are indeed motility disturbances evident in the small intestine in patients with chronic idiopathic constipation when studied using a prolonged ambulant method of recording.

Clinical Implications

The detection of abnormalities in oesophageal, gastric or small intestinal function in patients presenting with chronic severe constipation implies that the individual patient may have a generalized disorder of gastrointestinal activity and therapy directed at improving colonic function alone is unlikely to be successful. Not all patients will necessarily show such generalized dysfunction and it is becoming increasingly apparent that, in centres with a special interest in coloproctology, tests of upper bowel function should be performed as part of routine assessment. It is conceivable that such patients constitute a subgroup of chronic idiopathic pseudo-obstruction or perhaps are suffering from an underlying systemic autonomic neuropathy (Waldron et al. 1989b).

Influence on Treatment

The concept of small intestinal malfunction contributing to the symptoms of chronic constipation has not had a major influence on therapy as yet. If this condition is indeed a diffuse disorder of gut motility in some patients, it may explain the relative resistance of certain patients to drug or surgical therapy.

Histological Studies

Findings

Definite histological abnormalities have been described and are considered diagnostic of certain conditions associated with constipation, particularly the absence of ganglion cells in either congenital (Hirschsprung's disease) or acquired (Chagas' disease) aganglionosis. It is in the less well defined chronic functional constipation syndromes that, until recently, histological assessment of colonic tissue has been generally unhelpful as routine H&E stains have not shown any obvious abnormality. The concept of laxative-induced damage to the intrinsic nerve plexus (Smith 1968) in patients with long-standing constipation is plausible but recent improvements in histopathological techniques have suggested that this is not the case (Smith et al. 1977; Schuffler and Jonak 1982). Krishnamurthy et al. (1985), using silver staining of colectomy specimens, showed abnormal morphology and reduced numbers of argyrophilic neurones, decreased numbers of axons and increased numbers of variably sized nuclei within ganglia in the majority of specimens, all of which were considered to be histologically normal colons, using conventional stains. These changes were not seen in a control group and were felt not to be laxative induced, as the history of laxative abuse did not correlate with the pathology and the destructive changes associated with laxative damage were not evident. A previous report (Gilbert et al. 1984) also documented abnormal pathology in colectomy specimens in three cases which were considered normal using H&E stains. Further evidence against a laxative abuse origin comes from a study relating the incidence of melanosis coli to the pattern of colonic transit (Badiali et al. 1985). While the presence of melanosis coli bore a definite relationship to those patients using laxatives regularly, it was not a sensitive marker of impaired transit. An additional technical improvement, immunohistochemical staining using monoclonal antibodies against neurofilaments, allows for even greater accuracy in detecting abnormalities in the colons of patients with this condition. Kluck and his colleagues (Kluck et al. 1984) reported that those few patients with residual complaints following a definitive operation for Hirschsprung's disease could be shown to have abormal innervation in the retained proximal bowel, which was previously shown to be normal on routine H&E staining. This was in contrast to those who obtained complete recovery following surgery. In a later study, this staining technique was used in a group with chronic idiopathic constipation and a lack of axonal staining was detected in the intramural plexus (Kluck et al. 1987). From the authors' previous work it was possible to deduce that this indicated a disturbance in the extrinsic nerve network. Immunohistochemical techniques were also used (Kock et al. 1988) to determine the concentration and localization of specific neuropeptides in descending colon tissue from controls and patients with chronic constipation. These techniques demonstrated significantly reduced levels of VIP in constipated colons. This substance is considered to be a non-cholinergic, non-adrenergic inhibitory neurotransmitter in the colon, suggesting that an overactivity of the circular muscle may have a role in the constipating process.

Clinical Implications

The histological abnormalities described using silver staining techniques have implications in the pathophysiology of chronic idiopathic constipation. These changes are similar to those previously described in colonic tissue following section of the pelvic nerves of humans and animals (Devroede and Lamarche 1974) and following traumatic damage to the lower spinal cord (Devroede et al. 1979). Taken in conjunction with Kluck's work showing nonstaining of extrinsic nerve axons in the wall of the affected colon (Kluck et al. 1987), this strongly suggests that chronic functional constipation is a result of pathology originating in the lower spine or pelvic nerves. Functionally, these findings are supported by evidence of diminished acetylcholine release as a result of electrical field stimulation in in vitro specimens of constipated colonic muscle wall (Burleigh 1988). It is possible that the abnormal neurological innervation affects the control of inhibitory neuropeptide release, therefore allowing circular muscle overactivity with resultant constipation.

Influence on Treatment

Coupled with an earlier reference to pelvic nerve function and lower spinal cord lesions (Varma and Smith 1988), the histological data support the need for a thorough investigation of the lumbosacral cord in the initial examination of patients with constipation. Anti-neurofilament antibody studies may be used both in proven cases of Hirschsprung's disease to exclude proximal abnormality and in difficult conditions such as severe constipation of young women. Prevention of problems by the avoidance of prolonged labour in obstetric practice and extreme caution relating to potential pelvic nerve trauma during low pelvic operations such as hysterectomy may lead to a lesser incidence of these disorders.

Conclusion

The severity of symptoms relating to chronic intractable constipation dictates that all efforts must be made to both define an aetiological factor, where possible, and provide partial, if not complete, relief of symptoms. Having excluded underlying structural disease and well-recognized neurological and endocrine disorders, there are now considerable therapeutic advantages to be gained from referring a patient to a specialized unit where there is now available a considerable armamentarium of functional studies which can help to clarify the problems responsible for this distressing disorder. Perhaps more importantly, these tests can allow selection of patients from this heterogeneous group to appropriate treatment regimens. At a time when surgical resection of the whole malfunctioning colon is frequently being offered as the only method of alleviating symptoms in a disorder where the extent and aetiology of the disease is uncertain, it is mandatory that patients should have reached a stage where medical and dietary treatment have been fully exhausted, symptoms are severe enough to interfere substantially with quality of life and isolated outlet obstruction syndrome has been excluded. All patients considered for surgery should also have small bowel motility measured and have a full explanation of the potential postoperative functional difficulties and the risk of failure and recurrence of their original symptoms.

References

Akervall S, Fasth S, Nordgren S, Dresland T, Hulten L (1988) The functional results after colectomy and ileo-rectal anastomosis for severe constipation (Arbuthnot-Lane's Disease) as related to rectal sensory function. Int J Colorect Dis 3:96–101

Arhan P, Devroede G, Jehannin B et al. (1981) Segmental colonic transit time. Dis Colon Rectum 24:625–629

Badiali D, Marheggiano A, Pallone F (1985) Melanosis of the rectum in patients with chronic constipation. Dis Colon Rectum 28:241–245

Bannister JJ, Timms JM, Barfield L, Read NW (1986) Physiological studies in young women with chronic constipation. Int J Colorect Dis 1:175–182

Bannister JJ, Lawrence WT, Smith A, Thomas DG, Read NW (1988) Urological abormalities in young women with severe constipation. Gut 29:17–20

Barnes PRH, Hawley PR, Preston DM, Lennard-Jones JE (1985) Experience of posterior division of the puborectalis muscle in the management of chronic constipation. Br J Surg 72:475–477

Bartolo DCC, Roe AM, Virjee J, Mortensen NJ McC (1985) Evacuation proctography in obstructed defaecation and rectal intussusception. Br J Surg (supp) S111–116

Berman IR, Manning DM, Dudley-Wright K (1985) Anatomic specificity in the diagnosis and treatment of internal rectal prolapse. Dis Colon Rectum 28:816–826

Bueno L, Fioramonti J, Ruckebusch Y, Frexinos J, Coulom P (1980a) Evaluation of colonic myoelectrical activity in health and functional disorders. Gut 21:480–485

Bueno L, Fioramonti J, Frexinos J, Ruckerbusch Y (1980b) Colonic myoelectrical activity in diarrhoea and constipation. Hepatogastroenterology 27:281–289

Bueno L, Frexinos J, Fioramonti J (1988) Role of motility in pathogenesis of constipation and diarrhoea. Pharmacology 36 (supp): 15–22

Burleigh DE (1988) Evidence for a functional cholinergic deficit in human colonic tissue resected for constipation. J Pharm Pharmacol 40:55–57

Cann PA, Read NW, Brown C, Hobson N, Holdsworth CD (1983) The irritable bowel syndrome (IBS), relationship of disorders in the transit of a single solid meal to symptom patterns. Gut 24:405–411

Capps WF Jr (1975) Rectoplasty and perineoplasty for the symptomatic rectocele: a report of fifty cases. Dis Colon Rectum 18:237–243

Chowdhury AR, Dinoso VP, Lorber SH (1976) Characterisation of a hyperactive segment at the rectosigmoid junction. Gastroenterology 71:584–588

Connell AM, Avery-Jones F, Rowlands EN (1965) Motility of the pelvic colon. Part IV. Abdominal pain associated with colonic hypermotility after meals. Gut 6:105–112

Couturier C, Roze C, Couturier-Turpin MH, Debray C (1969) Electromyography of the colon in situ. An experimental study in man and in the rabbit. Gastroenterology 56:317–322

Cucchiara S, Coremans G, Staiano A et al. (1984) Gastrointestinal transit time and anorectal manometry in children with faecal soiling. J Ped Gastroenterol Nutr 3:545–550

Devroede G, Lamarche J (1974) Functional importance of extraparasympathetic innervation to the distal colon and rectum in man. Gastroenterology 66:273–280

Devroede G, Arhan P, Duguay C, Tetreault L, Akoury M, Percy B (1979) Traumatic constipation. Gastroenterology 77:1258–1267

Durdey P, Weston PM, Williams NS (1987) Colonoscopy or barium enema as initial investigation of colonic disease. Lancet ii:549–551

Eastwood MD (1972) Bowel transit studies in the elderly: radiopaque markers in the investigation of constipation. Gerontol Clin 14:154–159

Editorial (1986) Constipation in young women. Lancet i:778–779

Gilbert KP, Lewis G, Billingham RP, Sanderson E (1984) Surgical treatment of constipation. West Med J 140:569–572

Hallan RI, Williams NS, Melling J, Waldron DJ, Womack NR, Morrison JFB (1988) Treatment of anismus in intractable constipation with botulinum-A toxin. Lancet ii:714–717

Henry MM, Parks AG, Swash M (1982) The pelvic floor musculature in the descending perineum syndrome. Br J Surg 69:470–72

Hinton JM, Lennard-Jones JE, Young AC (1969) A new method for studying gut transit times using radiopaque markers. Gut 10:842–847

Howard RJ, Davis RH, Clench MH, Mathias JR (1985) Subtotal colectomy as a therapeutic consideration in patients with chronic obstipation refractory to medical therapy. Gastroenterology 88:1423

Kamm MA, Hawley PR, Lennard-Jones JE (1988a) Lateral division of the puborectalis muscle in the management of severe constipation. Br J Surg 75:661–663

Kamm MA, Hawley PR, Lennard-Jones JE et al. (1988b) Dynamic scanning defines a colonic defect in severe idiopathic constipation. Gut 29:1085–1092

Kerlin P, Zinsmeister A, Phillips S (1983) Motor responses to food of the ileum, proximal colon and distal colon of healthy humans. Gastroenterology 84:762–770

Kiff ES, Barnes PRM, Swash M (1984) Evidence of pudendal neuropathy in patients with perineal descent and chronic straining at stool. Gut 11:1279–1284

Kluck P, Van Muijen GNP, Van der Kamp AWM et al. (1984) Diagnosis of Hirschsprung's disease with monoclonal anti-neurofilament antibodies on tissue sections. Lancet i:652–653

Kluck P, ten Kate FWJ, Schouten WR et al. (1987) Efficacy of antibody NF2F11 staining in the investigation of severe long-standing constipation. Gastroenterology 93:872–875

Kock TR, Carney JA, Go L, Go VLW (1988) Idiopathic chronic constipation is associated with decreased colonic vasoactive intestinal polypeptide. Gastroenterology 94:300–310

Krevsky B, Malmud LS, D'Ercole F, Maurer AH, Fisher RS (1986) Colonic transit scintigraphy. A physiological approach to the quantitative measurement of colonic transit in humans. Gastroenterology 91:1102–1112

Krevsky B, Malmud LS, Maurer AH, Siegel JA, Fisher RS (1988) Cisapride accelerates colonic transit in constipated patients with colonic inertia. Gastroenterology 94:A293

Krishnamurthy S, Schuffler MD, Rohrmann CA, Pope CE (1985) Severe idiopathic constipation is associated with a distinctive abnormality of the colonic myenteric plexus. Gastroenterology 88:26–34

Kuijpers HC, de Morree H (1986) Intussusceptie van het rectum: fantasie of werkelijkheid? Med Tijdschr Genfsskd 130:590–592

Kuijpers HC, Bleijenberg G, de Morree H (1986) The spastic pelvic floor syndrome. Large bowel outlet obstruction caused by pelvic floor dysfunction: a radiological study. Int J Colorect Dis 1:44–48

Kumar D, Williams NS, Waldron DJ, Wingate DL (1989a) Prolonged manometric recording of anorectal motor activity in ambulant human subjects: evidence of periodic activity. Gut 30:1007–1011

Kumar D, Waldron D, Williams NS, Wingate DL (1989b) Slow transit constipation: a pan-enteric motor disorder? Gastroenterology 96:A277

Lanfranchi GA, Bazzocchi G, Brignola C, Campieri M, Labo G (1984) Different patterns of intestinal transit time and anorectal motility in painful and painless chronic constipation. Gut 25:1352–1357

Lesaffer L (1989) Pelvic floor support in constipation. Lancet i:674

Martelli H, Devroede G, Arhan P, Duguay C (1978) Mechanisms of idiopathic constipation: outlet obstruction. Gastroenterology 75:623–631

Melkersson M, Andersson H, Bosaeus I, Falkheden T (1983) Intestinal transit in constipated and non-constipated geriatric patients. Scand J Gastroenterol 18:593–597

Menardo G, Bausano G, Corazziari E et al. (1987) Large bowel transit in paraplegic patients. Dis Colon Rectum 30:924–928

Meunier P (1986) Physiological study of the terminal digestive tract in chronic painful constipation. Gut 27:1018–1024

Muller-Lissner SA and the Bavarian constipation group (1987) Treatment of chronic constipation with Cisapride and placebo. Gut 28:1033–1038

Patriquin H, Martelli H, Devroede G (1978) Barium enema in chronic constipation: is it meaningful. Gastroenterology 75:619–622

Preston DM, Lennard-Jones JE (1985a) Anismus in chronic constipation. Dig Dis Sci 30:413–418

Preston DM, Lennard-Jones JE (1985b) Pelvic motility and response to intraluminal bisacodyl in slow transit constipation. Dig Dis Sci 30:289–294

Preston DM, Lennard-Jones JE (1986) Severe chronic constipation of young women: 'idiopathic slow transit constipation'. Gut 27: 41–48

Preston DM, Lennard-Jones JE, Thomas BM (1984) The balloon proctogram. Br J Surg 71:29–32

Read NW, Timms JM, Barfield LJ, Donnelly TC, Bannister JJ (1986) Impairment of defaecation in young women with severe constipation. Gastroenterology 90:53–60

Reynolds JC, Ouyang A, Lee CA, Baker L, Sunshine AG, Cohen S (1987) Chronic severe constipation. Prospective motility studies in 25 consecutive patients. Gastroenterology 92:414–420

Roe AM, Bartolo DCC, Mortensen NJMcC (1986) Diagnosis and surgical management of intractable constipation. Br J Surg 73:854–861

Roe AM, Bartolo DCC, Mortensen NJMcC (1988) Slow transit constipation. Comparison between patients with or without previous hysterectomy. Dig Dis Sci 33:1159–1163

Schang JC, Devroede G (1983) Fasting and postprandial myoelectric spiking activity in the human sigmoid colon. Gastroenterology 85:1048–1053

Schuffler MD, Jonak Z (1982) Chronic idiopathic intestinal pseudoobstruction caused by a degenerative disorder of the myenteric plexus: the use of Smith's method to define the neuropathology. Gastroenterology 82:476–486

Sehapayak (1985) Transrectal repair of rectocele: an extended armamentarium of colorectal surgeons. A report of 355 patients. Dis Colon Rectum 28:422–433

Shouler P, Keighley MR (1986) Changes in colorectal function in severe idiopathic chronic constipation. Gastroenterology 90:414–420

Skomorowska E, Henrichsen S, Christiansen J, Hegedus V (1987) Videodefaecography combined with measurement of the anorectal angle and of perineal descent. AcTA Radiol 28:559–562

Skomorowska E, Hegedus V, Christiansen J (1988) Evaluation of perineal descent by defaecography. Int J Colorect Dis 3:191–194

Smith B (1968) Effect of irritant purgatives on the myenteric plexus in man and the mouse. Gut 9:139–143

Smith B, Grace RH, Todd IP (1977) Organic constipation in adults. Br J Surg 64:313–314

Snooks SJ, Barnes PRH, Swash M, Henry MM (1985) Damage to the innervation of the pelvic floor musculature in chronic constipation. Gastroenterology 89:977–981

Stanghellini V, Camilleri M, Malagelada JR (1987) Chronic idiopathic intestinal pseudo-obstruction: clinical and intestinal manometric finding. Gut 28:5–12

Sullivan MA, Snape WJ, Matarazzo SA, Petrokubi RJ, Jeffries G, Cohen S (1977) Gastrointestinal myoelectrical activity in idiopathic intestinal pseudoobstruction. N Engl J Med 297:233–238

Turnbull GK, Lennard-Jones JE, Bartram CI (1986) Failure of rectal expulsion as a cause of constipation: why fibre and laxatives sometimes fail. Lancet i:767–769

Turnbull GK, Bartram CI, Lennard-Jones JE (1988) Radiological studies of rectal evacuation in adults with idiopathic constipation. Dis Colon Rectum 31:190–197

Varma JS, Smith AN (1988) Neurophysiological dysfunction in young women with intractable constipation. Gut 29:963–968

Varma JS, Bradnock J, Smith RG, Smith AN (1988) Constipation in the elderly. A physiological study. Dis Colon Rectum 31:111–115

Verburon A, Devroede G, Bouchoucha M et al. (1988) Megarectum. Dig Dis Sci 33:1164–1174

Wald A (1986) Colonic transit and anorectal manometry in chronic idiopathic constipation. Arch Intern Med 146:1713–1716

Waldron DJ, Bowes KL, Kingma YC, Cote K (1988) Colonic and anorectal motility in young women with severe constipation. Gastroenterology 95:1388–1394

Waldron DJ, Kumar D, Hallan RI, Windgate DL, Williams NS (1989a) Reproducibility and measurement of segmental colonic transit using radiopaque markers. Gut 30:A1479

Waldron DJ, Kumar D, Williams NS, Hallan RI, Swash M (1989b) Is intractable constipation associated with a systemic autonomic neuropathy? Br J Surg 76:645

Waldron DJ, Kumar D, Williams NS, Hallan RI, Wingate DL (1990) Evidence for motor neuropathy and reduced filling of the rectum in chronic intractable constipation. Gut (in press)

Watier A, Devroede G, Duranceau A et al. (1983) Constipation with colonic inertia: a manifestation of systemic disease? Dig Dis Sci 28:1025–1033

Womack NR, Williams NS, Holmfield JHM, Morrison JFB, Simpkin KC (1985) New method for the dynamic assessment of anorectal function in constipation. Br J Surg 72:994–998

Yoshioka K, Keighley MRB (1987) Anorectal myectomy for outlet obstruction. Br J Surg 74:373–376

8 · Faecal Incontinence

N. S. Williams

Faecal incontinence has been estimated to have a prevalence of 4.2 per 1000 and may be twice as high in people over 65 years of age. Many adult patients are women and many are extremely embarrassed about their disability. Consequently, considerable tact and sensitivity are required when evaluating them. Children may suffer from faecal incontinence secondary to congenital abnormalities of the nervous system and anorectum. More commonly, childhood incontinence occurs in relation to behavioural disturbance and social deprivation, the children presenting with chronic constipation, soiling and encopresis. It is our intention in this chapter to concentrate on the investigation of faecal incontinence in adults, but before doing so, it is necessary briefly to review the pathophysiology of the problem.

Pathophysiology

In broad terms, incontinence may be classified in four categories: neurological, local sphincter pathology, enteric or multifactorial (Table 8.1).

Neurological Causes

Defaecation, being part of normal social behaviour, is under conscious control and is served by efferent and afferent pathways. The upper motor neurones for the voluntary sphincter muscles lie close to those for the lower limb musculature in the parasagittal motor cortex. They communicate by a fast conducting oligosymptomatic pathway with the Onuf nucleus, which is sited in the sacral and ventral grey matter mainly in the S2 and S3 segments of the cord (Merton et al. 1982). The frontal cortex is important for the conscious awareness of the need to defaecate and appropriate social behaviour.

The striated muscles of the pelvic floor, including the urethral striated sphincter and the external anal sphincter muscles, are innervated by the pelvic and pudendal nerves. The lower motor neurones innervating these sphincters arise in the Onuf nucleus.

Upper Motor Neurone Lesions

The common neurological diseases which affect the central nervous system are likely to disturb continence. However, many of these diseases, such as cerebrovascular accidents, multiple sclerosis and the dementias, cause multifocal lesions, making clinicopathological correlations of sphincter disturbance difficult. Patients with central nervous system disease affecting the upper motor neurone pathway to the sphincters will often suffer from urgency and urge incontinence. Provided the peripheral innervation of the sphincter mechanism is intact, reflex micturition and defaecation are still possible, and resting anal

Table 8.1. Classification of causes of faecal incontinence

Neurological
Upper motor neurone pathway lesions
1. Cerebral
   Dementia
   Cerebrovascular disease
   Hydrocephalus
   Cerebral tumours (especially frontal lobe)
   Multiple sclerosis
2. Spinal cord
   Trauma
   Spinal cord compression (spinal tumours, cervical spondylitic myelopathy, etc.)
   Multiple sclerosis
   Spinal cord ischaemic lesions

Lower motor neurone pathway lesions
1. Onuf's nucleus – conus medullaris lesions
   Structural
   Multiple sclerosis
   Conus medullaris ischaemia
   Degenerative: multisystem atrophy, primary autonomic failure
2. Cauda equina
   Lumbosacral spinal trauma
   Lumbar intervertebral disc prolapse
   Lumbar canal stenosis
   Ankylosing spondylitis
3. Peripheral (intrapelvic) nerves
   Diabetic peripheral neuropathy or plexopathy
   Intrapelvic tumour
   Endometriosis
   Pudendal/pelvic stretch induced neuropathy related to childbirth or chronic straining due to constipation

Local sphincter pathology
Congenital anorectal anomalies
Obstetric anal sphincter tears
Sphincter trauma
Perianal suppuration (e.g. Crohn's disease)
Rectal or anal neoplasms

Multifactorial
Faecal incontinence in elderly or cognitively impaired subjects
   Acute or chronic confusional states
   Drug intoxication
   Faecal impaction
   Physical immobility
   "Neural ageing"

Enteric
Acute or chronic diarrhoeal illness

Nathan 1974). They are often incontinent without warning. As the lesion becomes more widespread, they show an increasing indifference to their problem.

Lower Motor Neurone Lesions

If the lower motor neurone pathway is damaged or interrupted, the pelvic floor and sphincter muscles become weak and atrophic. The pelvic floor bulges on standing and straining, a condition which is termed perineal descent. These patients frequently develop faecal impaction when the stool is hard and incontinence when it is soft; when impacted, they may also suffer from overflow incontinence. The commonest cause of a lower motor neurone lesion in an adult is chronic stretching of the pudendal nerve over a long period of time. This situation tends to arise in multiparous women or those who suffer from chronic constipation and who strain continually. These two factors, i.e. childbirth and constipation, may well be interlinked in that some degree of neuropathic damage is inflicted on the sphincter during childbirth. This results in some weakness of the pelvic floor and perineal descent during straining, and may be perceived as an increased tendency to constipation. Over a long period of persistent straining, the terminal part of the pudendal nerve becomes damaged, and the sphincter eventually shows some degree of denervation and reinnervation. This explains why most of these patients present with their incontinence in later life.

About 10% of patients with pelvic floor weakness and incontinence will have a more proximal lesion affecting the conus medullaris, cauda equina or intrapelvic course of the pudendal and perineal nerves. They usually have other symptoms or neurological signs in the lower limbs, and such findings help in the diagnosis.

sphincter tone is normal. Voluntary inhibition of these processes is, however, impaired. Reflex relaxation of the internal anal sphincter muscle is also exaggerated in response to rectal filling, and reflex contraction in the external anal sphincter is poorly sustained. Voluntary contraction of the sphincter is weak, and this allows automatic defaecation to ensue.

The clinical presentation, however, is often more complex. Patients with a frontal lobe lesion show poor awareness of a full bladder or of an increasing desire to defaecate (Andrews and

Complex Neurological Lesions

Most incontinent subjects with a neurogenic basis for their disability have a sensory deficit in addition to their motor defect. Sometimes, the sensory deficit is predominant, and such patients may have reasonable resting tone within the sphincter and be able voluntarily to contract the external sphincter satisfactorily; they are, however, unable to appreciate the imminent passage of faeces and cannot pre-empt it. Some patients have a mixed upper and lower motor neurone pathology. Patients with multiple sclerosis often fall into this category. As expected, such individuals often have a mixed clinical presentation. They may present with frequency, urgency and urge incontinence, indicative of an upper motor neurone lesion, but also may have atonicity of the bladder and lower colon and sphincter weakness, often accompanied by a perineal sensory deficit characteristic of a conus lesion (Taylor et al. 1984). The latter presents with impaired bladder emptying, constipation, overflow incontinence and impotence.

Local Sphincter Pathology

The sphincter may be absent as a result of a congenital anomaly or be damaged due to trauma, sepsis or neoplastic infiltration. In traumatic cases, the incontinence usually dates from the injury and progressively becomes worse. In cases of obstetric trauma, continence may gradually improve in the first few years after parturition, only to deteriorate 15–20 years later. The assumption in these patients is that the remainder of their damaged sphincter is able to compensate for a long period of time. However, during the intervening period, perineal descent occurs and the pudendal nerve becomes stretched, resulting in denervation of the external anal sphincter. Patients who are incontinent as a result of trauma but do not have evidence of neuropathy will retain sensation, whereas those with concomitant neuropathy will often have some degrees of sensory deficit. Patients whose sphincters are damaged by pelvic sepsis (e.g. due to Crohn's disease) or are infiltrated by neoplasm will, in addition to their incontinence, invariably have symptoms and signs suggestive of their underlying disease.

Enteric Causes

In these patients the sphincter functions normally, but the intestine is so diseased that the patient is unable to control the copious amounts of loose or liquid faeces so produced. The patient may have an acute or chronic disease responsible for the condition.

Multifactorial Causes

The incontinence of elderly or disabled people tends to be mutifactorial in nature. Thus, the sphincteric mechanism becomes weaker with age. Any therapy for concomitant disease may affect the smooth muscle of the gut and urinary tract, as well as affecting the control of the peripheral nervous system. Faecal impaction may result from acute or chronic confusional states and physical immobility. The latter results in soiling due to overflow, but the presence of hard stool in the rectum will also stimulate the secretion of large volumes of mucus, which merely exacerbates the problem.

Investigation of Faecal Incontinence

An understanding of the pathophysiology is a prerequisite for evaluating patients with incontinence. As can be seen, the aetiology is complex and sophisticated investigations may be required to reach a final diagnosis. Before embarking on such studies, however, much can be gleaned from a comprehensive clinical examination.

History

The onset of incontinence may be acute or chronic. The investigator should elicit symptoms of bowel, bladder or sexual disturbance. Any associated backache or pain and sensory impairment of the legs and perineum must be enquired into. The characteristics of the incontinence also need detailed enquiry. The presence and degree of sensory loss, the presence of urgency and the severity and timing of incontinence are all important factors. Similarly, comprehensive drug, family, and past medical histories are vital. The relevant factors in the past medical history include previous pelvic or pelvic floor surgery, a neurological or neurosurgical history or trauma to the neuroaxis or pelvis. Other systemic disorders, such as diabetes, alcoholism or connective tissue disease, are important. Details of the obstetric history are required, particularly parity, the duration of the second stage of labour, forceps delivery and the incidence and degree of perineal tears.

Physical Examination

A general examination is required, paying particular attention to the neurological system. Inspection of the anus and perineum should be performed. The normal perianal skin has a corrugated appearance, which may be absent if the sphincters are lax. Any scars suggestive of previous trauma should be noted. The anal canal is usually closed when the buttocks are gently parted; any gaping is suggestive, although not diagnostic, of sphincter deficiency. The normal anus will react if the perianal skin is stimulated, and the sphincter will contract. This is known as the anal reflex, and can be elicited by scratching the skin gently with a neurological pin or similar object. Loss of the reflex indicates the reflex arc has been interrupted at some level. The patient should be asked to strain, and the degree of perineal descent should be noted. This examination is usually conducted in the left lateral position, with the patient's hips flexed to a right angle. It may be more accurate and physiological for the patient to strain in the squatting position, although this obviously makes observation more difficult. Normally, the perineum does not descend below the ischial tuberosities; any bulging below this level is defined as perineal descent. The degree of perineal descent can be quantified by using the perineometer described by Henry et al. (1982). This consists of a perspex crosspiece, which has two feet attached at either end which fit on the ischial tuberosities. In the centre of the crosspiece is a cylindrical rod which moves when the perineum comes in contact with its base. The degree of perineal descent is assessed by noting the distance the rod moves during straining. This is a useful research tool, which is not required in routine clinical practice. The relevance of perineal descent in the assessment of incontinent patients is that the greater the degree of descent, the greater the amount of neurogenic damage to the sphincter mechanism. In addition to perineal descent, there may be rectal or uterine prolapse, and its degree needs to be noted. Apart from uterine prolapse, there may be the presence of a rectocoele or cystocoele. The patient should be asked to cough, and any leakage of faeces or urine should be noted.

Digital examination of the rectum should next be undertaken. Resting tone corresponds mainly to the function of the internal anal sphincter. In the conscious person, it should not be possible to open the anal canal by pulling gently backwards with one finger towards the coccyx, since the normal anus continues to close on to the finger. The patient should be asked to squeeze the examining finger as tightly as possible, to give an indication of the strength of the puborectalis and the external anal sphincter. Deficiencies of the external anal sphincter and their position in relation to the circumference and longitudinal depth in the anal canal should be noted. The latter observations will

obviously be crude – accurate assessment requires the use of EMG mapping (see p. 49).

Digital examination also allows an appreciation of the anorectal angle. At rest, the angle normally approximates to 90°, but straightens out on straining and becomes more acute with voluntary contraction. In many incontinent patients in whom the puborectalis is weak, the anorectal angle is wider than 90°, and this may be detected on clinical examination. However, clinical measurement of the angle can only be considered as a rough approximation, and if it is considered to be useful in assessment, and this is debatable, more accurate data can be obtained by a lateral radiograph. Rectal examination should detect the presence or absence of a low rectal carcinoma or other space-occupying lesion, which may or may not be infiltrating the sphincter mechanism.

Proctosigmoidoscopy

It is usual to perform a rigid sigmoidoscopy before a proctoscopy. In incontinent patients, the value of this investigation is to rule out an enteric cause for the problem. Thus, proctitis should be obvious by the appearance of the rectal mucosa. Similarly, a large villous adenoma or carcinoma should be detected. Occasionally, a solitary rectal ulcer may be found in a patient who has suffered from evacuation problems before the development of incontinence.

Proctoscopy may detect the presence of an occult intussusception or anterior mucosal prolapse, the latter being the genesis of the former. To view these abnormalities, the proctoscope, having been inserted through the anal canal and directed towards the umbilicus, is angled backwards to look directly up into the lumen of the rectum. The patient is then asked to strain as the instrument is slowly withdrawn, and the anterior rectal wall mucosa fills the instrument until the anorectal ring is approached. If a complete intussusception is present, there is a circumferential infolding of the rectal wall, which may appear as a concentric ring of rectal mucosa prolapsing into the instrument. Such an intussusception may progress through the anal canal and become exteriorized as a full or partial thickness rectal prolapse.

Physiological Investigations

Up to the present time, little reliance has been placed on the results of sophisticated physiological tests. However, with increasing knowledge and the availability of more varied treatment options, it is becoming clear that some degree of physiological investigation of incontinent patients is required. Colorectal units will vary as to which investigations they regard as essential and which they consider are useful. It is the purpose of this section to describe the range of tests available, and their aims, and to indicate those which our group routinely use for diagnostic purposes, and those which at present we regard as research investigations.

Static Manometry

This is performed in the left lateral position using either a microtransducer or a perfused tube, during which the probe is pulled through the high pressure zone as part of a station pull-through technique. The maximum resting pressure and length of the high pressure zone are recorded. The resting anal pressure is an indication of internal anal sphincter (IAS) strength. With the probe positioned in the midanal canal, the patient is encouraged to exert a maximum voluntary contraction of the sphincter mechanism. The increase in pressure above resting basal pressure is a measure of the strength of the external anal sphincter (EAS). Measurement of anal pressures should also be combined with rectal distension (Fig. 8.1). With a distending balloon positioned at 10 cm above the anal sphincter, and the pressure probe within the high pressure zone, the anorectal reflexes can be elicited. At low distending volumes a transient reduction in anal pressure is observed (Meunier and Mollard 1977). At higher volumes an initial increase in pressure, caused by contraction of the external anal sphincter, is followed by a reduction in pressure caused by relaxation of the internal anal sphincter. As the rectal balloon is distended with larger volumes, the amplitude and duration of the relaxation increases (Schuster et al. 1965; Arhan et al. 1972; Meunier and Mollard 1977). These recto-anal reflexes may permit the sensitive anal epithelium to sample rectal contents without fear of incontinence (Duthie and Bennett 1963). Relaxation of the IAS allows rectal contents to enter the anal canal and stimulate the sensory anal mucosa, which is not exposed to rectal contents under resting conditions. The sensory epithelium can discriminate between solid, liquid and gaseous contents.

Findings in Incontinence

Patients with idiopathic faecal incontinence (IFI) have low resting and squeeze sphincter pressures (Read et al. 1979). Studies in which anorectal pressures have been recorded using a multilumen probe suggest the existence of two different abnormalities of sphincter function in these patients. In one group, resting pressures are very low, and

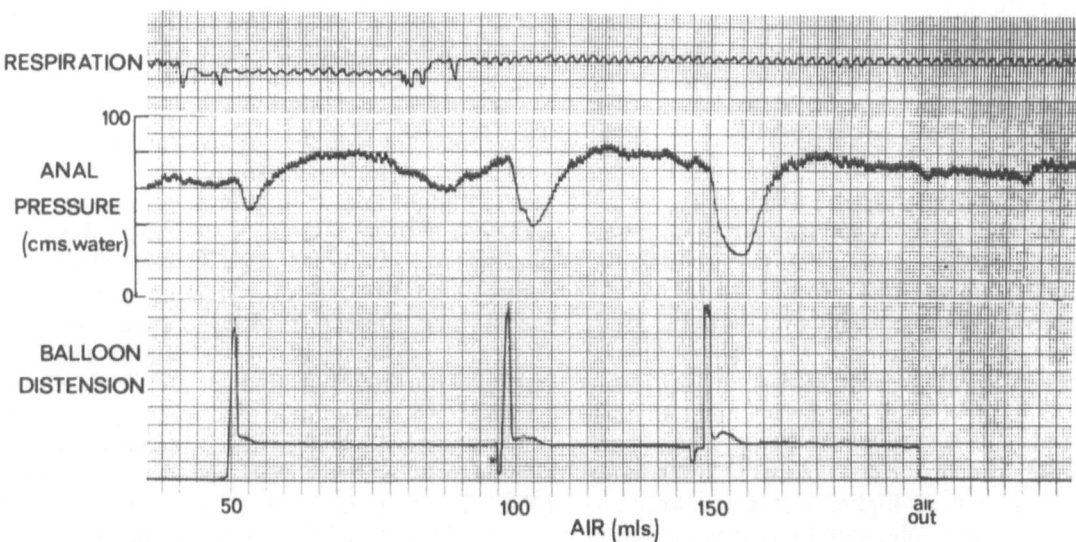

Fig. 8.1. Elicitation of the recto-anal distension reflex in a normal subject. Rectal distension produces an initial increase in anal canal pressure due to contraction of the external anal sphincter followed by a reduction in pressure due to relaxation of the internal anal sphincter. In incontinent patients, resting anal pressure is often so low, this reflex is absent.

rectal distension involves external anal sphincter contraction, but no internal anal sphincter relaxation. These patients presumably have a marked weakness of their internal sphincter. The second group of patients exhibit normal sphincter relaxation to rectal distension, although the external sphincter response is very small. These patients presumably have marked weakness of the external sphincter (Read and Bannister 1985).

Patients whose incontinence is due to trauma of the external anal sphincter may have normal resting pressure, but a markedly reduced voluntary contraction. Often, however, they have some degree of neuropathic damage in addition, which produces a low resting anal pressure.

The incontinence associated with diabetes produces changes in anorectal manometry. Both maximum basal and squeeze pressures are reduced in incontinent diabetics compared with continent diabetics (Schiller et al. 1982; Erckenbrecht et al. 1984). In addition, the rectal volume which induces anal relaxation in incontinent diabetic patients is often less than that which can be perceived by the continent patient (Wald 1983; Wald and Tunuguntla 1984). This may be an important factor in causing incontinence, because it means that the stimulus for the voluntary protective contraction of the EAS and puborectalis may not occur prior to soiling.

Resting anal pressure is reduced in patients with low spinal cord lesions, such as meningocoele (Meunier and Mollard 1977). In addition, the rectum in patients with low spinal and cauda equina lesions is large and compliant, and shows little contractile activity (White et al. 1940). Rectal sensation to balloon distension is blunted and felt as abdominal discomfort rather than a perineal sensation (Frenckner and Ihre 1976). The recto-anal inhibitory reflex is present in such patients, but the degree of relaxation does not necessarily bear a direct relationship to the distending volume (Meunier and Mollard 1977).

High spinal cord damage also causes impaired rectal sensation (Frenckner 1975). Although the compliance of the rectum is often normal, it may be increased in some patients (White et al. 1940; Frenckner and Von Euler 1975). The recto-anal inhibitory reflex is present, although the relaxation is more profound and lasts longer than in normal individuals (Frenckner 1975). Reflex contraction of the external sphincter is usually present, although at higher distension volumes than controls, but sphincter pressures are often normal (Denny-Brown and Robertson 1935; Frenckner 1975).

As can be seen, manometry is useful for diagnostic purposes. In those patients with a low resting anal pressure or poor squeeze pressure, or both, it gives a good indication of the degree of incontinence which the patient experiences. The latter may not be so clear on clinical examination, and manometry is therefore a good objective measurement. The investigation is also useful during follow-up, particularly after operation.

Although we regard manometry as an essential measurement in incontinent patients, we believe that the static technique of measurement in the laboratory provides only limited information. Our initial work with ambulatory techniques has provided us with a wealth of data not previously available. Although these techniques are at present research tools, we believe they will soon become routine.

Ambulant Manometry

As mentioned earlier, static anorectal manometry provides limited information on the sphincter complex and evoked reflex activity in the laboratory. We have developed an ambulant method of recording anorectal manometry in ambulant subjects. This method of recording is not only more physiological, it also provides valuable information on anorectal function in the patient's own environment away from the laboratory setting. The details of ambulant manometry have been described in the chapter on manometry. In a pilot study, we used this technique to evaluate the role of internal and external sphincters in six patients with idiopathic faecal incontinence. The patients were studied for a mean duration of 21 hours per subject. Anorectal pressure was measured by a two channel pressure sensitive probe with sensors positioned in the rectum and mid-anal canal respectively. All subjects were completely ambulant and were able to eat normal meals and sleep at home. We have previously shown that healthy subjects show 7.5 ± 2.0 (mean+SEM) episodes of anal relaxation per hour. Patients with faecal incontinence showed significantly more ($P<0.01$) episodes of anal relaxation (11.6 ± 1.8 episodes per hour) (Kumar et al. 1989). We also measured the duration of anal relaxation, which in patients with idiopathic faecal incontinence were significantly longer than in healthy controls (48 ± 3.1 seconds versus 28.4 ± 3.9 seconds) ($P<0.001$) (Fig. 8.2). Thus, using this technique it appears that anal relaxation occurs more frequently and for a prolonged period of time in patients with idiopathic faecal incontinence.

Control

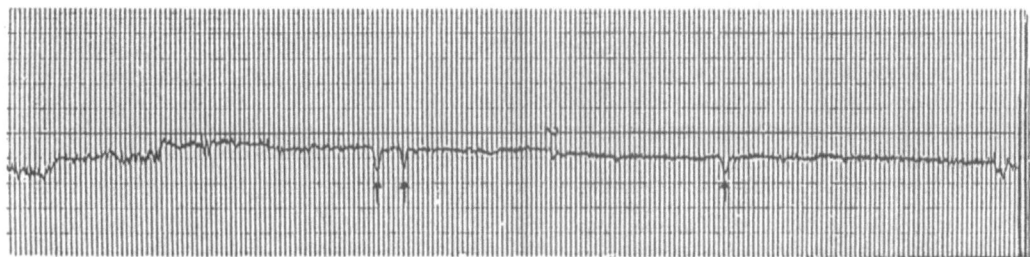

Incontinence

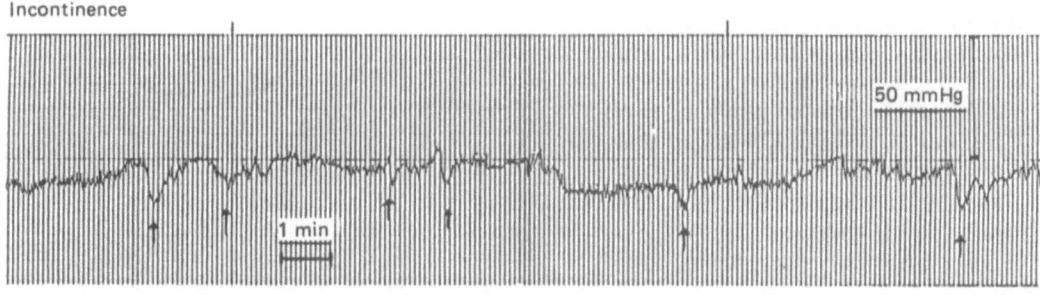

50 mmHg

1 min

Fig. 8.2. Ambulant recordings from a healthy volunteer (*upper trace*) and a patient with idiopathic faecal incontinence (*lower trace*). Note the short, sharp and less frequent episodes of anal relaxation in healthy controls. In contrast, patients with faecal incontinence have prolonged and more frequent anal relaxations.

These observations lend support to the hypothesis that incontinence in these patients is the result of internal anal sphincter dysfunction. We believe that ambulant monitoring of anorectal function in patients with idiopathic faecal incontinence will become an important part of their assessment and should make a significant contribution to our understanding of the pathophysiology of this disorder. It provides us with an opportunity to integrate the function of the anal canal, rectum and sigmoid colon (an assessment which cannot be easily made by left lateral manometry) and hopefully therapy can, as a result, be planned in a more physiological and meaningful way.

Electrophysiological Tests

A variety of electrophysiological tests are available for the investigation of incontinence. Many of these are primarily research tools. However, the coloproctologist should have electromyographic facilities available. There are two types of EMG measurement, which are invaluable in evaluating the incontinent patient: concentric needle EMG and single fibre EMG.

Concentric Needle EMG

This is the standard method of EMG measurement available in most units. The patient lies on an electrically insulated mat in the left lateral position on a couch in a warm room. The ground electrode is strapped to the thigh. Digital examination is then performed, and if possible the puborectalis ring is palpated. In order to localize the muscle, it is usually necessary to ask the patient to squeeze the anus as tightly as possible. After cleaning the perineal skin and warning the patient, the needle electrode is inserted approximately 10 cm posterior to the anal verge at an angle of 45° to the skin. By inserting the needle to its hilt and guided by the finger in the rectum, it can usually be inserted into the puborectalis. A few minutes must be allowed to elapse after needle or patient movement, so that the muscle activity can settle to a resting level. Recordings are then taken with the patient at rest, after maximal squeeze and after maximal straining. The needle is then withdrawn slightly so that it enters the external anal sphincter, and repeat recordings are made.

The important parameters in the study of motor unit action potentials are amplitude, duration, number of phases and firing rate. The range of these normal parameters is discussed in Chapter 3. It is, however, convenient to summarize here the salient features. The external anal sphincter shows continuous low-frequency activity at rest, and even during sleep (Floyd and Walls 1953). The activity consists of contractions of individual motor unit potentials at low firing rates and of low amplitude (<500 µV). A potential with more than four phases is termed a polyphasic motor unit potential. Normal skeletal muscles contain up to 12% polyphasic motor unit action potentials. Voluntary activity, as when the individual is asked to squeeze the anal sphincter as tight as possible, produces an interference pattern. Summation of individual motor unit action potentials occurs so that the oscilloscope is filled with activity. The motor unit potentials reach 2–3 mV in amplitude, although the mean amplitude is somewhat lower (200–600 µV) (Jesel et al. 1973). The mean duration of motor unit potentials is 5–7.5 ms (Petersen and Franksson 1955; Chantraine 1966), and this increases with age (Bartolo et al. 1983). In addition, the percentage of polyphasic units increases with age.

Findings in Incontinence

Patients with idiopathic (neurogenic) incontinence display characteristic concentric EMG findings in both the puborectalis and external anal sphincters. In severe cases, EMG activity is decreased, and zones of the sphincter muscles may be electrically silent. The motor unit action potentials are of larger amplitude and longer duration than normal. Polyphasic action potentials are numerous. In less severe cases, the maximal amplitude during the voluntary contraction is increased, and the major abnormality consists of polyphasic motor unit action potentials (Fig. 8.3). Increased neuromuscular jitter between components of these polyphasic potentials may be present, indicating instability of innervation.

Mapping of the anal sphincter with a concentric EMG needle electrode is very useful where a traumatic aetiology is suspected. Not only will it confirm the diagnosis, but by determining the area and extent of fibrosis and the degree of normal functioning sphincter that remains, the investigation is invaluable in planning the operative approach. Mapping is performed by inserting a concentric needle electrode into the external anal sphincter in the four quadrants of the muscle. Without removing the needle from the skin, it can be readjusted repeatedly so that the distribution of muscle fibres can be accurately mapped. Whereas posterior insertion usually produces abundant

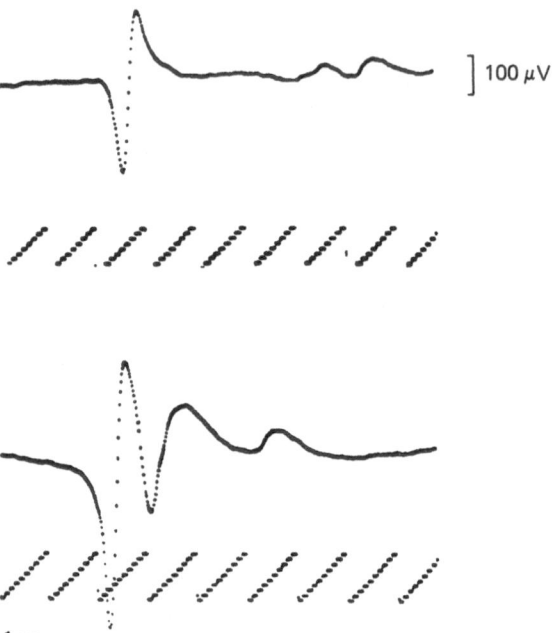

]100 µV

1ms

Fig. 8.3. Concentric needle EMG. *Upper trace*: normal recording. The motor unit potential is biphasic and of short duration (<2 ms). *Lower trace*: incontinent patient. The motor unit potential is complex and of longer duration (4 ms).

EMG activity, it should be realized that anterior insertion in women is painful and the muscle is often very thin, even in normal subjects.

Mapping can be quantified. We carry out sphincter mapping analysis by measuring the amount of EMG activity occurring during 1 s periods. This requires the use of rectified EMG activity during 1 s activation periods.

As well as detecting areas of fibrosis within the sphincter muscle, mapping can be used to locate the sphincter in infants with anorectal agenesis. One cause of incontinence following pull-through procedures in such patients is a failure to bring the colon down through the sphincteric ring. We have seen incontinent adult patients who had pull-through operations in childhood in whom sphincter mapping has subsequently correctly located a normal sphincter, and who have been rendered continent after a second procedure rerouted the colon through the intact, although rudimentary, sphincter mechanism.

Single Fibre EMG

Concentric needle electrodes are unable to detect individual muscle fibre action potentials, but this can be achieved using single fibre electrodes. Such electrodes can usually identify within normal muscles one or two single muscle fibre action potentials within the uptake area of the electrode. The mean duration of motor unit action potentials consisting of more than one component recorded by this method is less than 8 ms.

Single fibre EMG can be quantified by calculating mean fibre density (MFD) which has specific value in patients with idiopathic faecal incontinence (IFI) (Fig. 8.4). MFD is defined as the mean number of single muscle fibre action potentials recorded within the uptake area of the electrode in 20 different positions within the muscle (Stalberg and Thiele 1975). In the normal external anal sphincter, the MFD is 1.5±0.16 (Neill and Swash 1980). The calculation of MFD is dependent on the acquisition of recordings of sufficient clarity to allow measurement. By convention in limb muscles, components used for triggering must be greater than 150 μV in amplitude, but because of the smaller size of the muscle fibres of the pelvic floor potentials of 100 μV are accepted.

Denervation of the sphincter as occurs in IFI results in a process of reinnervation and fibre type groupings. As a consequence, there is an increasing compaction of muscle fibres within individual motor units, which results in an increase in mean fibre density, because there are more fibres within the uptake area of the electrode innervated by a single axon or its branches. Thus, an increased MFD confirms the presence of denervation and reinnervation, which are hallmarks of IFI. Single fibre EMG also allows the abnormalities seen on concentric needle EMG to be seen more clearly.

In patients with IFI, the activity in the resting sphincter muscle may be of such low intensity that it cannot be detected. It is usual to induce activity in these cases by the insertion of a balloon into the rectum. It should be realized that damage or disease of the lower motor neurone may lead to a denervation–reinnervation pattern, hence an increase in MFD is not pathogenic of IFI. However, in the absence of other neurological signs IFI is the most likely diagnosis.

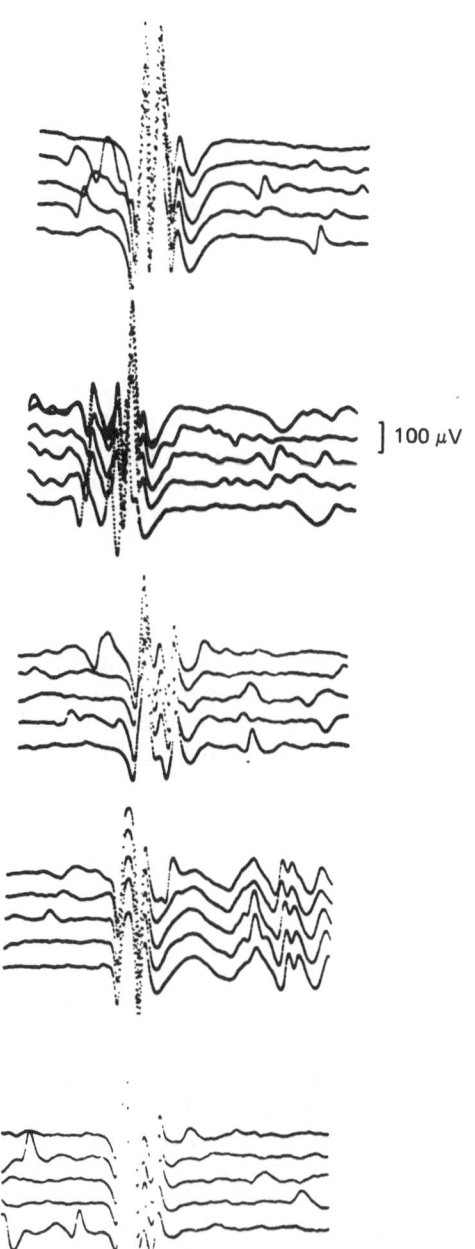

] 100 μV

1 ms

Fig. 8.4. Single fibre EMG. Faecal incontinence: five consecutively recorded traces of five different motor units in the muscle displayed as part of the calculation of the fibre density. In the first motor unit potential there are three components, in the second four components, etc. The mean number of components in 20 such positions is the mean fibre density (MFD). (From Snooks and Swash (1985), with kind permission.)

Nerve Stimulation Tests

Nerve stimulation techniques may be useful in pinpointing the exact site of nerve or muscle lesion causing incontinence. In the vast majority of cases, however, the combination of clinical findings, manometry and EMG, will establish the diagnosis. Nevertheless, in a minority of cases, more sophisticated investigations may be required. From a research point of view, such studies are most interesting, and it may be that in time these relatively simple tests will contribute more to the routine examination.

Pudendal and Perineal Nerve Stimulation

The pudendal nerve consists of inferior rectal branches which innervate the external anal sphincter and perineal branches that innervate the peri-urethral striated sphincter musculature. If the pudendal nerve is stimulated, and the response recorded selectively from both these muscles, it is possible to assess conduction in the motor fibres innervating them. Pudendal nerve stimulation is achieved using a specially designed glove (Kiff and Swash 1984; see Chap. 3), on the index finger of which is mounted stimulating electrodes at its tip and recording electrodes at its base; the index finger is inserted into the rectum and by stimulating close to the pudendal nerve at the ischial spine, and by recording the response in the external anal sphincter, the pudendal nerve terminal motor latency can be measured. Similarly, with an intra-urethral electrode positioned within the peri-urethral striated sphincter, the perineal nerve terminal motor latency can be measured. The latter may be useful in patients with both urinary and faecal incontinence. The normal values for these latencies are shown in Table 8.2 (Snooks and Swash 1985).

Table 8.2. Distal nerve latencies in control subjects

Nerve	n	Age (mean and range)	Terminal nerve motor latencies (ms)
Pudendal	40	50 (25–75)	21 ±0.2
Perineal	20	42 (25–60)	2.4±0.2

Eighty per cent of patients with IFI have been shown to have prolonged pudendal nerve terminal motor latency. These measurements are of little value on their own, but when combined with the measurement of latencies resulting from transcutaneous cervico-lumbar stimulation, may be very informative.

Transcutaneous Cervico-lumbar Stimulation

These techniques have been modified from those originally described by Merton et al. 1982). Transcutaneous stimulation can be performed over the lumbar spine at the level of the cauda equina or over the cervical spine at the level of the sixth cervical vertebra. The responses to stimulation in the puborectalis, external anal sphincter and peri-urethral striated sphincter can all be recorded, and

thus the spinal latencies to these muscles can be measured. By determining the distance between the stimulus sites and by a process of subtraction, it is possible to determine the conduction velocity in each part of the spinal pathway involved in the control of the sphincteric mechanism.

In patients with IFI, the spinal latencies from L1 and L4 stimulation to the puborectalis and external anal sphincter muscles are increased (Snooks and Swash 1984). In the majority of patients, motor conduction is normal between L1 and L4, i.e. in the cauda equina, the delay occurs in the pudendal nerve (Kiff and Swash 1984; Snooks and Swash 1984). However, in approximately 20% of patients, there is both proximal (cauda equina) and distal (pudendal nerve) conduction delay (Snooks and Swash 1984), indicating a proximal cause for the incontinence. Delay in the cauda equina may, for example, be due to lumbar canal stenosis, cauda equina tumour, arachnoiditis or sacral agenesis. These investigations can thus help select patients who should undergo myelography or magnetic resonance imaging of the spinal cord.

Sensory Investigations

Response of the anal canal mucosa to an electrical stimulus can be measured using a bipolar constant current stimulator probe (Roe et al. 1986). The technique is described in Chapter 3. Certain patients with IFI have been demonstrated to have a reduced threshold electrosensitivity when measured in this way. Similarly, a reduced appreciation of temperature as measured by a thermocouple has been recorded in these patients (Miller et al. 1987). It is considered that those receptors that respond to a temperature stimulus are those which are responsible for discrimination between solid, fluid and gas. However, although many patients with IFI complain of varying degrees of sensory loss, it has been difficult to correlate these symptoms with the objective sensory measurements. The exact role that these measurements play in the evaluation of patients with incontinence remains to be determined. At present, they can only be regarded as research investigations, but in the future they are likely to be an important part of assessment.

Radiological Evaluation

We regard radiological study of the anorectum as being an important part of the evaluation of patients with incontinence. While static films may

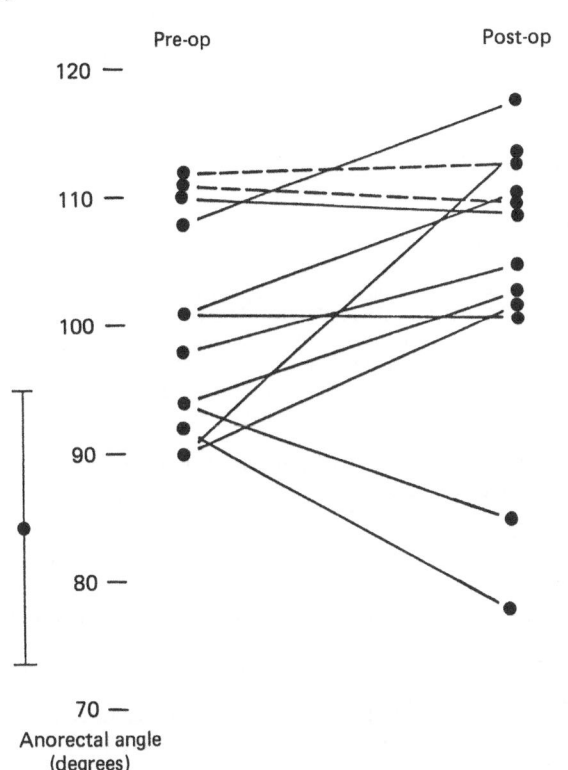

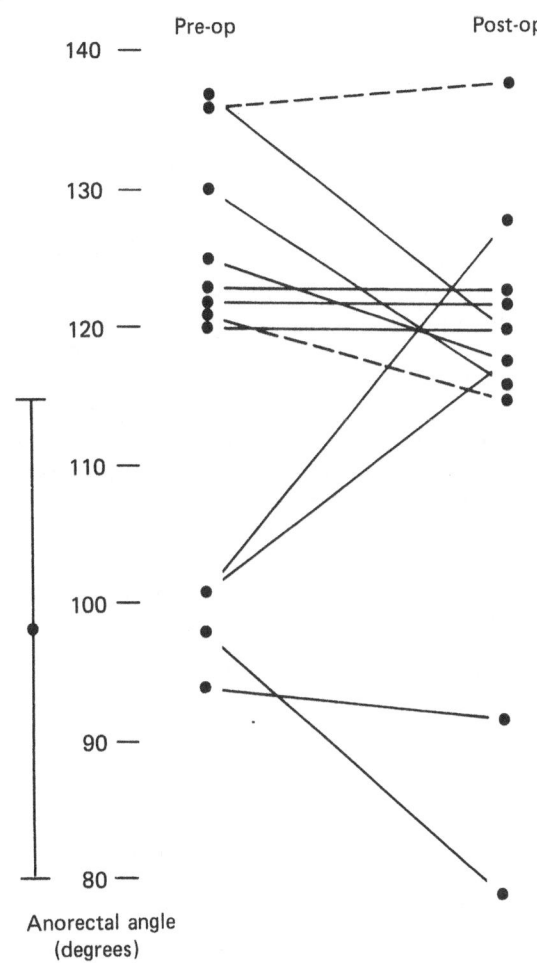

Fig. 8.5. Measurements of the anorectal angle at rest (**a**) and during straining (**b**) before and after postanal repair (*dashed lines*, failure; *continuous lines*, success) in patients with IFI. Note that not all patients pre-operatively have an abnormally wide angle and postanal repair does not significantly change the angle. The normal range is depicted to the left of the ordinate.

provide some useful information, some form of evacuation proctography is invaluable. In IFI a lateral proctogram will usually show that the anorectal ring is displaced below the pubococcygeal line (>1.8 cm), the anorectal angle is increased with shortening of the anal canal, and there is a significant increase in the anopubic distance (Hardcastle and Parks 1970). Much interest has concentrated on the widening of the anorectal angle since the operation of postanal repair was designed to make it more acute. Indeed, it has been recommended by some authorities that the operation should only be offered to those patients who are found to have a wide anorectal angle. Several studies (Womack et al. 1988; Miller et al. 1988), however, have recently shown that some IFI patients have anorectal angles within normal values and that postanal repair produces no significant change (Fig. 8.5a, b). The benefit of postanal repair would appear to be due to a lengthening of the high pressure zone, as opposed to a change in the anorectal angle. Thus, the latter

should not be used as an indication for this operation.

We prefer to perform evacuation proctography in an integrated fashion, whereby intrarectal pressure and sphincter EMG are measured simultaneously with the visualization of the anorectum (Womack et al. 1985; see Chap. 3). In patients with incontinence, useful clinical data, however, can be obtained by the proctogram alone. Proctography may demonstrate overt rectal prolapse, which has not been previously demonstrated on clinical examination. Often, however, it shows an occult intussusception or anterior rectal wall prolapse. In patients with IFI, it is difficult to know whether these radiological abnormalities are the cause or the effect of the incontinence. In certain patients with a particularly marked intussusception, consideration may be given to repairing the defect by some sort of rectopexy. In some patients, the proctogram shows a marked rectocoele in which the contrast pools during attempted defaecation. We have seen some incontinent patients with this defect who void satisfactorily, only to leak for a period after defaecation. They usually have an impaired sphincter mechanism as well, but this on its own is insufficient to produce the incontinence. In such patients, we believe that should surgery be indicated, the rectocoele needs to be repaired in conjunction with the appropriate sphincter procedure.

Integrated proctography may demonstrate associated anismus. This finding is not infrequent in patients with IFI, and presumably the chronic straining during evacuation results in stretching of the pudendal nerve and eventual denervation of the sphincter. Patients with this dual problem are extremely difficult to treat. Postanal repair may improve their continence, but they will invariably continue to strain, and thus the incontinence is likely to return. Clearly, any manoeuvre to relieve their anismus is likely further to weaken the sphincter mechanism. All that can usually be offered is advice about straining and a suppository regime.

References

Andrews J, Nathan P (1974) Lesions of the anterior frontal lobes and the disturbances of micturition and defaecation. Brain 87:233–262

Arhan P, Faverdin D, Persoz B et al (1972) Relationship between viscoelastic properties of the rectum and anal pressure in man. J App Physiol 41:677–682

Bartolo DCC, Jarratt JA, Read NW (1983) The use of conventional electromyography to assess external sphincter neuropathy in man. J Neurol Neurosurg Psychiat 46:1115–1118

Chantraine A (1966) Electromyographie des sphincters striés uretral, cerebral et anal humains: étude descriptive et analytique. Rev Neurol 115:396–403

Denny-Brown D, Robertson EG (1935) An investigation of the nervous control of defaecation. Brain 58:256–310

Duthie HL, Bennett RC (1963) The relation of sensation in the anal canal to the functional anal sphincter: a possible factor in anal continence. Gut 4:179–182

Erckenbrecht JF, Winter HJ, Cicmiri I, Berger H, Berges W, Wienbeck M (1984) Is incontinence in diabetes mellitus due to diabetic autonomic neuropathy. In: Gastrointestinal motility. MTP Press, Lancaster, pp 483–484

Floyd WF, Walls EW (1953) Electromyography of the sphincter ani externus in man. J Physiol (Lond) 122:599–609

Frenckner B (1975) Function of the anal sphincters in spinal man. Gut 16:638–644

Frenckner B, Ihre T (1976) Influence of autonomic nerves on the internal anal sphincter in man. Gut 17:306–312

Frenckner B, Von Euler C (1975) Influence of pudendal block on the function of the anal sphincters. Gut 16:482–489

Hardcastle JD, Parks AJ (1970). A study of anal incontinence and some principles of surgical treatment. Proc R Soc Med 63:116–118

Henry MM, Parks AG, Swash M (1982) The pelvic floor musculature in the descending perineum syndrome. Br J Surg 69:470–472

Jesel M, Isch-Treussard C, Isch F (1973) Electromyography of striated muscles of anal and urethral sphincters. In: Desmedt JE (ed) New developments in electromyography and clinical neurophysiology, vol 12. Karger, Basel, pp 406–420

Kiff ES, Swash M (1984) Slowed conduction in the pudendal nerves in idiopathic (neurogenic) faecal incontinence. Br J Surg 71:614–616

Kumar D, Waldron D, Williams NS (1989) Home assessment of anorectal motility and external sphincter EMG in idiopathic faecal incontinence. Br J Surg 76:635–636

Merton PA, Morton HB, Hill DK, Marsden CD (1982) Scope for a technique for electrical stimulation of human brain, spinal cord and muscle. Lancet ii:597–600

Meunier P, Mollard P (1977) Control of the internal anal sphincter (manometric study with human subjects). Pflügers Arch ges Physiol 370:233–239

Miller R, Bartolo DCC, Cevero F, Mortensen NJMcC (1987) Anorectal temperature sensation: a comparison of normal and incontinent patients. Br J Surg 74:511–515

Miller R, Bartolo DCC, Locke-Edmunds JC, Mortensen NJMcC (1988) Prospective study of conservative and operative treatment for faecal incontinence. Br J Sur 75:101–105

Neill ME, Swash M (1980) Increased motor unit fibre density in the external sphincter muscles in anorectal incontinence: a single fibre EMG study. J Neurol Neurosurg Psychiat 43:343–347

Petersen I, Franksson EE (1955) Electromyographic study of the striated muscles of the male urethra. Br J Urol 27:148–153

Read NW, Bannister JJ (1985) Anorectal manometry: techniques in health and anorectal disease. In: Henry MM, Swash M (eds) Coloproctology and the pelvic floor. Butterworth, London, pp 65–87

Read NW, Harford WV, Schmulen AC, Read MG, Santa Ana C, Fordtran JS (1979) A clinical study of patients with faecal incontinence and diarrhoea. Gastroenterology 76:747–756

Roe AM, Bartolo DCC, Mortensen NJMcC (1986) New method for assessment of anal sensation in various anorectal disorders. Br J Surg 73:310–312

Schiller LR, Santa Ana CA, Schmulen AC, Hendler MV, Fordtran JS (1982) Pathogenesis of faecal incontinence in diabetes mellitus. Evidence for internal anal sphincter dysfunction. N Engl J Med 307:1666–1671

Schuster MM, Hendrix TR, Mendeloff AI (1965) The internal anal sphincter response: manometric studies on its normal physiology, neural pathways and alteration in bowel diseases. J Clin Invest 42:196–207

Snooks SJ, Swash M (1984) Perineal nerve and transcutaneous spinal stimulation: new method for investigation of the urethral striated sphincter musculature. Br J Urol 56:406–409

Snooks SJ, Swash M (1985) Nerve stimulation techniques. In: Henry MM, Swash M (eds) Coloproctology and the pelvic floor. Butterworth, London

Stalberg E, Thiele B (1975) Motor unit fibre density in the extensor digitorum conmunis muscle. J Neurol Neurosurg Psychiat 386:874–880

Taylor MC, Bradley WE, Bhatia N, Glick M, Halderman S (1984) Theconus demyelination syndrome in multiple sclerosis. Act Neurol Scand 69:80–89

Wald A (1983) Biofeedback for neurogenic faecal incontinence: rectal sensation is a determinant of outcome. J Ped Gastroenterol Nutr 2:302–306

Wald A, Tunuguntla AK (1984) Anorectal sensation dysfunction in faecal incontinence and diabetes mellitus. N Engl J Med 310:1288–1287

White JC, Verlot MG, Ehrentheil D (1940) Neurogenic disturbances of the colon and their investigation by the colon metrogram. Ann Surg 112:1042–1057

Womack NR, Williams NS, Holmfield JHM, Morrison JFB, Simpkins KC (1985) New method for dynamic assessment of anorectal function in constipation. Br J Surg 72:994–998

Womack NR, Morrison JFB, Williams NS (1988) A prospective study of the effects of post-anal repair in neurogenic incontinence. Br J Surg 75:48–52

9 · Neurological Disorders

A. N. Smith and N. R. Binnie

Neurological lesions

Lesions associated with colonic and rectal dysfunction and with problems of the pelvic floor of neurological causation will be considered in the following order: central, spinal, nerve roots, peripheral nerves and ganglion nerve cells, with functional disorders which have neurological involvement but cannot be classified anatomically.

Central Lesions

In most central lesions the colon is most affected but there is a general inhibition of gastrointestinal motor function (Wilson 1976). Whether this is an exaggeration of the normal inhibitory factors modulating colonic motility or because excitatory factors are suppressed due to the withdrawal of vagal stimuli or the absence of gastro-colic reflex is unknown.

Central neurological lesions have many features in common with paralytic ileus. The right colon is most commonly affected; the dominant slow wave frequency falls from 11/min to 3/min in the right colon. Spike bursts are of low amplitude initially but later become normal by increasing in amplitude and propagating distally. The recovery phase is associated with the passage of flatus and faeces (Condon et al. 1986). In addition, there is delayed gastric emptying and involvement of the small intestine suggesting a lack of vagal activity. In postoperative ileus, however, the recovery is rapid especially in the stomach and small bowel, whereas in the colon it is delayed and less predictable (Rothnie et al. 1963).

Patients with major head injuries, raised intracranial pressure or posterior fossa tumours commonly exhibit delayed gastric emptying, atonic abdominal distension and evidence of absent colonic motor activity which fluctuates with the depth of unconsciousness.

Central neurological lesions such as in Parkinson's disease are often associated with constipation. Micturition is usually more severely affected than bowel function, which is partly due to incoordination of pelvic floor muscle activity. This is a direct effect on the extra-pyramidal control of muscle activity in the levator ani plates and thus not associated with any changes in the pelvic floor reflexes which are slightly prolonged. Drugs used for the treatment of Parkinson's disease may also produce intestinal pseudo-obstruction because of the hypomotility resulting from their anticholinergic activity.

Colonic ileus occurs in the treatment of depression by psychotropic drugs such as the tricyclic antidepressant compounds, for example amitriptyline (Burks 1988) and imipramine. These compounds prevent re-uptake of catecholamine centrally and at peripheral nerve endings and also have pronounced anticholinergic action at both sites. The effect is reversible and intestinal motility returns within 24–48 hours of withdrawal of the compound.

The internal ionic movement of all cells is

closely regulated for the maintenance of normal function. Potassium depletion suppresses the function of neurones and affects acetylcholine transmission from central cells to their peripheral counterparts. Conduction delay causes ileus, which predominantly affects the colon by altering transmission to intestinal smooth muscle. The ileus resolves when the hypokalaemia is treated. There is usually a delay in bowel transit because of decreased acetylcholine stimulation of smooth muscle. There is also an accompanying bladder atony which can be measured on cystometrograms.

The effect of a cerebrovascular accident on gut and pelvic floor function is variable. There is an initial ileus which resembles spinal shock or pseudo-obstruction (Reynolds and Elliasson 1977) and is thought to represent temporary cessation of the conduction of the central impulses from the hypothalamus and basal nuclei to the periphery.

The subsequent development of any colorectal disorder depends on the degree and extent of the central nervous system lesion and the relative sparing of autonomic centres necessary for the recovery of function. Other important factors are the effect of antihypertensive drugs, the general level of consciousness and the degree of disturbance of cerebral arterial perfusion. With clinical improvement the abnormal motility pattern improves; a deterioration in the clinical state usually leads to prolonged hypomotility and constipation and suggests progressive neural damage with little possibility of recovery.

Geriatric patients without stroke may have similar abnormalities as stroke patients since they commonly have severe cerebrovascular disease. Both a central and a peripheral neurogenic aetiology can be represented in the bowel disturbance. Clinically, the patients present in two groups (Varma et al. 1988), one with a megarectum and faecal impaction and the other showing colonic hypertonicity which may precipitate faecal incontinence if the sphincters are inadequate.

This has been investigated in a group of elderly patients (Fig. 9.1) with chronic constipation who were compared with an asymptomatic group. Proctometrograms were performed to measure initial rectal volume, maximal tolerable volume and rectal compliance. Anal sphincter pressure and reflexes were measured by conventional techniques. There was significant impairment of rectal sensory threshold in the elderly constipated patients.

A third of the patients in the group studied showed a megarectum which probably contributed to rectal impaction and dyschezia (Read and

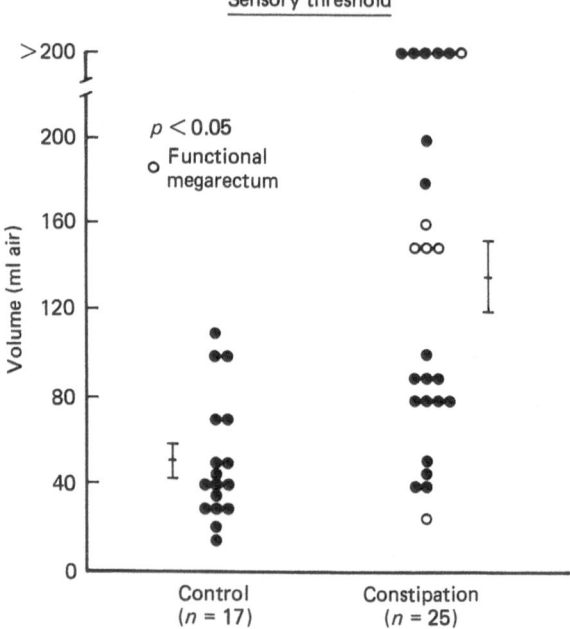

Fig. 9.1. In elderly patients with constipation one group was shown to have severely disturbed sensory function and an increased compliance (5 had a functional megarectum). A second group, not shown, had reduced compliance (mean 5.5 ± 0.5 ml/cm H_2O; normal 8.7 ± 0.4) ($p < 0.01$) and a reduced mean tolerable volume of 350 ± 28 (normal 509 ± 19) ($p < 0.01$). (Reproduced with permission from Varma et al. (1988).)

Abouzekry 1986). Two-thirds showed the opposite and had a significant reduction of maximal rectal volume and rectal compliance to the point of extruding the measuring balloon. There was no difference in the sphincter length and the rectosphincteric responses. Some patients had an absent or prolonged pudendo-anal reflex indicating delay in neural transmission through the S2, S3 and S4 segments of the spinal cord or its efferent supply to the pelvic floor. Oro-anal transit times were prolonged mainly due to rectal stasis.

The classification of two main groups presenting with chronic constipation, one with a functional megarectum and possible megacolon and the other with a hypertonic irritable bowel type of syndrome, similar to that observed in young patients, is compatible with a central lesion allowing escape of two separate spinal cord patterns of activity. Both groups appear to suffer additionally from defects of anorectal proprioception, probably mediated by receptors in the striated muscle of the pelvic floor or in the pararectal tissues. Anorectal sensory deficits (Read et al. 1985) may also compromise the sampling reflex involved in defaecation (Duthie 1975). The patients are best treated by suppositories to empty the rectum, high-fibre diets and the prokinetic agent cisapride, which improves smooth muscle tone in the hypotonic form, or by drugs such as mebeverine which relax smooth muscle activity in the hypertonic form.

Spinal Lesions

Spinal Cord Injury

Spinal cord injury leads to faecal incontinence in the phase of spinal shock. Classically, the resting anal canal pressure is low (Meunier and Mollard 1977) and the anal reflex is absent at this stage, but is the first reflex to return in the recovery phase (Riddoch 1917; Pedersen et al. 1978). Faecal incontinence is later followed by intractable constipation, often associated with the development of an acquired megacolon and megarectum.

Guttman (1970) and Connell et al. (1963) and later Meshkinpour et al. (1985) found that motility returned to the pelvic colon after a phase of inhibition during the period of spinal shock. The pelvic colon then develops greater motor contractions than the proximal colon, reversing the normal motility gradient. There is some doubt as to whether these contractions are peristaltic, since the distal bowel is only occasionally emptied spontaneously and the clinical picture has some of the elements of a pseudo-obstruction.

Meshkinpour and colleagues (1983) also found a marked absence of gastro-colic reflexes after spinal cord injury. The colon exhibits non-propulsive segmentation contractions which lead to a functional obstruction. At an early stage the colon shows an increased compliance and dilates. Many patients need suppositories and enemas to empty the lower bowel and find it preferable to continuous constipation with bypass incontinence. With improved general care and survival of spinal cord injury patients, late problems of bowel dysfunction are often encountered (Guttman 1973).

To improve bladder function and regain control over bladder emptying, Brindley introduced implantable electrodes with a system of radio frequency stimulation of the sacral nerve roots which carry the motor pelvic parasympathetic nerves to the bladder (Brindley et al. 1982). Since the pelvic parasympathetic nerves are also distributed to the left colon and anorectum, this implant promotes stimulation of the distal bowel as well as the bladder (Fig. 9.2). Peristaltic contractions of the entire left colon are evoked by stimulation of the sacral parasympathetic outflow S2, S3 and S4. The effects are maximal with S3

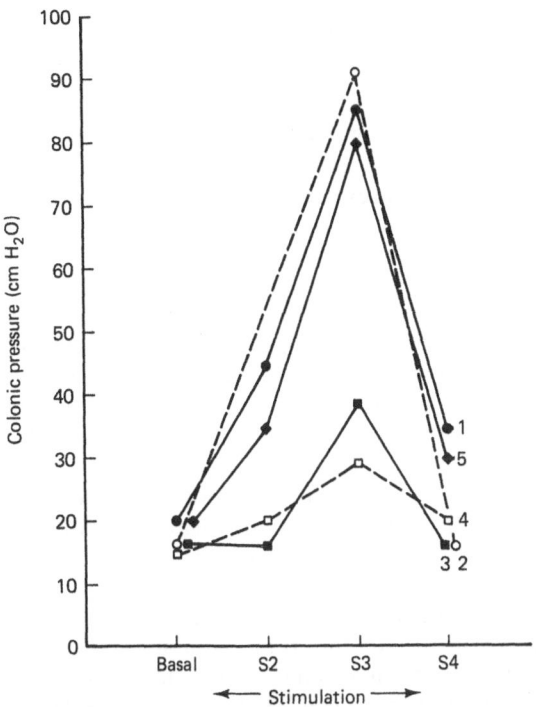

Fig. 9.2. Maximal pressure response in the sigmoid colon (cm H_2O pressure) in response to stimulation of sacral anterior nerve roots S2, S3 and S4 sequentially in 5 paraplegic subjects, compared with basal figures in response to the activation of an implanted Brindley stimulator. (Reproduced with permission from Varma et al. (1986).)

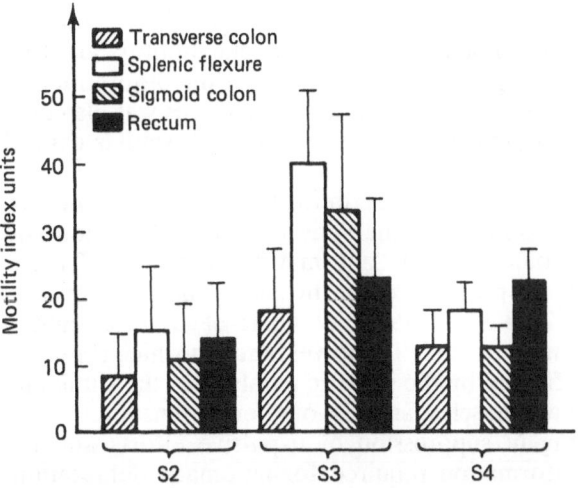

Fig. 9.3. Mean motility indices in the transverse colon, splenic flexure, sigmoid colon and rectum after individual sacral root stimulation. The S3 root produces the greatest response at the splenic flexure, while S4 produces a marked rectal pressure rise. (Reproduced with permission from N. R. Binnie et al. (1990) Motility effects of electrical anterior sacral nerve root stimulation of the parasympathetic supply of the left colon and anorectum in paraplegic subjects. *Journal of Gastrointestinal Motility* 2:12–17.)

stimulation and are most intense at the splenic flexure (Fig. 9.3) with the motility response gradually decreasing in the distal colon. These contractions are propulsive and promote emptying. S4 effects are greater on the anorectum but they also contract the pelvic floor and tend to be obstructive in nature. However the effects on the pelvic floor may be important in maintaining continence. The effect of S2 stimulation is weak but always above basal levels (Varma et al. 1986).

The Brindley stimulator is presumed to produce these effects by acting directly on the parasympathetic innervation, and by relaying impulses to nerve endings in the left colon and rectum, but the effect might equally follow the activation of a pacemaker in the left colon. The colon is thought to have several pacemaker sites throughout its length with a dominant site residing in the left colon below the splenic flexure (Christensen et al. 1974).

Spinal injuries above the level of the conus medullaris isolate the brain and higher centres from local control which is maintained by independent activity of nerve cells in the sacral spinal cord. Low injuries affect the end of the spinal cord at the S2, S3 and S4 level and annul independent activity of cells in this area. Whatever the level of the lesion, all injuries tend initially to have faecal incontinence but later the lack of motility of the left colon in both groups leads to intractable constipation. Weber et al. (1985) suggested that the pons was a possible supraspinal area for control of colonic and anorectal motility, and that when pontine control was lost the differentiation between high and low spinal lesions was also lost, resulting in a tendency towards a similar clinical state.

High lesions theoretically should allow preservation of the innervation of the distal colon and should lead to "automatic" evacuation. This is more pronounced in the case of bladder function (Klein et al. 1969; Wyndale et al. 1985) and is rarely possible for bowel function which is further affected by the somatic paralysis of the trunk and limb muscles, and loss of afferent sensation resulting in suppression of expulsive efforts and the information required for automatic defaecation. Rectal sensation to balloon distension is lost in both high and low lesions, and is felt as a vague abdominal discomfort rather than localized to the low pelvis or perineum (Frenckner and Ihre 1976a, b).

Many spinal injury patients learn to predict when the rectum and bladder are nearing maximum distension by recognizing the signs and features of autonomic dysreflexia (Crawford and Frankel 1971; Lindman et al. 1980) such as pounding headache, hypertension, hemifacial sweating or even piloerection in one forearm. Some have been successful in using these manifestations as reliable indicators of the need for bowel or bladder emptying. Changes in electrical resistance of the skin surface have also been used in such predictions. Most patients gradually develop severe constipation, occasionally associated with overflow faecal incontinence requiring stimulant drugs, repeated enemas, suppositories and manual evacuation.

Paraplegic subjects show a marked delay in oroanal transit, mainly due to prolonged colonic transit (Menardo et al. 1984). The maximal rectal capacity and compliance is increased in proctometrograms and is accompanied by a loss of sensory awareness of the distending balloon (Barnes and Lennard-Jones 1985). Absence of the cortical somatosensory evoked potentials suggests complete cord transection.

Electrophysiology studies show an intact pudendo-anal reflex arc when the lesion is above the level of the first lumbar vertebra, the conus medullaris is spared and therefore there is no peripheral nerve conduction defect (Binnie 1990). There is a normal MUPD and a normal cauda equina conduction velocity. A normal sacral reflex arc confirms the integrity of the efferent nerves and is important in selecting patients for a Brindley neuroprosthetic device to aid micturition and defaecation (Brindley et al. 1982).

A delayed pudendo-anal reflex latency (Table 9.1) suggests inter alia damage at the level of the conus medullaris and thus a low lesion. Some of these patients have delayed cauda equina conduction as tested by direct stimulation over the lumbosacral nerve roots and recording the ensuing electrical events in the external anal sphincter. The pudendo-anal reflex may be absent or delayed, indicating either complete or partial damage respectively. The mean motor unit potential duration is prolonged by reinnervation of the sphincters and pelvic floor (Bartolo et al. 1983). Direct examination shows a reduced maximal resting pressure and an x-ray proctogram shows a widened anorectal angle. Patients with high lesions may show the same changes despite having an intact S2, 3 and 4 arc and a degree of spontaneous EMG activity at rest in the anal sphincter, suggesting that higher influences other than the intact sacral reflexes are required to maintain normal resting tone in the striated muscle part of the anal sphincter.

A summary of tests done for high and low lesions is given in Table 9.1, with the reservation

Table 9.1. Investigations performed in 79 spinal cases[a]

Investigation	Upper	Lower	Patients mean/range	Control mean/range
Oral anal transit time	Both prolonged		10.4 (3.5–25 days)	3.5 (2–4.5 days)
Faecal water centres	Both reduced		57% (48%–63%)	67% (58%–74%)
Anal sphincter length	Unaffected		2.7 (2–4) cm H_2O	2.5 (2–4.5) cm H_2O
Maximum resting pressure	"Normal"	Reduced	60 (50–85) cm H_2O	95 (70–130) cm H_2O
Pudendo-anal reflex	Unaffected high lesion	May be absent in low lesion	37.4 (284–46 ms)	38 (31–45 ms)
MUPD external sphincter	Normal	Prolonged	5.3 (4.7–10.6 ms)	4.6 (4–6.8 ms)
Cauda equina conduction velocity	Normal	Prolonged	68 (58–76 m/s)	57 (46–69 m/s)
Somatosensory evoked potentials from anus to cortex	Absent	Absent	Not recordable	78 (65–88 ms)
Anorectal angle on x-ray	At first normal	Wide angle	107 (85–130°)	87 (78–105°)

[a] Upper motor neurone lesions: tetraplegia (C3–8), 20; paraplegia, 26. Lower motor neurone lesions: lumbosacral abnormalities, 23; spina bifida, 5; sacrococcygeal, 5.

that many of the patients with high or low lesions ultimately show the same defects. However, the value of the tests is threefold:

1. Those which assess the severity of the physiological disturbance: oro-anal transit is a useful indicator of the extent of colonic motor function impairment. Measurement of small bowel transit (Bond et al. 1975) allows a corrected caeco-anal transit but since small bowel transit is only on average 3.5 hours compared with the many days of caeco-anal transit, in practice the oro-anal measurement is the one most often used (Hinton et al. 1969). The faecal moisture is assessed by comparing the weight of aliquots of wet and dried stool. Since water absorption occurs during transit and is roughly proportional to it, the extent of the change of the faecal moisture may be used to assess the degree of constipation (Eastwood et al. 1984). In spinal injury patients this may fall from the normal moisture of around 70% to 55% in severe cases with difficulty in faecal evacuation (Binnie et al. 1988a).

2. Those indicating deranged bowel control. An important clinical indicator of low lesions affecting the conus medullaris is the absence of reflex contraction of the external anal sphincter. Sphincter pressure has often been reported as normal in paraplegia (Denny-Brown and Robertson 1935). The mean resting pressure measured in the anal canal can be low in both high and low lesions in the initial spinal shock phase. Thereafter, the mean resting pressure tends to settle above 60 cm H_2O for high lesions, as a result of the continued contraction of the internal sphincter

made possible through continuing activity in the myenteric nerve plexus and from continued reflex activity of the external sphincter ani (Gowers 1877). Pressures recorded with modern transducers, however, show that these tend to be reduced below the normal range, and may fall further, below the 60 cm H_2O necessary for the control of continence in low level lesions as a result of the paralysis of the external sphincter, which contributes approximately 20% of the maximum resting pressure (Bennett and Duthie 1964).

3. Differentiation between high and low lesions may be initially possible on a proctometrogram. Patients with a high lesion have a hypertonic response (White et al. 1940) while patients with lesions involving the sacral spinal cord or cauda equina exhibit a hypotonic response. As a result of loss of afferent impulses reaching higher centres because of the cord transection and chronic distension, high level lesions subsequently become hypotonic like the low lesions.

Connell et al. (1963) found that the resting and stimulated motility of the pelvic colon was also diminished in patients with high cord transection but was significantly increased in those with low cord lesions. It is often not feasible to use this information in diagnosing individual patients.

The majority of patients with paraplegia respond to cisapride, a prokinetic agent, which enhances motility by redressing the balance of the autonomic nervous system tone in favour of parasympathetic stimulation to the bowel (Binnie et al. 1988a). It reduces the oro-anal transit time and increases the frequency of defaecation in 10 paraplegic patients without producing diarrhoea or continuous incontinence. Cisapride also reduces the maximal rectal capacity and decreases the compliance of the colon through an improvement in rectal tone.

Some patients have a diminished awareness of the stimulus of anorectal contents which is in keeping with an incomplete spinal injury (Binnie et al. 1988b). The reduction of filling sensation results in sudden urgency of defaecation if the rectum fills before an awareness of this is appreciated. Rectal filling promotes relaxation of the internal sphincter and the consequences of this are faecal soiling. The internal anal sphincter particularly relaxes reflexly in the presence of distension by rectal contents (Gowers 1877). The volume of rectal contents necessary to produce this may be less than the volume at which the rectal sensation is registered and the need for defaecation appreciated.

Using biofeedback techniques the patient can be trained to use the relaxation produced by balloon distension of the rectum to reinforce voluntary control and reflexes (Constantinides and Cywes 1983). This allows time to contract the external sphincter to offset the fall in pressure due to relaxation of the internal anal sphincter, thus avoiding soiling and incontinence. During training, when manometry shows a fall in anal canal pressure (Engel et al. 1974), the patient tries to oppose impending rectal evacuation by voluntary contraction of the external anal sphincter (Cerulli et al. 1979). Biofeedback training can be successful in partial lesions when the patient can voluntarily contract his muscles and restore the pressure necessary for bowel control (Wald 1981). The volume of the rectal balloon is gradually reduced to a level that can be perceived by the subject. Over the course of a few weeks he should acquire a more normal limit for rectal sensation before defaecation and can dispense with the device at a point at which he has the assurance of greater sphincter control.

Cauda Equina

Cauda equina lesions are often incomplete and differ greatly in their effect on bowel function. The sacral parasympathetic fibres run with the anterior sacral nerve roots and may be damaged as one or several of the roots are compressed in their vertical course in the spinal canal before emerging through the sacral foramina. The arrangement of the roots and their accompanying parasympathetic

fibres favours partial rather than complete involvement by compression or traction. Some roots may be spared even in severe lumbosacral injuries as it is rare to have actual severance of the entire cauda equina. Both the parasympathetic innervation to the sphincter and the motor innervation

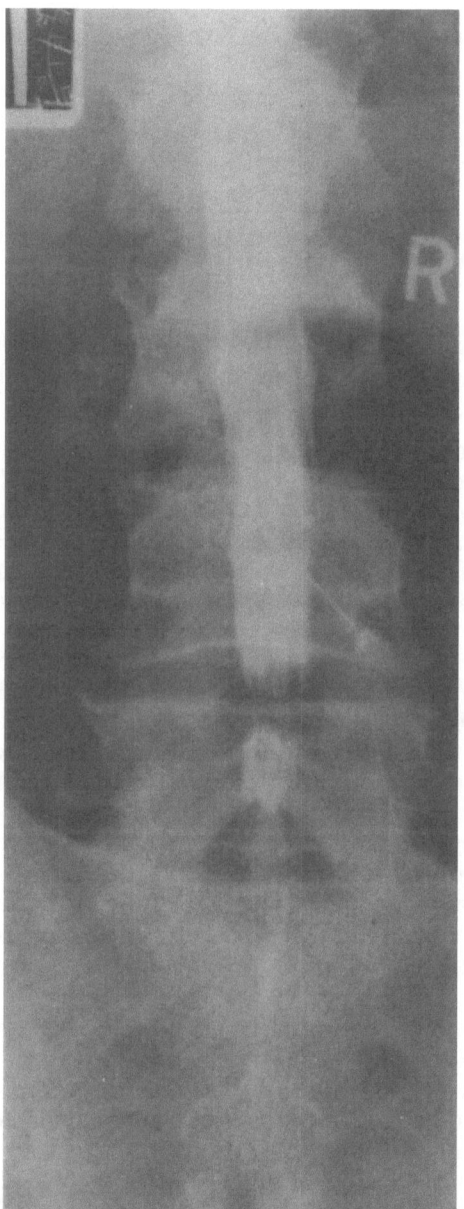

Fig. 9.4. Filling defect in a myelogram from a patient with a central lumbar protrusion. The patient had a reduced maximal anal resting pressure, a prolonged pudendo-anal reflex latency and a delayed cauda equina conduction velocity following stimulation over LV1 but not LV4, thus localizing the lesion to between these vertebral levels.

of the anorectum and pelvic floor may thus escape the more severe problems which occur at the slightly higher level of the conus medullaris. There may be preservation of some sensory awareness of rectal distension but this may have an abnormal quality as a dysaesthesia. Other causes of the cauda equina syndrome include pressure lesions from prolapsed intervertebral discs, lumbosacral fractures and haematomas.

Central lumbar disc protrusion (Fig. 9.4) causes compression of nerve roots as the spinal cord ends at the lower limit of the first lumbar vertebra. The lower the level of the lesion, the greater is the incidence of faecal incontinence because of the compression of S2, S3 and S4 roots. Damage at this site would cut off most of the nerve supply to the pelvic viscera (so that the bladder is affected as well as the bowel), pelvic floor and external sphincters. The sensory loss to the skin is restricted to the saddle area and may be asymmetrical because of the varying nerve root involvement. The reflex contraction of the external anal sphincter is lost. The mean internal anal sphincter resting pressure is usually low (Meunier and Mollard 1977). Paralysis of the external sphincter through loss of the S2, S3 and S4 contribution also contributes to the reduction in the overall mean resting pressure. The proctosphincteric (recto-anal inhibitory reflex) reflex is present, though the relaxation of the internal sphincter provoked by rectal distension is deeper and lasts longer (Frenckner 1975).

The barrier to incontinence requires a sphincter response of approximately 60 cm H_2O, and reduction below this level increases the likelihood of faecal soiling. There is also an increased maximal tolerable rectal volume with increase of compliance as measured by the proctometrogram (White et al. 1940). The latency in the cauda equina nerve conduction times following skin stimulation over LV1 and LV4 sites is detected by the EMG response to the external anal sphincter (Swash and Mathers 1988). This shows:

1. Conduction delay or complete absence of response when an electrical stimulus is administered at the LVI, with a normal LV4 conduction if the lesion is between the sites of stimulation. The spinal latency ratio will be increased:

$$\frac{\text{latency to external anal sphincter after stimulation at L1}}{\text{latency to external anal sphincter after stimulation at L5}}$$

(after Snooks and Swash 1984)

2. In asymmetric lesions one side may have its innervation response retained and thus partial preservation of its function and nerve conduction.

3. The test may also be used to observe any recovery in instances where the initial appraisal erroneously suggested a complete cauda equina lesion due to a compression haematoma, oedema or temporary bony compression, or from displaced vertebral fractures which have undergone early reduction.

An electrical stimulus of the order of 750 to 1000 volts is given as a shock impulse over 100 μs directly over the LV1 and LV4 skin. The conduction time and velocity of the impulses are calculated from the distance between the stimulation site at LV1 and LV4 and the difference in the latency times to the external anal sphincter EMG response.

Occasionally during investigation of patients with faecal incontinence the electrophysiological features of cauda equina lesions emerge in patients with no clinical signs of cauda equina disease (Snooks et al. 1985). If the anal reflex is absent in patients with anorectal incontinence, it suggests a spinal lesion and merits further neurological investigation, including myelography to localize potentially surgically remediable lesions.

Measurement of the mean motor unit potential duration gives an indication of reinnervation in individual cases of the cauda equina syndrome. Because the proctometrogram only gives secondary information about sensory awareness to distension and may be abnormal due to the degree of rectal dilatation or megarectum already present, electromucosal sensitivity is a better determinant for defective sensation and conduction in the afferent neural pathway from the rectum. Somatosensory testing can be used to check the afferent pathways from the sacral and lumbar sensory root levels to the cortex and may be absent or delayed in cauda equina lesions. By varying the level at which the skin stimulus is applied to the sacral and lumbar region, an indication may be obtained of the site of the lesion according to the arrival or absence of impulses initiated in the lumbosacral region, recognized at a cortical level with scalp electrodes. Repeat examination may show a degree of recovery indicating the presence of a partial lesion. Patients with a cauda equina syndrome are prone to constipation as well as faecal incontinence, which may in fact be an overflow incontinence.

It is not uncommon for some of these patients with cauda equina syndrome to develop a partial or complete rectal prolapse. When faecal incontinence is the dominant problem, and the pelvic floor can be shown to retain some innervation, postanal repair is the treatment of choice.

Developmental Anomalies of the Spine

Spina bifida patients have the features of a severe cauda equina lesion with lower limb paralysis and loss of sphincter control of the bowel and bladder. Spina bifida occulta is not so readily recognizable and poses a diagnostic difficulty due to the general nature of the symptoms. There is usually a latent period between a normal childhood and the appearance of symptoms in late adolescence. Furthermore, the bladder complaints tend to be more severe than the bowel symptoms which are often overlooked.

The anomalies producing features of both bowel and bladder disturbance have been described as spinal dysraphism, which is the failure of fusion of the spinal arches which normally mature to protect the soft tissues of the spinal cord and roots at the lumbar and sacral levels. Whether the clinical features result from the bony deformity or associated malalignment and tethering of the nerve roots or a failure of development of the distal cord is not known. It is difficult to determine the exact nature of the soft tissue deformity which is probably responsible for the lack of neurological control. There is no doubt, however, that the bony deformity serves as a guide to the bowel or bladder involvement and is strongly associated with symptoms (Alva et al. 1967). It is difficult to explain the late onset of symptoms when the structural deformity has obviously been present since birth. It has been suggested that the symptoms are precipitated by unrecognized neurogenic damage during childbirth or by toxic factors such as alcohol (Fidas et al. 1989).

Furthermore, there is no correlation between the bony defect and a single neurological abnormality. The degree of traction on nerve roots or compression from associated lesions such as lipomas and dermoids appears to determine the nature of the abnormality (James and Lassman 1981).

The single most useful investigation of patients with the fully established syndrome causing intractable constipation is radiological examination of the lumbosacral area, especially of L4 to L5, to determine the state of fusion of the bony arches. If three normal sacral segments are not seen on a child's x-ray, the likelihood of development

symptoms as a result of failed neurological maturation is high.

The severity of the problem in patients with comparable arch defects also varies widely. Patients with severe bony defects can be symptom free whereas others with minimal bony abnormality have severe symptoms (Fidas et al. 1987). A myelogram may reveal root tethering in such cases.

In symptomatic patients, anorectal assessment is directed at external sphincter function and motility in the distal colon, which show a low resting pressure and a megarectum with faecal retention respectively. The common end result of faecal soiling and frank incontinence is due to sphincter incompetence and loss of sensory conduction. The maximum squeeze and cough pressures are reduced or absent, while the internal sphincter relaxes in the presence of rectal distension through a preserved recto-anal inhibitory reflex allowing faecal soiling to occur. The pudendo-anal reflex is absent or has a prolonged latency. Decreased sensory awareness can be measured by the proctometrogram which shows a raised maximal capacity, rectal distension and increased compliance. There may also be variable cauda equina nerve conduction defects depending upon the extent of the lesion (Fig. 9.5).

Sometimes, instead of pelvic floor paralysis, there is outlet obstruction or anismus. It is possible that in the incontinent group the efferent motor fibres to the pelvic floor are damaged while in the anismus group there is a sensory nerve abnormality of the pelvic floor muscles through the motor neurones in Onuf's nucleus which increases the contractile activity (Onuf 1901).

Fidas et al. (1989) came to the conclusion, when considering spina bifida occulta and its associated urodynamic abnormalities, that these were not directly related to anomalous bone growth per se and suggested abnormal development of the tail bud in early gestation. It is perhaps in this area that an explanation might be found for the severe constipation of young women who have no radiological bony structural abnormality in their distal spine. Their constipation is severe and intractable, necessitating enemas, suppositories and purgatives after the failure of all simple measures such as a high-fibre diet and stool softners. The colonic problems interfere with their work, their careers and their social lives. The pudendo-anal reflex is absent in some or grossly delayed in others, which tends to suggest a conus medullaris anomaly (Varma et al. 1988). The condition has been strongly associated with concomitant urinary evacuation problems (Bannister et al. 1988).

colectomy with ileorectal anastomosis which affords relief of symptoms, but this should only be done if sphincter function is normal.

Spinal Cord Disease

The commonest spinal cord disease causing bowel dysfunction is multiple sclerosis, and constipation in this disease can equal the severity of the "constipation of young women syndrome", but faecal incontinence may be equally distressing. The diagnosis of multiple sclerosis may be clinically obvious but occasionally the first presentation is with bowel symptoms. The increasing constipation has been attributed to diminished colonic motility (Glick et al. 1982) and absent postprandial stimulation of the sigmoid colon but a secondary megacolon may also supervene. Rectal prolapse is not uncommon especially if there is pelvic floor paresis. Pudendo-anal reflex is lost if the conus is involved but this is a rare finding. As the condition worsens there is a severe loss of sensation of rectal filling which can be detected on a proctometrogram.

Confirmation of the spinal involvement and the presence or absence of afferent sensation can be determined directly by electromucosal sensitivity tests or by tests of afferent conduction upwards through the spinal cord to cortical levels.

A few patients with normal sphincter control have been treated by surgery for the megacolon by a subtotal colectomy and ileosigmoid anastomosis. Two patients with severe constipation in our series were treated in this manner. Two years later, one requested an ileostomy because of progressive faecal incontinence. The other has a satisfactory result thus far. Three other multiple sclerosis patients without a secondary megacolon have been treated conservatively with cisapride with clinical improvement.

Poliomyelitis which affects the anterior motor neurones of the spinal cord was formerly a condition which caused serious bowel problems and it still does so in some parts of the world, notably Africa, India and the Far East. Bowel symptoms are commonly the result of a severe attack which paralyzes the abdominal musculature. This results in defaecation impairment due to inability to raise the intra-abdominal pressure necessary for expulsion through an otherwise paralysed pelvic floor.

Conduction in the spinal cord may be abnormal in the diabetic patient but the more dominant picture is that of an autonomic or peripheral neuropathy (Battle et al. 1980).

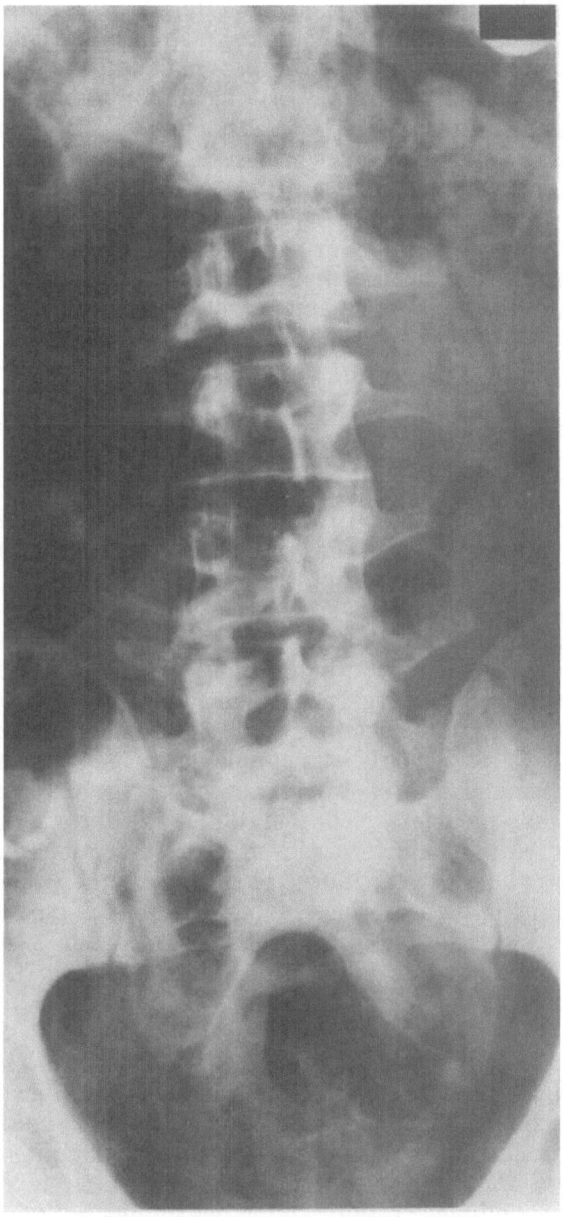

Fig. 9.5. Spina bifida occulta and partial sacral agenesis causing a variable picture of bowel upset. The sphincter pressure was reduced as the motor component of the lesion was detectable at stimulation over LV1, and caused by the dysraphism at the lumbar level. A sensory component was caused by the sacral agenesis and was in turn associated with a gross megarectum.

Other investigations in the same group of patients have sought anomalous secretion of prolactin, varying disturbance of oestrogen or progesterone or even a visceral autonomic neuropathy. Many of these young women come to subtotal

The Effect of Spinal Anaesthesia and Other Anaesthetic Agents

Local anaesthetic agents may be injected into the spinal canal either intradurally or extradurally (epidural anaesthesia). In each type the sensory anaesthesia and paresis produced follows the level to which the local anaesthetic is instilled and is commonly intended to affect the thoracic cord so that the abdomen and lower thoracic area as well as the lower limbs will have sensory and motor loss.

The effect on bowel function resembles the acute stage of spinal cord injury since the distal sympathetic outflow is paralysed and the unopposed parasympathetic stimulation of the vagus produces hypermotility in both the small and proximal large intestine. The mean resting pressure in the anal canal falls as a result of paralysis of the external anal sphincter (Frenckner and Ihre 1976b).

An advantage of epidural anaesthesia is that it may be used to produce restricted anaesthesia for lower abdominal procedures such as Caesarean section and some bowel and bladder operations. The motility effects of blockade of the sacral parasympathetic innervation include periods of atony at suture lines during surgery and hypermotility on recovery.

Reversal of neuromuscular blocking agents by anticholinesterase drugs also requires careful consideration in relationship to colonic motility because of their effects on anastomoses. The normal intracolonic pressure is much higher than in the stomach, jejunum and ileum and may rise to as much as 30–90 cm H_2O. Anticholinesterase agents used to reverse neuromuscular blockade potentiate cholinergic activity in the gut and have been incriminated as a cause of anastomotic breakdown (Bell and Lewis 1968). Rises in colonic pressure may equal the diastolic blood pressure, rendering the anastomosis ischaemic for short periods. Atropine given prior to neostigmine does not reliably reverse the rise in intracolonic pressure (Wilkins et al. 1970).

Anticholinesterase agents have conversely been used for the stimulation of colonic motility, both in paralytic ileus (Marsden and Williamson 1939) and to relieve the faecal stasis and intractable constipation (Catchpole 1969) of pseudo-obstruction and idiopathic megacolon. The physiological effect on the colon in these patients is predominantly one of hypomotility. Marker studies show a very protracted slow transit form of constipation (Preston and Lennard-Jones 1986).

Spina bifida occulta must be excluded by radiology of the lumbosacral spine and other diseases of the spinal cord and neuropathies by appropriate clinical examination. Some of these patients have their symptoms improved by a combination of prostigmine anticholinesterase stimulation of the colon and a sympathicolytic drug such as a beta blocker (Neeley and Catchpole 1971).

Catecholamines secreted into the circulation are known to be inhibitory to colon motility since one of the rarer but accepted features of phaeochromocytoma is severe and intractable constipation.

Nerve Lesions

The commonest nerve lesions are to fibres from the S2, S3 and S4 roots which supply the pelvic floor and external anal sphincter muscle as well as the striated muscle of the urethral sphincter. The pudendal nerve is susceptible because its length and extrapelvic course effectively tether it at the ischial spine before returning to the pelvis to supply the external anal sphincter and the striated portion of the external urethral sphincter muscle. It is particularly susceptible to damage in its terminal portion where it supplies the external anal sphincters (Neill et al. 1981). The fibres to the urethral sphincter are even more susceptible due to their longer course. Early EMG studies and muscle biopsies suggested a neuropraxial type of denervation disorder (Parks and Swash 1979; Beersiek et al. 1979) of the pudendal nerve. The descending perineum results in damage to the fibres which supply the pelvic floor from S2, S3 and mainly S4 directly on its superior surface. This may follow lifelong straining at stool but in female patients the onset may be as a result of nerve traction at parturition (Kiff et al. 1983; Snooks et al. 1984). In both aetiologies neurogenic faecal incontinence results. In the descending perineum syndrome, this follows a previous period of gross constipation associated with straining which in turn produces a descent of the pelvic floor (Fig. 9.6). This can be measured in centimetres by measuring the downward movement of the perineum during a Valsalva manoeuvre. As much as 4 cm of movement may be detected and a descent of more than 0.5 cm or a 13% increase imposes traction forces on the distal part of the pudendal nerve. This in turn leads to nerve damage, and denervation can be confirmed by single fibre density electromyography and also by delayed conduction in the terminal section of the pudendal nerve. The conduction of this portion of the nerve

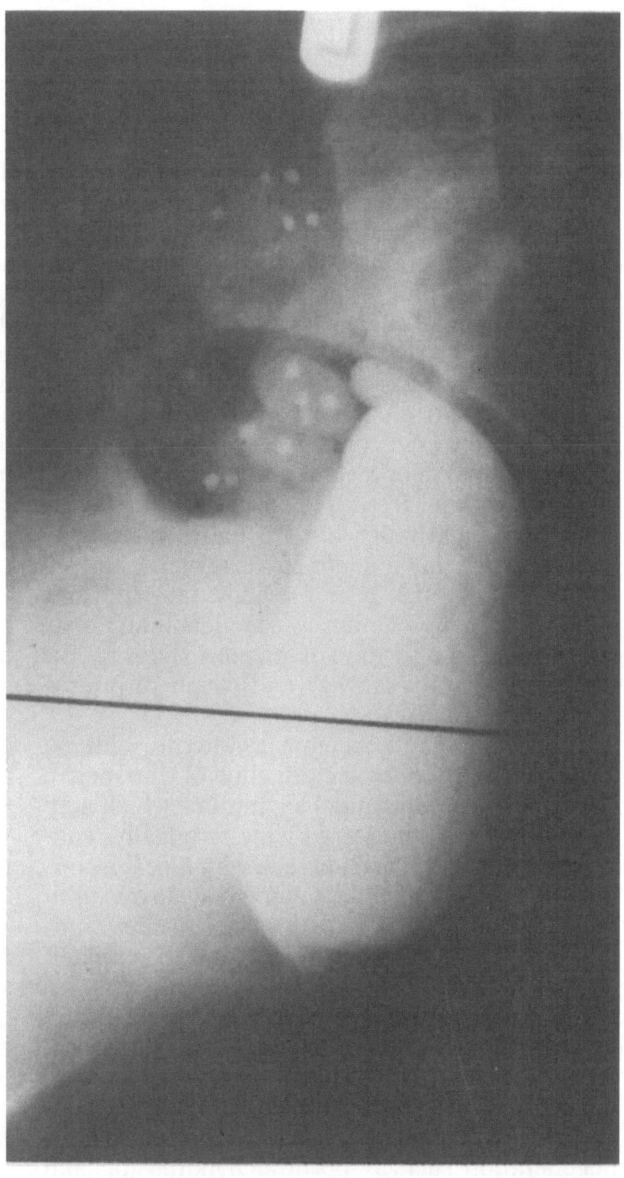

Fig. 9.6. X-ray proctogram of patient with descending perineum syndrome. The normal acute anorectal angle is undone and there is descent of the perineum (and rectum) below the pubococcygeal line. The transit markers which are present recorded a gross delay in the colonic transit time.

may be tested by transrectal stimulation using a finger-glove electrode devised by Brindley for electro-ejaculation and adapted for this purpose by Snooks and Swash (1985). Snooks and his co-workers (1984) have shown that a stretch neuro-pathy occurs in childbirth during the second stage of labour. Serious nerve lesions of the pelvic floor were strongly associated with such problems as disproportion and forceps delivery. In the major-ity spontaneous recovery was the rule, but the more severe the lesion, the greater the chance of faecal incontinence.

In others with multiparity and recurrent mild damage, faecal incontinence may supervene a decade or so later, perhaps because of a general failure of pelvic floor function and continuing denervation and muscle atrophy. The bowel problem is often accompanied by a significant incidence of genuine stress incontinence of urine. These patients can be investigated by studying the latency of pelvic floor reflexes such as the urethro-sphincteric reflex and the pudendo-anal reflex which are prolonged. The mean motor unit poten-tial duration is also prolonged, which indicates that there has been a denervation injury. There is a diminution in the maximal resting pressure of the external anal sphincter. Although the puborectalis muscle is innervated separately from the external anal sphincter, both are affected in neurogenic incontinence of obstetric causation and by the descending perineum syndrome (Henry et al. 1985).

The pudendal nerve supplying the external anal sphincter is more often and more severely affected. Denervation of the puborectalis muscle alters the anorectal angle which becomes wider because of the weakness in the pull of the puborectalis sling (Fig. 9.6). The anorectal angle can be corrected by postanal repair. Since many of these patients are elderly, nonoperative methods have been explored. In our experience, physiotherapy produces minimal change (Varma 1987).

Another approach harnesses the pudendo-anal reflex arc and uses electrical stimulation to send trains of stimuli on the afferent side from the genital nerve to the conus medullaris and on the efferent side to puborectalis and the external anal sphincter muscle. Repeated electrical stimulation of the pudendal reflex arc results in reflex contraction of the puborectalis and external sphincter muscle. This reflex is not readily fatigued and repeated stimulation improves the maximum resting pressure, the position of the pelvic floor at rest and the voluntary squeeze and cough responses (Binnie et al. 1988c).

The descending perineum syndrome with its tendency to produce neuropathy of the pelvic floor may be accompanied by anismus which may explain why so many patients originally constipated because of anismus end with faecal incontinence. The continued straining may also lead to rectal prolapse which in turn causes further diminution of sphincter competence due to repeated anal dilatation.

Diabetes may cause a similar neuropathy of the pelvic floor (Henry and Swash 1985) with faecal incontinence. A co-existent intestinal autonomic neuropathy may contribute to slow transit constipation with other systemic aspects of autonomic degeneration such as postural hypotension and diminished afferent sensory conduction problems in the spinal cord. This may also be seen in tabes dorsalis and suspected in multiple sclerosis and degenerative diseases such as subacute combined degeneration of the cord associated with vitamin B_{12} deficiency.

A denervation injury of the parasympathetic nerve supply of the distal colon has been proposed for the dysfunction which may follow anterior resection of the rectum (Catchpole 1988). Hysterectomy is a common operation involving deep pelvic dissection known to have relatively few sequelae, but its urological consequences such as bladder dysfunction are well known (Green et al. 1973). Urologists accept that the motor nerves of the bladder are at risk in the presacral region, in

the lateral wall of the pelvis and close to the bladder neck. The possibility of interruption of the parasympathetic innervation of the left colon and rectum which is derived from the same S2, S3 and S4 sacral segments as supply the bladder is less well known (Varma and Smith 1985). Parasympathetic fibres run from the sacral roots to the inferior hypogastric plexus and then pass forwards to innervate the bladder and rectum. Others run upwards and outwards from the pelvis to the left colon as far as the distal transverse colon. This innervation is thought to be of paramount importance in the coordinated contractions of the smooth muscle of the distal colon. The same fibres also carry sensory information from these viscera. It is conceivable that damage during pelvic surgery could result in functional disorders of the evacuation of the distal colon. During hysterectomy the inferior hypogastric or pelvic plexus which in the female is placed on either side of the rectum, uterus, vaginal fornix and posterior aspect of the urinary bladder and extends into the base of the broad ligament of the uterus is susceptible to injury.

Thirty-four post-hysterectomy patients have been investigated in Edinburgh, all with severe constipation dating from the time of their operation. They were collected over a five-year period from many different clinicians during a time in which as many as 5000 women had hysterectomies performed in the hospitals of this medical centre.

The sigmoid colon motility exhibited hypomotility (Smith et al. 1990). Rectal compliance and sphincter function remained relatively normal, suggesting that the damage to the plexus and its distributing fibres is mainly at a higher level in the pelvis and that the fibres supplying the rectum at a lower level mainly escape (Fig. 9.7). This motor abnormality can be shown to follow both abdominal and transvaginal hysterectomy; in the latter case a traction injury is the most likely cause.

The parasympathetic motor fibres passing upwards from the pelvis to the left colon run close to the inferior mesenteric artery which is often tied in aortic aneurysm surgery. The ligation of this vascular bundle may result in an ileus further promoted by any extensive retroperitoneal dissection and haematoma accumulating postoperatively. Spinal ischaemia can result in severe ileus following aneurysm surgery. Somatic features such as lower limb paralysis and a sensory loss accompany functional disturbances such as bowel hypomotility and unawareness of bowel and bladder filling. This combination is due to spasm or damage to the exclusive blood supply to the lower thoracic and lumbar spinal cord which is derived from the arteria radicularis magna which

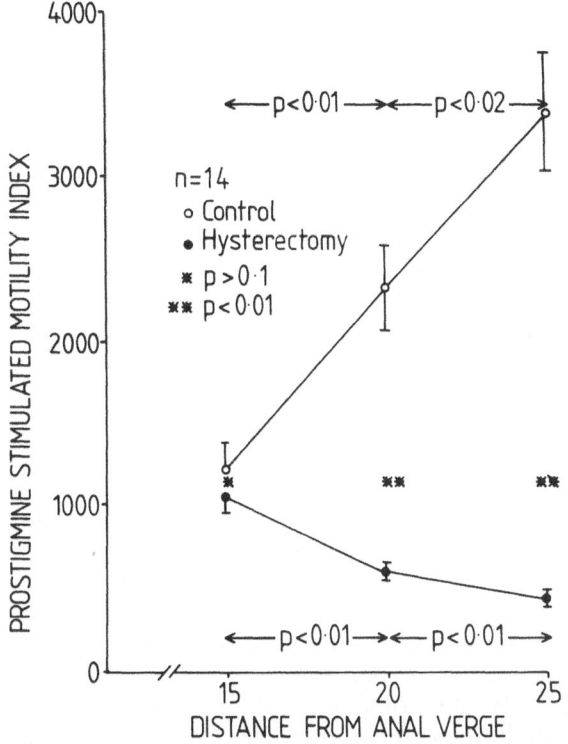

Fig. 9.7. Pressure response as mean motility indices after cholinergic stimulation of the colon with prostigmine, in control cases and controls: records at 25, 20 and 15 cm. There is a normal downward propulsive gradient with reversal to an "obstructive" type of gradient, with the highest pressures recorded distally in post-hysterectomy cases. (Reproduced with permission from A. N. Smith et al. (1990). Disordered colorectal motility in intractable constipation following hysterectomy. *British Journal of Surgery* 77.)

has its origin from the aorta between T8 and L4 (Suh and Alexander 1939). A more specific form of pseudo-obstruction follows the retroperitoneal spread of tumours known as Ogilvie's syndrome, but mechanical causes of obstruction should always be excluded.

Ganglion Cell Lesions

Infantile Hirschsprung's disease is considered elsewhere in this volume. When the condition presents in the adult slow transit constipation is always present and motility tests show little response to food and cholinergic stimulation. Patients who were undetected in the neonatal period sometimes reach adolescence or even adult life with minimal symptoms until an eventual decompensation of bowel motor function occurs. The features generally fit the hypothesis of a short segment of aganglionosis beyond which active bowel has managed to expel faecal contents but the local motility failure is difficult to prove. The proctosphincteric reflex is dependent on intact ganglion cells. The aganglionic defects of Hirschsprung's disease is confirmed by an absence of this recto-anal inhibitory reflex. Elicitation of this reflex is more valid than diagnosis by a mucosal biopsy to check cholinesterase activity in short segment Hirschsprung's cases as the site of the ganglionic anomaly may be easily missed on random biopsy. Many such patients have a gross secondary proximal dilatation of the colon and the preferred treatment in these late cases is a subtotal colectomy with ileosigmoid anastomosis, which leaves enough colonic reservoir function for water absorption to protect against faecal incontinence and removes the dilated, now inert, colon.

Similar aganglionic bowel with a gross megacolon and hypomotility and a patchy dilatation in other areas of the gastrointestinal tract occurs in South America in the infective disorder known as Chagas' disease resulting from infection by *Trypanosoma cruzi*. Absence of the proctosphincteric reflex may be found as well as multiple motor defects culminating in pseudo-obstruction. An absent proctosphincteric reflex is not invariably indicative of the aganglionosis of Hirschsprung's disease and Chagas' disease. The reflex may be missing in patients with an irradiation anorectal injury which has destroyed ganglion cells. Damage to ganglion cells may also follow the use of chemotherapeutic agents such as vincristine, and some formerly used anthelminthic agents had a sinister reputation for producing a lasting pseudo-obstruction.

Ganglion cell function is very sensitive to hypoxia and ischaemia. Maturation arrest may affect wide areas of the myenteric plexus and it is now recognized that the gut may be affected widely by familial, sporadic and developmental abnormalities presenting as a visceral neuropathy. The familial group may be associated with mental retardation and calcification of basal ganglia. Sporadic cases are mainly degenerative and result from noninflammatory and inflammatory agents, among which Chagas' disease and cytomegalovirus are included. The most common representative of the developmental visceral neuropathies is undoubtedly Hirschsprung's disease but various less well known forms exist, often more severe in their expression, with mental retardation presenting with a myenteric plexus disorder in which some neurones exist but are few in number and are argyrophilic. Other forms exist and are associated with neurofibromatosis and the multiple endocrine adenoma syndrome MEA2 (for review see Schuffler 1988).

Table 9.2. Comparison of manometric and rectal motility parameters in control subjects and post colo-anal sleeve anastomosis cases showing lowered rectal sensory threshold, low maximal tolerable volume and a diminished amplitude of rectosphincter reflex inhibition which combine to create increased frequency of defaecation and a sensation of obstruction

Parameter	Control (n=8)	Colo-anal sleeve anastomosis (n=8)	Statistical significance
Maximum resting anal pressure (cm H_2O, mean±s.e.m.)	104 ± 5.3	54 ± 7.7	P<0.01
Maximum anal squeeze pressure (cm H_2O, mean±s.e.m.)	159 ±15.9	120 ±17.9	P>0.1
Sphincter length (cm, mean±s.e.m.)	3.5± 0.25	2.4± 0.21	P<0.02
Amplitude of rectosphincteric reflex (cm H_2O, mean±s.e.m.)	47.5± 3.1	12.5± 5.6	P<0.02
Rectal sensory threshold (ml air, mean±s.e.m.)	58 ±10.2	29 ± 3.8	P<0.05
Maximal tolerable rectal volume (ml H_2O, mean±s.e.m.)	504 ±29	120 ±25	P<0.01
Rectal pressure at maximal tolerable volume (cm H_2O, mean±s.e.m.)	73 ± 2.8	86 ± 6.5	P>0.1

From Varma and Smith (1986a) with permission.

The ganglion cells of the bowel may be damaged by abuse of anthracene purgatives in the so-called cathartic colon syndrome. The typical brown staining of the mucosa is seen at sigmoidoscopy and there may be a dilatation of the lumen throughout the colon and rectum. These patients have mixed investigative details, the most outstanding of which is a slow transit form of constipation. They not uncommonly have other features among which are anismus, the descending perineum syndrome, a secondary megacolon or megarectum, an absent rectosphincteric reflex indicating damage to ganglion cells or nonpropulsive left colon and rectum as a result of colonic inertia.

Radiation damage is not only mucosal but may be accompanied by a visceral neuropathy, both of which contribute to frequent stools and dysmotility. The main physiological abnormality is a loss of internal anal sphincter function, with a significant reduction in the mean anal canal resting pressure and sphincter length (Varma and Smith 1986a). The rectosphincteric reflex may be absent with the maximal tolerable volume and the compliance severely reduced. The change in rectal compliance correlates well with the symptoms and the degree of mucosal abormality seen at sigmoidoscopy. Excised specimens show marked abnormalities of the myenteric plexus (Varma et al. 1985). Chronic irradiation of the colon and rectum usually follows radiotherapy for carcinoma of the cervix, prostate or urinary bladder. The symptoms are distressing, with urgency of micturition, frequency of defaecation and faecal incontinence. Although the mucosal damage may be severe with haemorrhage, stricture of the rectum and sigmoid colon and fistulae (Hatcher et al. 1985), studies show an abnormality consistent with damage to smooth muscle and its innervation. These patients can be successfully treated by removal of the damaged segment of the colon and restoring intestinal continuity by anastomosing the healthy tissue of the transverse or descending colon to the anal canal.

Physiological studies several years after this operation show persistence of some of the preoperative abnormalities such as a low rectal capacity (Varma and Smith 1986b). The persistence of altered sensory awareness and reduced rectosphincteric reflex may follow mucosectomy of the anorectal junction (Table 9.2). This in turn promotes a failure of the normal reflex responses of the internal sphincter to rectal ampullary distension and may explain the rectal obstructive symptoms. This is in contrast to the reinnervation and return of rectosphincteric reflex following colo-anal anastomosis for nonirradiated tissue, and indicates that the functional abnormality caused by the addition of radiation to the surgical management of carcinoma of the rectum is a lesion of ganglion cells.

Miscellaneous

Anismus is the severe constipation resulting from an obstruction syndrome of the anorectum. This is due to paradoxical contraction of the pelvic musculature during defaecation straining, instead of the relaxation seen in normal subjects (Preston and Lennard-Jones 1985). The cell bodies of the neurones controlling the striated muscle of the pelvic floor lie in the S2, S3 and S4 ventral horns in neurones known as Onuf's nucleus. Percutaneous concentric needle EMG of the external anal sphincter and puborectalis muscle shows continuous electrical activity of these muscles at rest.

The diagnosis of anismus is established by the loss of inhibitory reaction to straining with pronounced increase in motor activity in the pelvic floor, delayed left colonic transit and poor rectal filling with a high intrarectal pressure.

Severe anismus acts as a block to defaecation and straining against the obstruction may cause secondary pathological changes and damage to the anterior rectal wall. In mild cases the anterior rectal wall trauma results in mucoid discharge and abdominal pain but in severer forms rectal intussusception, external prolapse or solitary rectal ulcer result (Womack et al. 1987; Alexander-Williams 1977).

The phenomenon appears to be due to the loss of the normal inhibitory effect on the pelvic floor which follows straining by a pathway as yet unknown (Whitehead and Schuster 1981). This may be central, because EMG-induced biofeedback training (Binnie et al. 1989) can reverse the abnormal phenomenon and correct symptoms. For intractable cases, the alternative of partial muscle division of puborectalis has been practised (Keighley 1988) but could have the danger of inducing prolapse or incontinence. A recently reported method is the use of locally injected Botulinum A toxin (Hallan et al. 1988) which produces local paralysis of the puborectalis muscle of the pelvic floor.

Neural mechanisms are involved in the pain of proctalgia fugax, inflammatory lesions and advanced tumours; while the effects of tumours are mainly local, these are occasionally due to metastatic involvement of central nerve pathways or of the spinal cord.

References

Alva J, Nendeloff AI, Schuster MM (1967) Reflex and electromyographic problems associated with faecal incontinence. Gastroenterology 53:101–105

Alexander-Williams J (1977) Solitary ulcer syndrome of the rectum. Its association with occult rectal prolapse. Lancet i:170–171

Bannister JJ, Lawrence WT, Smith A, Thomas DG, Read NW (1988) Urological abnormalities in young women with severe constipation. Gut 29:17–20

Barnes PRH, Lennard-Jones JE (1985) Balloon expulsion from the rectum in constipation of different types. Gut 26:1049

Bartolo DCC, Jarratt JA, Read MG, Donnelly TC, Read NW (1983) The role of partial denervation of the pubo-rectalis in idiopathic faecal incontinence. Br J Surg 70:664–667

Battle WM, Snape WJ Jr, Alair A, Cohen S, Brainstem S (1980) Colonic dysfunction in diabetes. Gastroenterology 79:1217

Beersiek F, Parks AG, Swash M (1979) Pathogenesis of anorectal incontinence: a histometric study of the anal canal musculature. J Neurol Sci 42:111–127

Bell CMA, Lewis CB (1968) The effects of neostigmine on integrity of ileorectal anastomosis. Br Med J iii:587

Bennett RC, Duthie HL (1964) The functional importance of the internal sphincter. Br J Surg 51:355–357

Binnie NR (1990) The effect of spinal cord injury on the motor function of the human colon, and the assessment of the influence of implanted radiofrequency stimulating electrodes. MD Thesis, University of Edinburgh

Binnie NR, Creasey GH, Edmond P, Smith AN (1988a) The action of cisapride on the chronic constipation of paraplegia. Paraplegia 26:151–158

Binnie NR, Edmond P, Smith AN (1988b) Defining constipation: the value of ano-rectal function tests. Gastroenterol Int 1/1:338

Binnie NR, Kawimbe BM, Smith AN (1988c) Use of the dorsal genital nerve pudendoanal reflex for the treatment of neurogenic faecal incontinence. Gut 29/5:A734

Binnie NR, Kawimbe BM, Papachrysostomou M, Smith AN (1989) EMG feedback as a domiciliary treatment of anismus. Gut 30:A714

Bond JH, Levitt MD, Prentiss R (1975) Investigation of small bowel transit in utilising pulmonary hydrogen (H_2) measurements. J Lab Clin Med 85:546–555

Brindley GS, Polkey CE, Rushton DN (1982) Sacral anterior root stimulators for bladder control in paraplegia. Paraplegia 20:365–381

Burks TF (1988) Actions of pharmacological agents on gastrointestinal function. In: Kumar D, Gustavsson S (eds) Gastrointestinal motility. Wiley, Chichester, pp 272–290

Catchpole BN (1969) Ileus: use of sympathetic blocking agents in its treatment. Surgery.66:811–820

Catchpole BN (1988) Motor pattern of left colon before and after surgery for rectal cancer: possible implications in other disorders. Gut 29:624–630

Cerulli MA, Nikoomanesh P, Schuster MM (1979) Progress in biofeedback conditioning for faecal incontinence. Gastroenterology 76:742–746

Christensen J, Anuras S, Hauser RL (1974) Migrating spike bursts and electrical slow waves in the cat colon: effect of sectioning. Gastroenterology 66:240–247

Condon RE, Cowles VE, Schulte WJ, Frantzides CT, Mahouney JL, Sarna SK (1986) Resolution of post-operative ileus in humans. Ann Surg 203:574–581

Connell AM, Frankel H, Guttman L (1963) The motility of the pelvic colon following complete lesions of the spinal cord. Paraplegia 1:93–115

Constantinides CG, Cywes S (1983) Faecal incontinence: a simple pneumatic device for home biofeedback training. J Paed Surg 18:276–277

Crawford JP, Frankel HL (1971) Abdominal "visceral" sensation in human tetraplegia. Paraplegia 9:153–158

Denny-Brown D, Robertson G (1935) An investigation of the nervous control of defaecation. Brain 58:256–310

Duthie HL (1975) Dynamics of the rectum and anus. Clin Gastroenterol 4:467–477

Eastwood MA, Brydon WG, Baird JD et al. (1984) Faecal weight and composition, serum lipids, and diet among subjects aged 18 to 80 years not seeking health care. Am J Clin Nutr 40:628–634

Engel BT, Nicoomanesh P, Schuster MM (1974) Operant conditioning of rectosphincteric responses in the treatment of faecal incontinence. N Engl J Med 290:646–649

Fidas A, Galloway NTM, Varma JS, McInnes A, Chisholm GD (1987) Sacral reflex latency in acute retention in female patients. Br J Urol 59:311–313

Fidas A, MacDonald HL, Elton RA, McInnes A, Wild SR, Chisholm GD (1989) Prevalence of spina bifida occulata in patients with functional disorders of the lower urinary tract and its relation to urodynamic and neurophysiological measurements. Br Med J 298:357–359

Frenckner B (1975) Function of the anal sphincters in spinal man. Gut 16:638–644

Frenckner B, Ihre T (1976a) Function of the anal sphincters in patients with intussusception of the rectum. Gut 17:147–151

Frenckner B, Ihre T (1976b) Influence of autonomic nerves on the internal anal sphincter in man. Gut 17:306–312

Glick ME, Meshkinpour H, Haldeman S, Batta NN, Bradley WE (1982) Colonic dysfunction in multiple sclerosis. Gastroenterology 83:1002–1007

Gowers R (1877) The automatic action of the sphincter ani. Proc R Soc London 26:77–84

Green TH Jr, Meigs JV, Ulfelder H, Reder N, Aalder J, Abeler V (1973) Urological complications of radical Wertheim hysterectomy: incidence, etiology, management and prevention. Obstet Gynecol 115:81–87

Guttmann L (1970) Spinal shock and reflex behaviour in man. Paraplegia 8:100–110

Guttmann L (1973) Spinal cord injuries: comprehensive management and research. Blackwell Scientific, Oxford, pp 430–445

Hallan RI, Williams NS, Melling J, Waldron DJ, Womack NR, Morrison JFB (1988) Treatment of anismus in intractable constipation with botulinum A toxin. Lancet ii:714–717

Hatcher PA, Thomson HJ, Ludgate SN, Small WP, Smith AN (1985) Surgical aspects of intestinal injury due to pelvic radiotherapy. Ann Surgery 201:470–475

Henry MM, Swash M (1985) Pathogenesis and clinical features. In: Henry MM, Swash M (eds) Coloproctology and the pelvic floor. Butterworth, London, pp 222–227

Henry MM, Snooks SJ, Barnes PRH, Swash M (1985) Investigation of disorders of the anorectum and colon. Ann R Coll Surg Eng 67:355–360

Hinton JM, Lennard-Jones JE, Young AC (1969) A new method for studying gut transit times using radio-opaque markers. Gut 10:842–847

James CCM, Lassman LP (1981) Spina bifida occulta. Academic Press, London

Keighley MRB (1988) Surgery for constipation. Br J Surg 75:625–626

Kiff ES, Barnes PB, Henry MM (1983) Prolongation of pudendal nerve latency and increased single fibre density in patients with chronic defaecation straining and perineal descent. Br J Surg 70:681

Klein SJ, Omieczynski T, Reingold IM, Bors E (1969) Urinary tract disease in spinal cord injury patients. Paraplegia 7:6–9

Lindman R, Joiner E et al. (1980) Incidence and clinical features of autonomic dysreflexia in patients with spinal cord injury. Paraplegia 18:285–292

Marsden PA, Williamson EG (1939) The use of prostigmine methylsulfate in the prevention of post-operative intestine atony and urinary bladder retention. Surg Gynecol Obstet 69:61

Menardo G, Fazio A, Marangi A et al. (1984) Large bowel transit in patients with paraplegia. Gut 25:1314

Meshkinpour H, Nowroozi F, Glock ME (1983) Colonic compliance in patients with spinal cord injury. Arch Phys Med Rehab 64:111–112

Meshkinpour H, Harmon D, Thompson R, Yu J (1985) Effects of thoracic spinal cord transection on the colonic motor activity in rats. Paraplegia 23:272–276

Meunier P, Mollard P (1977) Control of the internal anal sphincter (manometric study with human subjects). Pflügers Arch ges Physiol 370:233–239

Neely JT, Catchpole BN (1971) The restoration of alimentary tract motility by pharmacological means. Br J Surg 58:21–28

Neill ME, Parks AG, Swash M (1981) Physiological studies of the anal sphincter musculature in faecal incontinence and rectal prolapse. Br J Surg 68:531–536

Onuf B (1901) On the arrangement and function of cell groups of the sacral region of the spinal cord in man. Arch Neurol 3:387–412

Parks AG, Swash M (1979) Denervation of the anal sphincter causing idiopathic faecal incontinence. Roy Coll Surg Edinb 24:94–96

Pedersen E, Harving H, Klenmar B, Torring J (1978) Human anal reflexes. J Neurol Neurosurg Psychiatry 9:813–818

Preston DM, Lennard-Jones JE (1985) Anismus in chronic constipation. Dig Dis Sci 30:413–418

Preston DM, Lennard-Jones JE (1986) Severe chronic constipation of young women: "idiopathic slow transit constipation". Gut 27:41–48

Read NW, Abouzekry L (1986) Why do patients with faecal impaction have faecal incontinence? Gut 27:283–287

Read NW, Abouzekry L, Read MG et al. (1985) Anorectal function in elderly patients with faecal impaction. Gastroenterology 89:959–966

Reynolds BJ, Elliasson FG (1977) Colonic pseudo-obstruction in patients. Ann Neurol 1:305

Riddoch G (1917) The reflex function of the divided spinal cord in man, compared with those associated with less severe lesions. Brain 40:264–402

Rothnie NG, Kemp-Harper RA, Catchpole BN (1963) Early post-operative gastrointestinal activity. Lancet ii:64–67

Rutter KRF (1974) Electromyographic changes in certain pelvic floor abnormalities. Proc R Soc Med 67: 53

Schuffler MD (1988) Chronic idiopathic pseudo-obstruction. In: Kumar D, Gustavsson S (eds) An illustrated guide to gastrointestinal motility. Wiley, Chichester, pp 383–399

Smith AN, Varma JS, Binnie NR, Maria Papachrysostomou (1990) Disordered colorectal motility in intractable constipation following hysterectomy. Br J Surg (in press)

Snooks SJ, Swash M (1984) Perineal nerve and transcutaneous spinal stimulation: new methods for the investigation of the urethral striated sphincter musculature. Br J Urol 56:406–409

Snooks SJ, Swash M (1985) Nerve stimulation techniques. A. Pudendal nerve terminal motor latency and spinal stimulation. In: Henry MM, Swash M (eds) Coloproctology and the pelvic floor. Butterworth, London, pp 112–124

Snooks SJ, Setchell M, Swash M, Henry MM (1984) Injury to innervation of pelvic floor sphincter musculature in childbirth. Lancet ii:546–550

Snooks SJ, Swash M, Henry MM (1985) Abnormalities in peripheral and central nervous conduction in ano-rectal incontinence. J R Soc Med 78:294–300

Suh TH, Alexander L (1939) Vascular system of the human spinal cord. Arch Neurol 41:659–687

Swash M, Mathers S (1988) Abnormalities of anorectal function. In: Kumar D, Gustavsson S (eds) An illustrated guide to gastrointestinal motility. Wiley, Chichester, pp 447–459

Varma JS (1987) Observations on some motility disturbances of the human distal bowel and pelvic floor. MD Thesis, University of Edinburgh

Varma JS, Smith AN (1985) Abnormalities of colorectal function in intractable constipation following hysterectomy. Gut 26:581–582

Varma JS, Smith AN (1986a) Anorectal function following colo-anal sleeve anastomosis for chronic radiation injury to the rectum. Br J Surg 73:285–289

Varma JS, Smith AN (1986b) Function of the anal sphincters after chronic radiation injury. Gut 27:528–533

Varma JS, Smith AN, Busuttil A (1985) Correlation of clinical and manometric abnormalities of rectal function following chronic radiation injury. Br J Surg 72:875–878

Varma JS, Binnie, NR, Smith AN, Creasey GH, Edmond P (1986) Differential effects of sacral anterior root stimulation on anal sphincter and colorectal motility in spinal man. Br J Surg 73:478–482

Varma JS, Bradnock JH, Smith RC, Smith AN (1988) Constipation in the elderly: a physiological study. Dis Colon Rectum 31:111–115

Wald A (1981). Biofeedback therapy for faecal incontinence. Ann Intern Med 95:146–149

Weber J, Denis P, Mihout B et al. (1985) Effect of brain stem lesion on colonic and anorectal motility. Study of three patients. Dig Dis Sci 30:419–425

White JC, Verlot MG, Ehrentheil O (1940) Neurogenic disturbances of colon and their investigation by colonmetrogram: preliminary report. Ann Surg 112:1042–1057

Whitehead WE, Schuster MM (1981) Behavioural approaches to the treatment of gastrointestinal motility disorders. Med Clin Am 65:1397–1411

Wilkins JL, Hardcastle JD, Mann CV et al. (1970) Effects of neostigmine and atropine on motor activity of ileum, colon and rectum of anaesthetised subjects. Br Med J i:793–794

Wilson JP (1976) Post-operative motility of the large intestine in man. Gut 16:689–692

Womack NR, Williams NS, Mist JH, Morrison JFB (1987) Anorectal function in the solitary rectal ulcer syndrome. Dis Colon Rectum 30:319–323

Wyndale JJ, De Sy WA (1985) Correlation between the findings of a clinical neurological examination and the urodynamic dysfunction in children with myelodysplasia. J Urol 133:638–640

10 · Rectal Prolapse, Solitary Rectal Ulcer Syndrome and Haemorrhoids

M. M. Henry

Rectal Prolapse

Introduction

Although the occurrence of complete prolapse is not usually associated with major constitutional disturbance, the condition can be a source of significant disability, particularly in the presence of anal sphincter and pelvic floor weakness. Detailed and complex investigation of patients with prolapse is generally unnecessary but the study of pelvic floor and anal sphincter function may be useful in predicting function after the prolapse has been successfully corrected by surgery.

Clinical Assessment

Examination of the patient will be principally directed towards the anorectum but a general examination should always be encouraged to assess general fitness and to exclude co-existent pathology. The detection of a complete prolapse is not always a simple process. Frequently patients find they are unable readily to produce the prolapse in the left lateral position; hence it may only be apparent after defaecation or on straining, with the patient adopting a squatting position. Once prolapse is observed it is important to delineate complete from partial or mucosal prolapse since the management of the two conditions differs substantially. The clinical distinctions between the two are listed in Table 10.1 and illustrated in Figs. 10.1 and 10.2. On inspection of the perineum abnormal pelvic floor descent may be observed and measured with the perineometer. The anus may be seen to gape with gentle retraction.

Table 10.1. Clinical markers of distinction between rectal mucosal prolapse and complete rectal prolapse

Complete prolapse	Mucosal prolapse
Concentric furrows	Radial grooves
Protrusion up to 40 cm	Protrusion <5 cm
Anus in normal position	Anus everted
Thickness of double rectal wall	Thickness of double mucosa

On digital examination, resting (internal anal sphincter) and squeeze (external anal sphincter) tone may both be markedly diminished. On sigmoidoscopy, the macroscopic appearances of the mucosa of the lower rectum may closely resemble those of acute proctitis with marked inflammation and contact bleeding. These are the appearances of traumatic proctitis, a direct consequence of eventration of the rectal wall and its mucosa. Where doubt exists a biopsy should always be considered.

On proctoscopy, redundant mucosa fills the lumen of the instrument, particularly when the patient is requested to strain. Sometimes the initiation of the prolapse can clearly be seen to arise from the anterior hemicircumference; the so-called anterior mucosal prolapse.

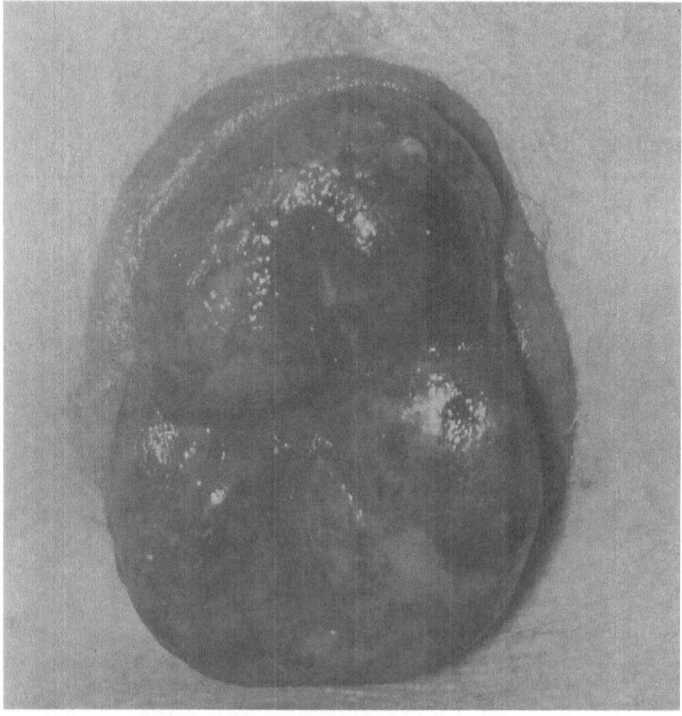

Fig. 10.1. An example of rectal mucosal prolapse.

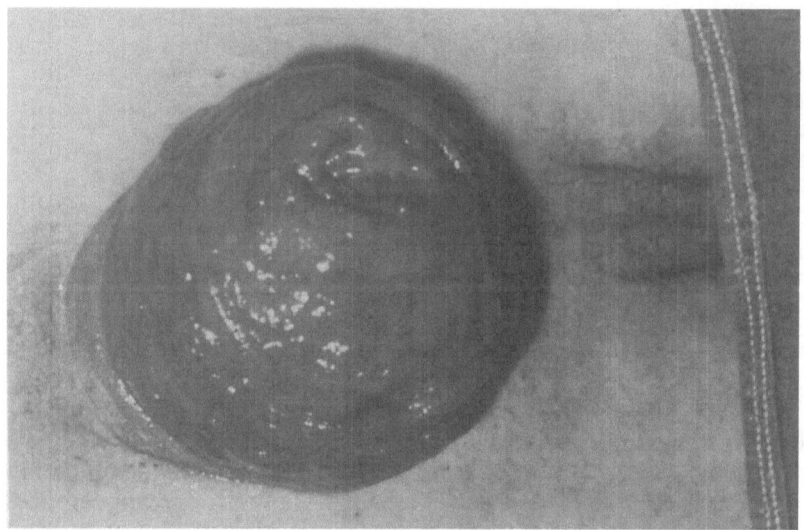

Fig. 10.2. An example of complete rectal prolapse.

Investigations

Proctography

Wherever doubt over the diagnosis exists either simple evacuation proctography (Bartram et al. 1988) or integrated proctography (Womack et al. 1985) will provide valuable information on whether or not there is a prolapse and delineate its anatomy and whether or not the prolapsing sac contains small bowel (enterocoele). Using these techniques it can be clearly seen that complete prolapses commence as an intussuscepting segment in the midrectum approximately 6–8 cm

above the anal canal (Broden and Snellman 1968). The perineum normally lies at a level 2 cm above that of the ischial tuberosities. During defaecation the perineal plane descends up to 3 cm radiologically; descent of greater than 3 cm is abnormal (Bartram et al. 1988; Skomorowska et al. 1988).

Anal Sphincter Function

The treatment of a complete prolapse should be considered with a degree of priority since persistent prolapse may cause sequential traumatic damage to the anal sphincters and pelvic floor; most notably to the internal anal sphincter. The methodology by which the anal sphincters and pelvic floor may be assessed objectively have been dealt with comprehensively in previous chapters.

Manometry

Patients with complete prolapse will usually display evidence of internal anal sphincter weakness; hence resting pressures will be significantly reduced and there may be a reduction in the length of the anal canal. Squeeze pressures may be similarly reduced.

Electromyography (EMG)

EMG evidence of denervation may be demonstrated in the external anal sphincter and pelvic floor muscles in the same manner as in some patients with idiopathic anorectal incontinence. Hence the fibre density may be raised if single fibre EMG techniques are employed (Fig. 10.3). Neill and colleagues (1981) demonstrated that the fibre density was raised in patients with complete rectal prolapse with incontinence but was not raised in those patients with rectal prolapse who were continent. These findings suggest that in some patients the prolapse may be directly related to pelvic floor denervation, but not in others. The aetiopathology in the latter group for the moment remains obscure but may be related to abnormalities in the structure of the supporting fascia; the evidence for this is scanty. If severe denervation of these muscles is found on testing, such patients may remain faecally incontinent after correction of the prolapse and therefore will require pelvic floor surgery as a secondary procedure.

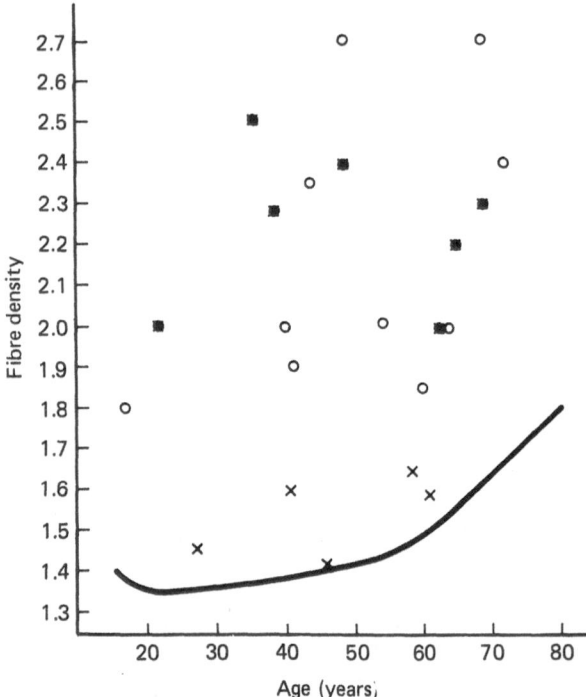

Fig. 10.3. Fibre density measurements from the external anal sphincter muscle plotted against age. The *continuous line* represents fibre density measurements recorded from a control population. O, fibre density in patients with anorectal incontinence alone ■, fibre density in patients with anorectal incontinence and complete rectal prolapse ×, fibre density in patients with complete rectal prolapse *without* anorectal incontinence.

Pudendal Nerve Terminal Motor Latency (PNTML)

Where there is established denervation within the external anal sphincter and pelvic floor muscles, patients may also display prolongation of the latency of the motor unit action potential associated with external anal sphincter contraction in response to electrical stimulation of the pudendal nerve. In patients with abnormal perineal descent the increase in latency has been found to be directly related to the degree of descent (Jones et al. 1987a).

Solitary Rectal Ulcer Syndrome (SRUS)

SRUS is a distinct histological and clinical entity which forms one aspect of the spectrum of functional disorders of the pelvic floor. Histologically the disorder is characterized by obliteration of the

lamina propria by fibrosis and by reorientation of smooth muscle fibres which grow towards the lumen from a thickened muscularis mucosae. Macroscopically the lesion can be identified on sigmoidoscopy as an area of zonal proctitis or as a superficial ulcer 0.5–5.0 cm in diameter and situated on the anterior wall 5–10 cm from the anus. The ulcer may cause profuse bleeding and mucous discharge and a history of excessive straining at defaecation is usual.

Clinical Assessment

The first consideration is the exclusion of malignancy, since the macroscopic appearances of a solitary ulcer on sigmoidoscopy may closely resemble those of an underlying malignancy, particularly if there is oedema of the mucosal edges of the ulcer. A full thickness rectal prolapse may be observed clinically but usually any prolapse is restricted to within the anal canal. Abnormal perineal descent may be present and sphincter tone is frequently reduced (Snooks et al. 1985).

Investigations

Proctography

The use of dynamic proctography (Womack et al. 1985) has resulted in a better understanding of the pathophysiology of SRUS. Womack and collea-

gues (Womack et al. 1987) have demonstrated significantly greater intrarectal pressures during defaecation in patients with SRUS and in 94% of cases this was associated with some degree of rectal prolapse. The prolapsed rectal muscosa becomes hyperaemic or ulcerated. It appears to be a combination of excessive intrarectal pressure during straining and rectal prolapse which causes SRUS. The fact that ulceration has a significantly greater incidence of associated anismus (inability to relax the anal sphincter musculature during straining) may explain why only some patients ulcerate. An earlier study (Mahieu 1986) also demonstrated the relationship between the presence of occult or clinical rectal prolapse and SRUS, the former being present in 79% of their patients. The beneficial effect of rectopexy in those patients with rectal prolapse (occult or clinical) associated with the SRUS (Mahieu 1986) highlights the place of proctography in the investigation of this syndrome.

Electromyography (EMG)

Using conventional EMG it has been shown that in many patients with SRUS there is a failure of inhibition of electrical activity in the pelvic floor muscles during straining and sometimes there may even be recruitment of motor unit activity (Rutter 1974) (Fig. 10.4). Womack and colleagues (1987) demonstrated that in patients with SRUS voiding was accompanied by overactivity of the external

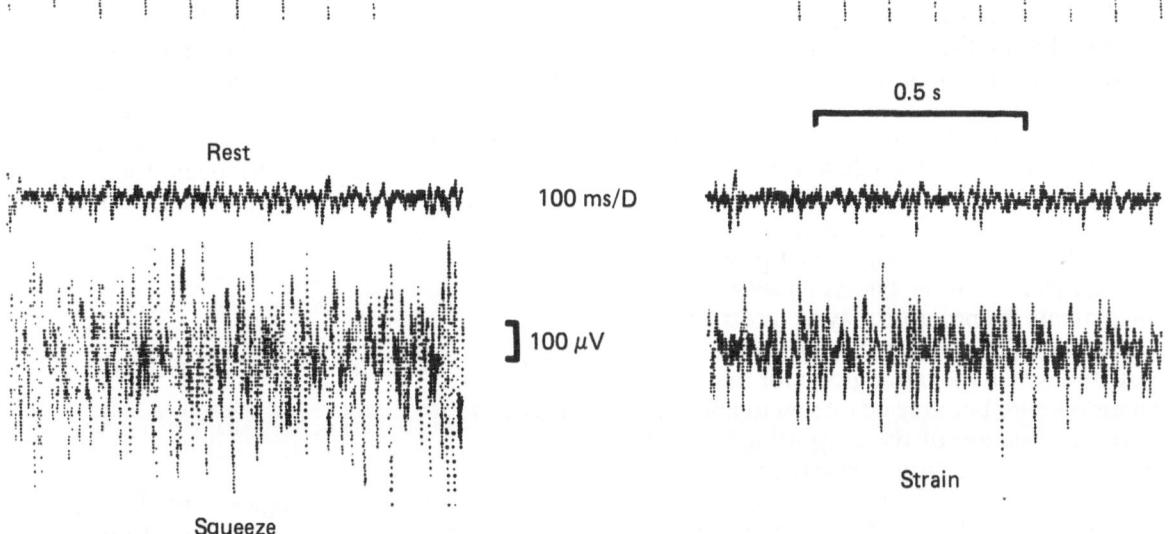

Fig. 10.4. Conventional EMG of puborectalis muscle in patient with solitary rectal ulcer syndrome. During a straining effort there has been marked recruitment of motor activity (i.e. paradoxical contraction) instead of inhibition.

anal sphincter to a median level of 30% of the activity of a maximum voluntary contraction.

The interpretation of paradoxical contraction needs to be made with caution since it is now recognized that this is a relatively non-specific finding. Jones and colleagues (1987b) found that paradoxical contraction on concentric EMG was observed in 76% of patients with simple constipation, 48% of patients with perineal pain and in only 50% of patients with SRUS.

By employing single fibre EMG and nerve stimulation techniques, Snooks and colleagues (1985) demonstrated that, in addition to paradoxical contraction, some patients also displayed evidence of denervation in the pelvic floor muscles. Fifteen of 20 patients with SRUS studied had raised fibre densities and 12 of 20 patients had an increase in their pudendal nerve latencies. The denervation presumably is the consequence of repeated straining, particularly if this is associated with perineal descent (Lubowski et al. 1988).

Haemorrhoids

This common condition has rarely been the subject of detailed scientific study other than in the comparison of different treatment regimens. Thomson (1975) undertook injection studies of the vascular supply and drainage of the anorectum and demonstrated that haemorrhoids were anal cushions richly supplied by vessels with numerous arteriovenous communications. Thomson considered these to be a constant finding in all subjects, but in some patients a lax anal mucosa permitted downward displacement of the anal cushions with all the sequelae commonly associated with haemorrhoids.

Investigations

The Internal Anal Sphincter (IAS)

Hancock and Smith (1975) have shown an increase in IAS activity in some patients with haemorrhoids. Although resting pressures were higher in patients with haemorrhoids than in normal subjects, there was considerable overlap. The pattern of slow wave activity was also reported to be abnormal in some patients in that ultra-slow wave activity was more frequently found in patients with haemorrhoids. Read and colleagues (1982) re-

ported similar findings and also demonstrated that a fall in resting pressure and cessation of ultra-slow wave activity occurred after haemorrhoidectomy.

The role of the IAS in the pathogenesis of haemorrhoids is far from clear. It is possible that the high pressures recorded are a direct consequence of local vascular hypertension in the anal cushions and this would explain why the pressure falls after haemorrhoidectomy.

The External Anal Sphincter (EAS)

Teramoto and colleagues (1981) demonstrated that fibre size was increased in muscle biopsies taken from patients with haemorrhoids and stained with ATPase. This may reflect an increased work hypertrophy as a consequence of straining, a factor long considered to be important in the aetiology of haemorrhoids. More recently Bruck and colleagues (1988) have addressed the problem of whether or not patients with haemorrhoids have denervation in the pelvic floor muscles and found that the fibre density was higher in the haemorrhoid group compared with a control group. The pudendal latencies were increased in patients with haemorrhoids but not to a level which achieved significance. Again, these findings are probably the consequence of a combination of perineal descent and straining.

Prolonged Ambulant Studies

Recently, more physiological home-based prolonged ambulant assessment of anorectal function has been applied to patients with prolapsing haemorrhoids (Waldron et al. 1989). Using microtransducers and surface electrode EMG recordings to monitor rectal and anal sphincter function over a 24-hour period, these authors were able to confirm earlier findings of abnormal internal sphincter motility, seen in static short-term laboratory studies (Hancock and Smith 1975). In addition, marked external sphincter overactivity was evident both during the day and at night, while the rectal motility pattern was normal. This study suggests that rectal motor function is not affected by the presence of prolapsing haemorrhoids, whereas the anal sphincter musculature shows continuous motility abnormalities, even during sleep. Further studies using such techniques may help elucidate the aetiology and long-term consequences of haemorrhoids on anorectal function.

References

Bartram CI, Turnbull GK, Lennard-Jones JE (1988) Evacuation proctography: an investigation of rectal expulsion in 20 subjects without defaecatory disturbance. Gastroint Radiol 13:72–80

Broden B, Snellman B (1968) Procidentia of the rectum studied with cineradiography: a contribution to the discussion of causative mechanisms. Dis Col Rec 11:330–347

Bruck CE, Lubowski DZ, King DW (1988) Do patients with haemorrhoids have pelvic floor denervation? Int J Colorect Dis 3:210–214

Hancock BD, Smith K (1975) The internal sphincter and Lord's procedure for haemorrhoids. Br J Surg 62:833–836

Jones PN, Lubowski DZ, Swash M, Henry MM (1987a) Relation between perineal descent and pudendal nerve damage in idiopathic faecal incontinence. Int J Colorect Dis 2:93–95

Jones PN, Lubowski DZ, Swash M, Henry MM (1987b) Is paradoxical contraction of the puborectalis muscle of functional importance? Dis Col Rec 30:667–670

Lubowski DL, Swash M, Henry MM (1988) Increase in pudendal nerve terminal motor latency with defaecation straining. Br J Surg 75:1095–1097

Mahieu PHG (1986) Barium enema and defaecography in the diagnosis and evaluation of the solitary rectal ulcer syndrome. Int J Colorect Dis 1:85–90

Neill ME, Parks AG, Swash M (1981) Physiological studies of the pelvic floor in idiopathic faecal incontinence and rectal prolapse. Br J Surg 68:531–536

Read MG, Read NW, Haynes WG, Donnelly TC, Johnson AG (1982) A prospective study of the effect of haemorrhoidectomy on sphincter function and faecal incontinence. Br J Surg 69:396–398

Rutter KRP (1974) Electromyographic changes in certain pelvic floor abnormalities. Proc R Soc Med 67:53–56

Skomorowska E, Hegedus V, Christiansen J (1988) Evaluation of perineal descent by defaecography. Int J Colorect Dis 3:191–194

Snooks SJ, Nicholls RJ, Henry MM, Swash M (1985) Electrophysiological and manometric assessment of the pelvic floor in solitary rectal ulcer syndrome. Br J Surg 72:131–133

Teramoto T, Parks AG, Swash M (1981) Hypertrophy of the external and internal sphincters in haemorrhoids: a histometric study. Gut 22:45–48

Thomson WHF (1975) The nature of haemorrhoids. Br J Surg 62:542–552

Waldron DJ, Kumar D, Hallan RI, Williams NS (1989) Prolonged ambulant assessment of anorectal function in patients with prolapsing haemorrhoids. Dis Colon Rectum 32:968–974

Womack NR, Williams NS, Holmfield JHM, Morrison JFB, Simpkins KC (1985) New method for the dynamic assessment of anorectal function in constipation. Br J Surg 72:994–998

Womack NR, Williams NS, Holmfield JHM, Morrison JFB (1987) Pressure and prolapse – the cause of solitary rectal ulceration. Gut 28:1228–1233

11 · The Irritable Colon

D. L. Wingate

The irritable colon is a topic of dubious relevance to a work devoted to measurement in coloproctology, since there is no clear evidence that any such entity can be substantiated by measurement. Even the term itself is fading into obsolescence, and in the UK and North America has been largely replaced by irritable bowel syndrome (IBS), although the French still prefer the term *colopathie fonctionelle*. However, even though eminent authorities such as Christensen (1983) have denied the existence of such a syndrome, it remains obstinately manifest in the form of large numbers of patients who present with symptoms suggestive of colonic or colorectal dysfunction.

There is general agreement that there is a large number of patients who can be distinguished by (a) the absence of evidence of organic colorectal disease and (b) the presence of two or more "cardinal" symptoms; these were defined by Manning et al. (1978) and subsequently confirmed by Kruis et al. (1985) as an erratic bowel habit, a feeling of inadequate evacuation after defaecation, lower abdominal pain temporarily associated with defaecation, abdominal distension, and the presence of mucus in the stool. The condition is chronic, with a tendency to relapse and remission, and is often exacerbated when the patient is subjected to stress. Every clinician with an interest in gastrointestinal disorders is familiar with such patients. The question to be posed in the present context is whether clinical coloproctological measurement has a place in the diagnosis and/or management of the condition. For the research oriented, there is also the question of whether

objective study of such patients is helpful in the elucidation of the (as yet unknown) pathophysiology, or in the design of effective therapeutic strategies.

There is no clear answer to these questions. A number of lines of enquiry have yielded data that are to a greater or lesser extent equivocal.

Hypersensitivity of the Colorectum

The classic studies of Ritchie (1973) showed that balloon distension of the pelvic colon in patients with IBS induced pain. Other workers have reported similar findings, and there are anecdotal accounts of apparent hypersensitivity to the insufflation of air during sigmoidoscopy in these patients. Unfortunately, even if the techniques of distension had been standardized (which has not happened) to allow multicentre studies, such tests do not appear to be diagnostic; the findings in a *single patient*, as opposed to groups of patients, do not have the discrimination which enables the clinician to make a confident diagnosis of a normal or irritable bowel/colon. Statistically significant differences between groups of controls and patients conceal the fact that unless there is a clear discrimination between normal and abnormal values of a variable, such differences are of little value to the clinician who must deal with patients as individuals rather than groups. Nor do most of the studies take into account variables such as intrapatient or interpatient variation; in this field replicate studies are rare.

Electromyographic Abormalities in the Colon and Rectum

Some hope of progress was offered when it was reported by two groups of workers (Taylor et al. 1978; Snape et al. 1977a) that there appeared to be an abnormality of slow activity in the smooth muscle of the sigmoid colon in patients suffering from IBS. However, there was no correlation between the presence of the abnormality – an excess of 3 wave/min activity – and the presence or absence of symptoms. Subsequently, another extensive study (Latimer et al. 1981) failed to confirm these findings.

Evidence of a different type of abnormality was produced when Snape et al. (1978) reported increased rectosigmoid spike activity in IBS patients in response to a meal when compared with healthy controls. In the technique used by these workers, which consisted of recording from a metal clip attached to the sigmoid mucosa, very few muscle spikes were detected (3–10 spikes per 10 minute recording period) and the myogenic origin of the high frequency components of the signal was not proven. Nor has the technique proved to be reproducible by other workers.

Contractile Abormalities in the Colon and Rectum

Contractile activity in the colorectum has been studied in IBS patients by manometry from perfused open tip tubes in the bowel lumen. Using such techniques, increased responsiveness of the colorectum in response to the ingestion of a meal (Snape et al. 1978) or after cholinergic challenge (Snape et al. 1977b) has been reported. These conclusions have been based largely on the calculation of motility indices; these derived values depend upon both the precise nature of the recording system used and the subjective judgement of different investigators as to what constitutes a "pressure wave". Such studies have not produced evidence that manometry can be used to diagnose

the presence of IBS. Other workers (Dinoso et al. 1983) have shown that the value of such studies is largely negated by the considerable intra-individual variability in colorectal motor activity.

Other Directions

The largely negative outcome of studies carried out so far does not disprove the presence of colorectal sensory hypersensitivity or motor inability in IBS. What is clear, however, is that no reliable method for the detection of these abnormalities has yet been devised; they cannot, as yet, be measured. The impetus for such studies derives from the notion that it would be surprising if these abnormalities were not present in IBS given that erratic and uncomfortable defaecation is one of the characteristic features of the condition. The implication of this idea is that IBS is, in fact, a disorder of the colorectum, and that if a lesion exists in this condition, it will be found in the colorectum. In fact there is no objective evidence that this is the case. It has been shown that there is very little correlation between the actual and the perceived location of a stimulus within the lumen of the bowel (Swarbrick et al. 1980). Moreover, pathology upstream from the colon can produce a symptomatology which is similar to IBS; Crohn's disease is, after all, one of the major differential diagnoses.

The change in terminology from "irritable colon" to "irritable bowel" mirrors a change in the perception of the syndrome from a condition localized in the colorectum to a more generalized disturbance of the entire intestine. While objective evidence of the former remains inconclusive, recent studies suggest that there is an associated disorder of the small bowel. Kellow and Phillips reported an increased incidence of clustered contractions in the proximal and distal small bowel of IBS patients (Kellow and Phillips 1987), particularly under cholinergic challenge. Kumar and Wingate (1985) showed that clustered contractions could be evoked in the proximal jejunum of most IBS patients under controlled psychological stress, but not in any controls. Kellow et al. (1987) have shown similar clustered contractions in freely ambulant patients; again, these did not occur in controls. One factor common to all of these studies was the temporal association between the small bowel motor abnormality and the incidence of symptoms. Finally, Trotman and Price showed that monitoring the transit of an isotope marker from ileum to caecum produced a very clear discrimination between IBS patients and controls (Trotman and Price 1986).

It would be foolish, on the basis of these studies, to assert that IBS is exclusively a small bowel motor disorder; it is likely that the whole bowel is affected and that the disorder is sensory as well as motor. What does seem to have been shown is that in the present state of technology, upstream studies in IBS yield more consistent data than downstream studies. Technology is not the only determinant of the outcome; one important factor in the success of the small bowel studies is that the normal motor activity of the small bowel is stereotypic and has been characterized in many studies, while this is not true for the colon. Given our relative ignorance of normal colonic function, the technique of ambulatory monitoring which has been so helpful in the small bowel seems cosiderably less so in the colon.

These new directions of study should eventually lead to standardized diagnostic protocols and to a better understanding of the pathophysiology. That is for the future; for now, it remains true to say that measurement of colorectal function in IBS has little to contribute either to our understanding of the problem, or to the diagnosis and the selection and monitoring of therapies.

References

Christensen JC (1983) In: Christensen JC, Wingate DL (eds) A guide to gastrointestinal motility.

Dinoso UP, Murthy SNS, Goldstein J, Rosner B (1983) Basal motor activity of the distal colon. A reappraisal. Gastroenterology 85:637–642

Kellow JE, Phillips SF (1987) Altered small bowel motility in irritable bowel syndrome is correlated with symptoms. Gastroenterology 92:1885–1893

Kellow JE, Gill RC, Wingate DL (1987) Proximal gut motor activity in irritable bowel syndrome (IBS). Patients at home and at work. Gastroenterology 92:1463

Kruis W, Azpiroz F, Phillips SF (1985) Contractile patterns and transit of fluid in canine terminal ileum. Am J Physiol 249:G264–270

Kumar D, Wingate DL (1985) The irritable bowel syndrome: a paroxysmal motor disorder. Lancet ii:973–977

Latimer PR, Sarna SK, Campbell D, Latimer M, Waterfall W, Daniel EE (1981) Colonic motor and myoelectric activity: a comparative study of normal subjects, psychoneurotic patients and patients with irritable bowel syndrome. Gastroenterology 80:893–901

Manning AP, Thompson WG, Heaton KW, Morris AF (1978) Towards positive diagnosis of the irritable bowel. Br Med J ii:653–654

Ritchie J (1973) Pain from distension of the pelvic floor by inflating a balloon in the irritable colon syndrome. Gut 14:125–132

Snape WJ, Carlson GM, Matarazzo SA, Cohen S (1977a) Evidence that abnormal myoelectric activity produces colonic dysfunction in the irritable bowel syndrome. Gastroenterology 72:383–387

Snape WJ, Carlson GM, Cohen S (1977b) Human colonic myoelectric activity in response to prostigmine and the gastrointestinal hormones. Am J Dig Dis 22:881–887

Snape WJ, Matarazzo SA, Cohen S (1978) Effect of eating and gastrointestinal hormones on human colonic myoelectrical and motor activity. Gastroenterology 75:373–378

Swarbrick ET, Bat L, Dawson AM, Hegarty JE, Williams CB (1980) Site of pain from the irritable bowel. Lancet ii:443–446

Taylor I, Derby C, Hammond P (1978) Comparison of rectosigmoid myoelectrical activity in the irritable colon syndrome during relapses and remissions. Gut 19:923–929

Trotman IF, Price CF (1986) Bloated irritable bowel syndrome defined by dynamic ^{99}Tc bran scan. Lancet ii:364–366

12 · Pseudo-obstruction

P. R. O'Connell

Introduction

The term pseudo-obstruction was introduced by Dudley et al. (1958) to refer to a group of patients with signs and symptoms of acute intestinal obstruction in whom a mechanical cause could not be found. The term was intended (Dudley and Patterson-Brown 1986) to refer to acute or sub-acute colonic dilatation, previously termed "ileus" (Murphy 1896) or "spastic ileus" (Zimmerman 1930) and, more recently, "Ogilvie's syndrome" (Ogilvie 1948). The term has been broadened to include chronic conditions previously known as "chronic ileus" (Faulk et al. 1978a). This has led some authors to specify whether the condition is acute or chronic, and whether it is generalized or confined to the colon (Schuffler et al. 1981; Anuras and Shirazi 1984; Vanek and Al-Salti 1985). Christensen (1986) suggested that, in the absence of a mechanical obstruction, the term ileus refer to an acute, potentially reversible, failure of gastrointestinal flow, whereas pseudo-obstruction refer to a chronic, irreversible and often progressive condition. In this article the broader view is taken and the term pseudo-obstruction is used to mean a clinical syndrome caused by ineffective intestinal propulsion, which may be acute or chronic and may be generalized or confined to one segment of the gastrointestinal tract.

Clinical Presentation

The clinical presentation of pseudo-obstruction usefully divides into acute and chronic, although a degree of overlap may be observed. Acute pseudo-obstruction most commonly affects the large bowel in older patients hospitalized for other illnesses. Chronic pseudo-obstruction affects younger patients and is characterized by a prolonged history, often punctuated by previous investigations and laparotomy.

Acute Pseudo-obstruction

Acute pseudo-obstruction presents with abdominal pain, nausea, vomiting and constipation. On examination the abdomen is distended and tympanic. Abdominal tenderness is usually not marked but a degree of rebound tenderness may be present. The bowel sounds are usually increased (Vanek and Al-Salti 1985). The differential diagnosis includes mechanical obstruction, ischaemic colitis and toxic megacolon. The diagnosis is suggested by the presence of a precipitating medical or surgical condition (Table 12.1) and the absence of an antecedent history of gastrointestinal disease. In a literature review of 400 cases, Vanek and Al-Salti (1985) found an associated surgical condition in 49% of cases and an associated medical condition in 45%. In 6% no

Table 12.1. Acute intestinal pseudo-obstruction: causes

Surgical
Caesarean section
Urological surgery
Orthopaedic surgery
Multiple trauma

Medical
Hypokalaemia
Uraemia
Cardiac failure
Respiratory failure
Drug related

Table 12.2. Chronic intestinal pseudo-obstruction: secondary causes

Diseases involving enteric smooth muscle
Scleroderma
Collagen vascular disease
Muscular dystrophies
Ceroidosis

Neurological diseases
Parkinson's disease
Chagas' disease
Paraneoplastic neuropathy
Achalasia
Hirschsprung's disease

Endocrine diseases
Myxoedema
Diabetes mellitus
Hypoparathyroidism
Phaeochromocytoma
Addison's disease

Pharmacological causes
Phenothiazines
Tricyclic antidepressants
Anticholinergics
Ganglion blockers
Clonidine
Cathartic drugs
Opiates

Miscellaneous
Amyloidosis
Radiation enteritis
Coeliac sprue
Jejunal diverticulosis

cause could be identified, and these were deemed idiopathic.

The pathophysiology of acute pseudo-obstruction is uncertain. Ogilvie (1948) proposed that colonic atony resulted from an imbalance of colonic autonomic innervation with diminished sympathetic activity, leading to relative para-sympathetic overactivity. This hypothesis was based on observations in two patients with retroperitoneal infiltration by tumour. An alternative hypothesis is that sacral autonomic, not lumbar sympathetic, innervation is temporarily interrupted, rendering the distal colon atonic and producing functional colonic obstruction (Vanek and Al-Salti 1985). The mechanism may involve prolonged activation of inhibitory non-adrenergic, non-cholinergic nerves which serve to suppress neuromuscular activity and produce neurogenic ileus. This would be in keeping with the clinical observation that acute pseudo-obstruction often follows lumbosacral or pelvic surgery.

Chronic Pseudo-obstruction

Chronic intestinal pseudo-obstruction may be usefully classified under the headings primary and secondary (Faulk et al. 1978a). Primary pseudo-obstruction, or chronic idiopathic intestinal pseudo-obstruction, defines a group of propulsive disorders of the gastrointestinal tract which have no recognized underlying disease. Secondary pseudo-obstruction defines a condition in which dysfunction of the enteric smooth muscle occurs as part of a multisystem disorder (Table 12.2).

The term chronic idiopathic intestinal pseudo-obstruction (CIIP) was introduced by Maldonado et al. (1970) to describe patients who had recurrent unexplained episodes of intestinal obstruction, diarrhoea, malabsorption and weight loss. Progressive deterioration occurred, with death from malnutrition. At least two types of CIIP exist. In the majority of cases, intestinal pseudo-obstruction is due to abnormalities of intestinal smooth muscle (Murley 1959; Naish et al. 1960; Schuffler and Pope 1977; Faulk et al. 1978b; Anuras et al. 1986a; Rodrigues et al. 1989). As these abnormalities are not confined to the gastrointestinal tract but regularly affect the urinary bladder, ureter and muscles of the eye, the syndrome is also known as visceral myopathy. There appears to be a strong familial incidence, with both autosomal recessive and autosomal dominant inheritance (Christensen 1986). Anuras et al. (1986a) have suggested that the small bowel is relatively spared in the autosomal dominant form and the long-term prognosis is good. By contrast, in the autosomal recessive form, the entire small intestine is affected and the prognosis is poor.

A second group type of familial CIIP has been recognized, characterized by a visceral neuropathy which primarily affects the myenteric plexuses, although a polyneuropathy may occur (Tanner et al. 1976; Schuffler et al. 1978; Roy et al. 1980; Faber et al. 1987). Both familial and sporadic cases of visceral neuropathy causing CIIP have been recorded. Visceral neuropathy has been recorded within a family known to have hereditary visceral myopathy (D. Windgate 1989, personal communication) so that the two conditions may not be mutually exclusive. The extent of visceral neuropathy is variable and, depending on the distribution of gastrointestinal tract involvement, chronic constipation or dysphagia may be prominant symptoms. A working diagnosis of Hirschsprung's disease or oesophageal achalasia is often made before small bowel manifestations become apparent. When this occurs, the more typical clinical picture of recurrent abdominal pain, malabsorption and diarrhoea emerges.

In addition to familial CIIP, sporadic cases occur (Faulk et al. 1978b; Anuras et al. 1986b; Schuffler et al. 1988). In these cases, the condition is usually extensive and progressive and the prognosis, particularly in children, is worse than in familial cases. The underlying pathological processes are variable and both neuropathy and myopathy have been described (Christensen 1986). There may also be an underlying genetic abnormality in patients with sporadic CIIP. Gottlieb and Schuster (1986) have shown a high incidence of a particular dermatoglyphic pattern in patients with sporadic CIIP, rarely found in healthy control subjects and patients with functional bowel disorders.

Chronic pseudo-obstruction may be a secondary feature of a wide spectrum of diseases. The causes may be grouped into those affecting enteric smooth muscle, those affecting myenteric nerves and a number of endocrine, pharmacological and miscellaneous causes which may affect either enteric smooth muscle or myenteric nerves (Table 12.2). The degree to which the gastrointestinal tract is involved is variable and treatment depends on ability to treat the underlying disease process.

Progressive systemic sclerosis is the most common disease to affect enteric smooth muscle producing atrophy and fibrosis. The majority of patients with systemic sclerosis have demonstrable abnormalities of gastrointestinal function. These abnormalities are clinically significant in approximately 50% of patients. In patients with diffuse small bowel involvement, malnutrition and death occur in up to 20% of cases (Cohen et al. 1980). Other collagen vascular diseases, particularly systemic lupus erythematosus, may rarely affect enteric smooth muscle (Christensen 1986). Progressive muscular dystrophy (Leon et al. 1986), dermatomyositis and polymyositis (Faulk et al. 1978a) may affect enteric smooth muscle in addition to skeletal muscle. The oesophagus and colon are particularly affected. In ceroidosis, lipofuscin pigment is deposited in the enteric smooth muscle. The condition has been found in several cases of

CIIP, but a cause and effect relationship has not been established (Christensen 1986).

Secondary enteric visceral neuropathy may occur as part of a systemic neurological disorder such as Parkinson's disease or as part of a disease process confined to the gastrointestinal tract, such as Chagas' disease. The latter, an infection with *Trypanosoma cruzi*, produces a progressive enteric neuropathy which primarily affects the oesophagus and colon. Paraneoplastic visceral neuropathy has been reported, particularly in association with small cell carcinoma of the lung (Chinn and Schuffler 1988). Myotonic dystrophy, an autosomal dominant progressive multisystem disorder, has recently been shown to produce pseudo-obstruction through a visceral neuropathy (Yoshida et al. 1988). Achalasia of the oesophagus and Hirschsprung's disease may also be included in this classification as both result in a functional intestinal obstruction in the absence of a mechanical cause (Christensen 1986).

Several endocrine disorders have been associated with intestinal pseudo-obstruction. Myxoedema may present with abdominal distension and constipation before other features are apparent. Oedema of the bowel wall with accumulation of mucopolysaccharide may account for defective intestinal motility. In diabetes mellitus, gastrointestinal symptoms are common. Constipation, diarrhoea and gastric stasis may occur and are thought to be part of an autonomic neuropathy. Disorders of gastric motility are particularly common and may take the form of gastroparesis or tachygastria, in which coordination of gastric motility is deranged (Camilleri and Malagelada 1984).

A large number of pharmacological agents affect gastrointestinal motility (Table 12.2). Severe constipation and megacolon are common in psychotic patients and may be due to a combination of phenothiazines and tricyclic antidepressants. Large doses of phenothiazines have an anticholinergic effect (Milner 1969) and decrease slow wave frequency in the cat colon, possibly by an effect on calcium binding to calmodulin, a calcium binding protein (Anuras and Shirazi 1984). Opiates have widespread effects on both enteric motility (Wienbeck and Korner 1981) and secretion (Beubler 1981). Narcotic analgesics have been implicated in acute colonic pseudo-obstruction (Strodel et al. 1983), but an association between opiates and CIIP is uncertain. Prolonged usage of laxatives may result in a dilated, atonic "cartharctic" colon. Anthraquinone purgatives have been particularly implicated (Smith 1973).

There remain a number of miscellaneous conditions which may produce secondary chronic intestinal pseudo-obstruction. In amyloidosis this is due to deposition of amyloid in enteric smooth muscle coupled with myenteric neuropathy (Wald et al. 1981). External beam radiation therapy may produce muscular and neuronal degeneration many years after treatment (Perino et al. 1986). A clinical picture of chronic pseudo-obstruction has been reported in a patient with coeliac disease (Dawson et al. 1984). Finally, jejunal diverticula are frequently observed in patients with CIIP. There is some evidence that the diverticula result from structural abnormalities of either the smooth muscle or myenteric plexus (Krishnamurthy and Schuffler 1987), but a cause or effect relationship has yet to be established (Christensen 1986).

Diagnosis

Diagnosis of pseudo-obstruction presents a challenge to the clinician because of the diversity of presentation and associated conditions. In the acute setting, distinction between acute intestinal pseudo-obstruction and acute mechanical intestinal obstruction is of utmost importance so that a laparotomy, which may prolong pseudo-obstruction, may be avoided. Likewise, early recognition of CIIP may prevent endless investigations and repeated needless laparotomies. The diagnostic and therapeutic approach to acute pseudo-obstruction and chronic pseudo-obstruction differ, and therefore the two conditions will be considered separately.

Acute Pseudo-obstruction

A supine abdominal x-ray is the single most useful investigation in diagnosis and management of acute intestinal pseudo-obstruction. The usual appearance is of greatly distended large bowel, with air fluid levels visible on erect or decubitus views. Small bowel dilatation is rarely seen, as the ileocaecal valve is usually competent to allow colonic dilatation of such degree (Vanek and Al-Salti 1985). A distinction between mechanical obstruction and intestinal pseudo-obstruction cannot be made on non-contrast radiological

studies alone; however, when examined in the light of the clinical background, plain abdominal x-rays are very useful. Some distinction may be drawn between the megacolon of chronic constipation and the dilated colon of chronic pseudo-obstruction as in megacolon, and in sigmoid volvulus, the sigmoid colon is grossly dilated, whereas in pseudo-obstruction dilatation of the caecum and transverse colon is more marked.

In the differential diagnosis of acute intestinal obstruction, a contrast enema study is valuable (Fig. 12.1). Koruth et al. (1985) found in a series of 91 patients that a diagnosis of pseudo-obstruction was missed in 18 of 79 patients considered on clinical grounds to have a mechanical intestinal obstruction, while carcinoma of the colon was present in two of 12 patients considered to have pseudo-obstruction. If gastrograffin, a water-soluble contrast material, is used to perform the contrast study, the effect is sometimes therapeutic as well as diagnostic (Vanek and Al-Salti 1985). Dudley and Patterson-Brown (1986) concluded that "a contrast enema will save a substantial number of patients from unnecessary and dangerous surgery, while disclosing a mechanical cause in a smaller number of patients".

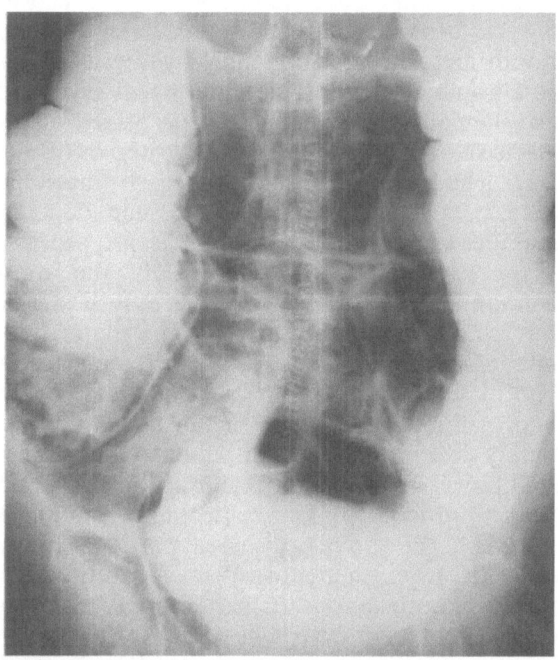

Fig. 12.1. A gastrograffin enema in a 60-year-old woman with acute colonic pseudo-obstruction 6 days following spinal decompression. The x-ray shows dilatation in the absence of a mechanical obstruction. Because the maximum caecal diameter was 12.5 cm, the patient underwent successful colonoscopic decompression.

Chronic Pseudo-obstruction

The first consideration in a patient presenting with
signs and symptoms of recurrent intestinal
obstruction is to determine whether a mechanical
obstruction is present and, if so, whether this can
be treated. As with acute colonic pseudo-
obstruction, the clinical history may raise the
possibility of pseudo-obstruction. A particularly
detailed family history and drug history must be
obtained. A careful physical examination must be
performed, looking for features of scleroderma,
endocrine or neuromuscular disorders. Only then
can a differential diagnosis be made and a logical
approach to investigation decided upon.

Radiological Investigations

When a diagnosis of chronic intestinal pseudo-
obstruction is entertained, radiological examination of the entire gastrointestinal tract should be
obtained. The initial radiological investigation
should be erect and supine abdominal x-ray.
These are likely to show a pattern of small bowel
dilatation similar to, but more symmetrical than,
that seen with mechanical obstruction (Fig. 12.2).
Small bowel diameters greater than 3 cm and
colonic diameters greater than 8 cm are abnormal
(Rohrmann et al. 1984). The colon, the oesophagus or the duodenum may be greatly dilated,
suggesting Hirschsprung's disease, achalasia or
megaduodenum. Approximately 15%–20% of
patients have normal findings on plain x-ray, the
abnormality being apparent only on contrast
radiography (Schuffler 1988). Using contrast
radiography, the following are the radiological
hallmarks of chronic intestinal pseudo-obstruction
(Byrne et al. 1981).

1. Absence of a mechanical obstruction
2. Absent, decreased or disorganized intestinal
   motility
3. Dilated loops of small bowel, including the
   proximal duodenum
4. Decreased or absent haustral markings

If a mechanical cause of obstruction is strongly
suspected or if the colon is dilated on plain
abdominal x-ray, a barium or water-soluble contrast enema should be performed as the next
investigation. Otherwise, a barium meal and intestinal follow-up through examination are likely to
yield most information. Screening of the oesophagus, stomach and proximal small bowel is import-

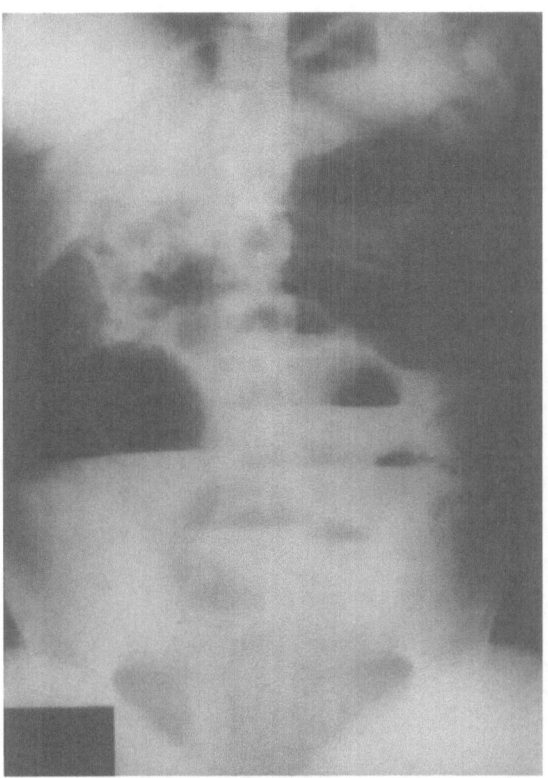

Fig. 12.2. An erect abdominal x-ray in a patient with familial
chronic idiopathic intestinal pseudo-obstruction showing distended small bowel with multiple air fluid levels.

ant to detect subtle abnormalities in motility. An
air-contrast small bowel enema technique is particularly useful in defining incomplete mechanical
obstruction (Christensen 1986). If pseudo-
obstruction is suspected, some inferences regarding the aetiology may be drawn from the radiographic findings. In general, visceral myopathies
produce hypocontractility and dilatation. Megaduodenum is common in the autosomal dominant
familial type (Fig. 12.3). By contrast, visceral
neuropathies produce increased, unco-ordinated
motility. In particular, the oesophageal findings
mimic achalasia (Schuffler 1988). Jejunal diverticula are associated with autosomal recessive visceral myopathy and systemic sclerosis, but a finding of diffuse small bowel diverticulosis is
nonspecific. Colonic abnormalities are nonspecific, except that the features of Chagas' disease and
Hirschsprung's disease are usually diagnostic. It is
important to remember that visceral myopathies
may also involve the urinary tract, therefore an
intravenous urogram should be obtained. If
abnormalities are present, a cystometrogram
should be performed.

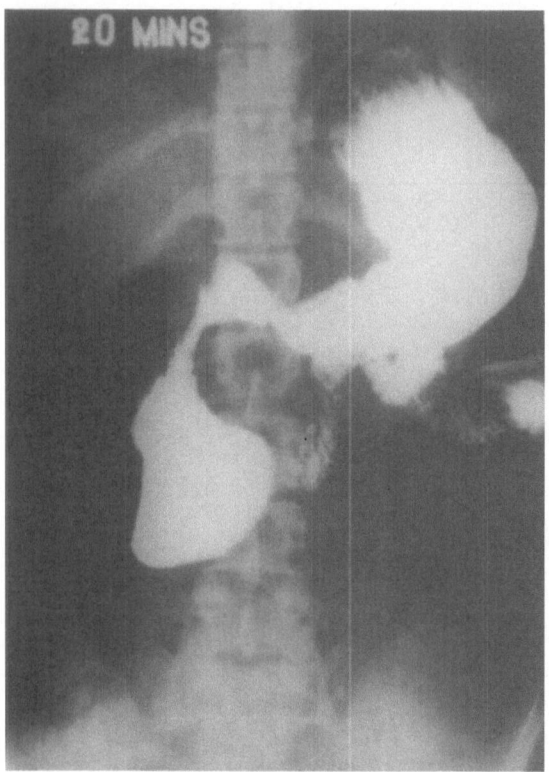

Fig. 12.3. A barium meal examination showing megaduodenum in a patient with familial visceral myopathy.

Manometry

Every patient in whom chronic intestinal pseudo-obstruction is suspected should undergo oesophageal manometry (Christensen 1986). Oesophageal manometry is now widely available and approximately 75% of patients with chronic intestinal pseudo-obstruction have abnormal manometric findings (Schuffler 1988). Abnormal manometry in addition to abnormal radiographic findings strongly supports a diagnosis of pseudo-obstruction.

Visceral myopathy is characterized in the oesophagus by low amplitude non-peristaltic contractions with preservation of lower oesophageal sphincter pressure. In systemic sclerosis the findings are similar, except that lower oesophageal sphincter pressure is reduced and if pH is also measured, acid reflux can be demonstrated. Visceral neuropathy is characterized by non-peristaltic simultaneous contractions, with raised lower oesophageal sphincter pressure, a pattern similar to that seen in achalasia.

Motility studies of the stomach and small intestine require elaborate equipment and are rarely performed outside a research laboratory setting. The most common abormalities seen in gastric antral motility recordings are reduced frequency or absence of migrating motor complexes (MMC) and diminished antral postcibal phasic activity (Mayer et al. 1988). The criteria for diagnosis of pseudo-obstruction using jejunal manometry are well defined (Summers et al. 1983; Stanghellini et al. 1987). The presence of at least two of the following is considered diagnostic:

1. Abnormal propagation or configuration of the MMC
2. Non-propagated bursts of phasic activity
3. Sustained incoordinated activity
4. Failure of a meal to induce a normal fed pattern

These abnormalities can be distinguished from the pattern of "clustered contractions" seen in the proximal small bowel of patients with mechanical intestinal obstruction (Summers et al. 1983). Two separate small bowel motility patterns are usually discernible in pseudo-obstruction. Visceral myopathy is characterized by low amplitude tracings, with abnormal MMCs and failure of a meal to induce a fed pattern. Visceral neuropathy is characterized by sustained incoordinate activity with non-propagated bursts of phasic activity (Fig. 12.4). Both sets of features may be found in patients with systemic sclerosis, which has been taken to indicate that both neuropathic and myopathic elements are present in the pseudo-obstruction of systemic sclerosis (Greydanus and Camilleri 1989). Analysis of gastric and intestinal motility tracings has been facilitated by use of computer integration analysis to derive a motility index. This measurement can be used to quantify motility responses to prokinetic drugs (Camilleri et al. 1989b).

Manometric studies of the stomach and small bowel are invasive and time consuming. Two experimental noninvasive techniques may find a role in investigation of enteric myoelectric activity. Electrogastrography detects gastric smooth muscle electrical activity in a way similar to recording cardiac smooth muscle electrical activity by electrocardiography. Data analysis and interpretation are complex. Computer techniques using frequency analysis may be a useful adjunct to simple visual analysis (Abell and Malagelada 1988). Electrogastrographic techniques have not yet been applied to analysis of small bowel myoelectric activity.

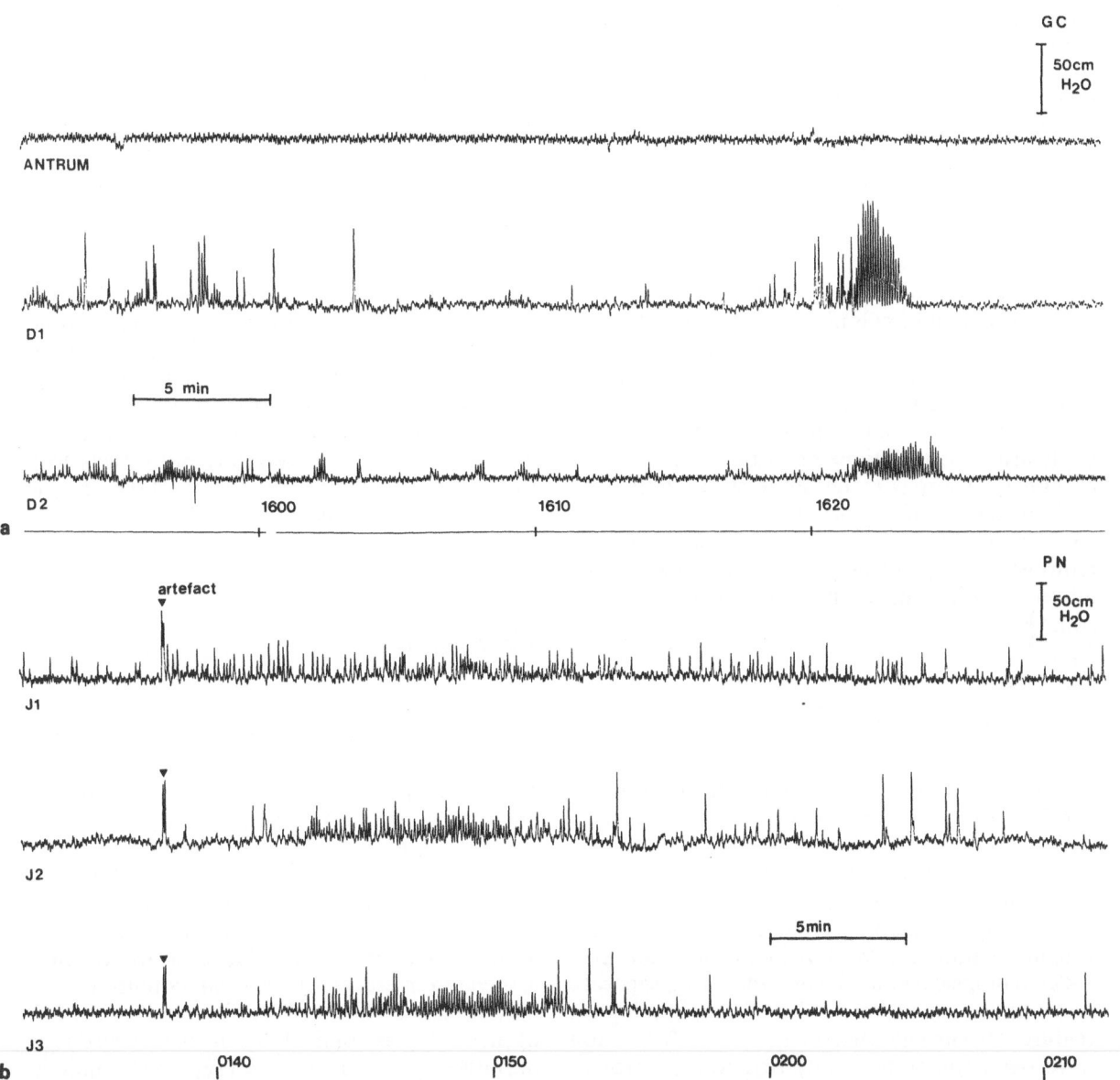

Fig. 12.4. a Antral and duodenal motility in a healthy volunteer showing a fasting motility pattern with a migrating motor complex appearing in the proximal duodenum at 1620. (Courtesy of Professor David Wingate.) b Jejunal motility pattern in a patient with familial visceral neuropathy showing sustained incoordinated activity and non-propagated bursts of phasic activity. (Courtesy of Professor David Wingate.)

Surface vibration analysis detects and quantifies vibrational energy generated by enteric contractions (Campbell et al. 1989). The technique has been applied in volunteers and patients with mechanical intestinal obstruction and a close correlation has been found between vibration analysis and "clustered contractions" measured by simultaneous intestinal manometry (Cullen et al. 1989). Application of surface vibration analysis in patients with intestinal pseudo-obstruction is awaited.

Transit Studies

Transit studies are useful in assessment of enteric function. Scintigraphy is particularly suitable as it is noninvasive, quantifiable and has a low radiation dosage. The main difficulties using scintigraphy are image resolution and separation of radio-isotope marker. Nevertheless, scintigraphy is a useful adjunct to oesophageal manometry in evaluation of motility disorders, particularly achalasia (O'Connell et al. 1984; Mughal et al.

1986). Improved methods of solid phase labelling, using either ^{99}Tc-labelled chicken liver (Wright et al. 1981) or ^{131}I-labelled fibre (Malagelada et al. 1984; Camilleri et al. 1989a), have allowed elaborate studies of gastric emptying in patients with intestinal pseudo-obstruction (Mayer et al. 1988; Camilleri et al. 1989b). These studies have confirmed a high prevalence of gastric emptying disorders in pseudo-obstruction. Scintigraphy is less useful in assessment of small bowel transit and such techniques remain experimental.

Measurement of colonic transit is difficult. The conventional technique is to record time taken for ingested barium pellets to traverse the colon, as measured on serial abdominal x-rays (Hinton et al. 1969). More elaborate calculations can be made using the technique described by Metcalf et al. (1987). There is recent interest in methods of radio-isotope delivery to the caecum either by naso-enteric intubation or enteric coated capsule. However, isotope dispersal and poor image resolution are difficulties which remain to be overcome.

Histopathology

In the majority of cases a confident diagnosis of chronic pseudo-obstruction can be made using a combination of clinical, radiological and manometric investigations. When the diagnosis remains uncertain, or when the diagnosis is suspected at laparotomy, a histological diagnosis should be sought. Schuffler (1988) recommends that two 2×2 cm biopsies should be obtained from separate areas of the small bowel. The histopathological features of chronic intestinal pseudo-obstruction have been comprehensively reviewed (Mitros et al. 1982; Krishnamurthy and Schuffler 1987) and the following is a summary of these accounts.

In visceral myopathy the enteric smooth muscle shows extensive degeneration, with a distinctive pattern termed vacuolar degeneration (Schuffler et al. 1981). This may affect predominantly the circular layer or the longitudinal layer, but abnormalities are invariably present in both. The myenteric plexus is normal.

Visceral neuropathy is characterized by degeneration of neurones and nerve fibres in the myenteric plexus. In contrast to visceral myopathy, muscular hypertrophy is often present. The changes of visceral neuropathy may be subtle and can be missed on conventional light microscopy unless a silver staining technique is used to visualize the myenteric plexus (Schuffler and Jonak

1982). Longitudinal as well as transverse sections are needed to demonstrate quantitative loss of neurones as well as fragmentation and degeneration of axons. Furthermore, it appears that the histological findings are not constant and different abnormalities have been found in several families reported with visceral neuropathy (Mayer et al. 1986). Recent elaborate histochemical techniques using monoclonal autoantibodies have suggested that a disturbance of extrinsic innervation may be also implicated in visceral neuropathy (Kluck et al. 1987). Using immunohistochemistry, Yoshida et al. (1988) have demonstrated that the myenteric neuropathy associated with myotonic dystrophy is due to degeneration of substance P and enkephalin immunoreactive fibres of the myenteric plexus. It is clear that there are many more facts to be elucidated before the pathogenesis of this complex family of disorders is understood.

Treatment

Acute Pseudo-obstruction

The treatment of acute colonic pseudo-obstruction is conservative, with surgery reserved for approximately 10% of patients who fail to respond to conservative measures. Treatment consists of nasogastric decompression, correction of fluid and electrolyte imbalances, discontinuance of narcotic analgesia, and treatment of associated medical or surgical conditions. The patients should be carefully observed for evidence of increasing abdominal distension, localized tenderness or perforation. Serial supine abdominal x-rays should be performed at least daily and the diameter of the caecum and transverse colon measured. A sigmoidoscopy should be performed to eliminate the possibility of a rectosigmoid tumour, sigmoid volvulus or inflammatory bowel disease. A rectal tube may be passed but it is seldom effective in relieving colonic dilatation. Phosphate or saline enemas are rarely helpful. The value of prokinetic drugs is controversial (Vanek and Al-Salti 1985). If a mechanical cause of intestinal obstruction cannot confidently be excluded, an urgent contrast enema should be obtained.

With close observation and serial x-rays, it will become apparent whether simple measures will suffice. If no improvement occurs within 48 hours or the caecal diameter increases then the colon should be decompressed to prevent ischaemic necrosis with perforation. The diameter of caecal dilatation at which active intervention should be considered is controversial. Most would agree that a diameter of 12 cm is an indication for intervention (Nivatvongs et al. 1982; Vanek and Al-Salti 1985), although some would argue that a diameter of 9 cm is a safer threshold (Dudley and Patterson-Brown 1986).

Colonoscopic decompression, introduced by Kukora and Dent (1977), has been found to be successful in over 80% of cases (Nivatvongs et al. 1982; Strodel et al. 1983; Vanek and Al-Salti 1985). Bowel preparation is unnecessary. Recurrent distension after colonoscopic decompression is frequently a problem and may occur several days following initial decompression. Repeated colonoscopy is often needed. To overcome this, long-term decompression has been advocated with a long catheter passed using a colonoscope (Bernton et al. 1982; Groff 1983). More recently Burke and Shellito (1987) have advocated the use of a fenestrated overtube placed at the time of initial colonoscopic decompression.

Failure of colonoscopic treatment is an indication for surgical decompression. Repeated colonoscopic decompression may be attempted and the timing of surgical intervention is a matter for individual judgement. Conventionally either a tube or formal caecostomy is performed (Vanek and Al-Salti 1985). Others have suggested that caecal exteriorization is perferable (Dudley and Patterson-Brown 1986).

Chronic Pseudo-obstruction

The treatment of chronic intestinal pseudo-obstruction is essentially palliative as no specific treatment has been shown to alter the disease process. In many patients, particularly those identified by family screening after identification of an affected proband, the symptoms are mild and intermittent. In others, the disease follows a progressive course resulting in malnutrition and death. For these, several treatment modalities are available and are discussed.

Prokinetic drugs have been extensively studied in patients with CIIP. Metoclopramide, bethanecol (Malagelada et al. 1981) and domperidone (Horowitz et al. 1985) all have prokinetic effects, yet none has been shown to be consistently of value. Cisapride increases both gastric emptying and small bowel transit and tends to normalize the abnormal manometric features of intestinal dysmotility (Camilleri et al. 1986). However, a recent double blind placebo controlled trial in 26 patients showed no overall symptomatic benefit in patients during a 6-week trial (Camilleri et al. 1989b). While it is reasonable to consider a therapeutic trial of a prokinetic agent, symptoms may wax and wane and, as Camilleri et al. (1989b) have noted, the placebo effect is pronounced.

Bacterial overgrowth in the small bowel may contribute to malabsorption and abdominal distension. Schuffler et al. (1981) found intermittent courses of tetracycline of value in patients with systemic sclerosis; however, treatment was of little value in patients with CIIP. Nevertheless, a few patients do respond and an empirical trial of antibiotics is usually worthwhile, particularly if malabsorption and small bowel bacterial overgrowth can be demostrated.

Dietary manipulations do not significantly affect the natural history of CIIP (Schuffler et al. 1981). Nevertheless, a low residue diet may reduce abdominal discomfort as impaired intestinal motility, particularly loss of the MMC, results in a tendency to form inspissated stool and bezoars. In some patients, chronic mucosal damage produces a relative lactase deficiency and a lactulose free diet may be considered. Fat malabsorption may occur due to bacterial overgrowth and bile salt deconjugation. Antibiotic treatment and dietary bile salt supplementation may help. Vitamin deficiencies occur, particularly of fat soluble vitamins and essential fatty acids, and appropriate dietary supplements should be given.

There remains a group of severely affected patients who are unable to maintain adequate enteral nutrition. For these, home parenteral nutrition (Levien et al. 1985) may provide an acceptable quality of life for many years (Pitt et al. 1985). Fourteen of 27 patients reviewed by Schuffler et al. (1981) eventually required parenteral nutrition, nine of whom continued at home. Once an optimal weight gain was achieved, parenteral infusions were decreased to a maintenance level which varied from three to seven overnight infusions per week, each infusion consisting of 2000 calories.

Surgery has a very limited role in the management of patients with CIIP. Palliative surgery directed at specific problems may be of value (Anuras et al. 1979; Schuffler and Deitch 1980; Pitt et al. 1985). Intractable gastric stasis may respond to gastrectomy and Roux-en-Y reconstruction. Megaduodenum can be treated by duodenojejunostomy. Intractable constipation may require subtotal colectomy. In extreme situations, large portions of the small bowel may require resection to palliate painful abdominal distension. A venting gastrostomy or jejunostomy allows decompression of the proximal small bowel, and may reduce the frequency of hospital admission (Pitt et al. 1985).

Conclusion

Intestinal pseudo-obstruction is a rare entity that presents a diagnostic challenge because of its diverse aetiology and presentation. The diagnosis may be suspected on the clinical history and examination. Clinical, radiological and manometric data must be combined to confirm the clinical suspicion and used to plan a treatment strategy.

References

Abell TL, Malagelada JR (1988) Electrogastrography: current assessment and future prospects. Dig Dis Sci 33:982–992

Anuras S, Shirazi SS (1984) Colonic pseudo-obstruction. Am J Gastroenterol 79:525–532

Anuras S, Shirazi S, Faulk DL et al. (1979) Surgical treatment in familial visceral myopathy. Ann Surg 189:306–310

Anuras S, Mitros FA, Milano A, Kuminsky R, Decanio R, Green JB (1986a) A familial visceral myopathy with dilation of the entire gastrointestinal tract. Gastroenterology 90:385–390

Anuras S, Mitros FA, Soper RT et al. (1986b) Chronic intestinal pseudo-obstruction in young children. Gastroenterology 91:62–70

Bernton E, Myers R, Reyna T (1982) Pseudo-obstruction of the colon: case report including a new endoscopic treatment. Gastrointest Endosc 28:90–92

Beubler E (1981) Opiates and intestinal secretion. Clin Res Rev 1:141–148

Burke G, Shellito PC (1987) Treatment of recurrent colonic pseudo-obstruction by endoscopic placement of a fenestrated overtube. Dis Colon Rectum 30:615–619

Byrne WJ, Cipel L, Ament ME et al. (1981) Chronic idiopathic intestinal pseudo-obstruction: radiologic signs in children with emphasis on differentiation from mechanical obstruction. Diagn Imaging 50:294–304

Camilleri M, Malagelada JR (1984) Abnormal intestinal motility in diabetics with the gastroparesis syndrome. Eur J Clin Invest 14:420–427

Camilleri M, Brown ML, Malagelada JR (1986) Impaired transit of chyme in chronic intestinal pseudo-obstruction: correction by cisapride. Gastroenterology 91:619–626

Camilleri M, Colemont LJ, Phillips SF et al. (1989a) Human gastric emptying and colonic filling of solids characterised by a new method. Am J Physiol 257:G284–G290

Camilleri M, Malagelada JR, Abell TL, Brown ML, Hench V, Zinsmeister AR (1989b) Effect of six weeks treatment with cisapride in gastroparesis and intestinal pseudo-obstruction. Gastroenterology 96:704–712

Campbell FC, Storey BE, Cullen PT, Cuschieri A (1989) Surface vibration analysis: a new non-invasive monitor of gastrointestinal activity. Gut 30:39–45

Chinn JS, Schuffler MD (1988) Paraneoplastic visceral neuropathy as a cause of severe gastrointestinal motor dysfunction. Gastroenterology 95:1279–1286

Christensen J (1986) Intestinal pseudo-obstruction and paralytic ileus. In: Moody FG, Carey LC, Jones RS, Kelly KA, Nahrwold DL, Skinner DB (eds) Surgical treatment of digestive disease, Year Book Medical, Chicago, pp 565–579

Cohen S, Laufer I, Snape W et al. (1980) The gastrointestinal manifestations of scleroderma: pathogenesis and management. Gastroenterology 79:155–166

Cullen PT, Storey BE, Cuschieri A, Campbell FC (1989) Detection of clustered gastrointestinal contractions in partial intestinal obstruction by surface vibration analysis. Ann Surg 210:234–238

Dawson DJ, Sciberras CM, Whitwell H (1984) Coeliac disease presenting with intestinal pseudo-obstruction. Gut 25:1003–1008

Dudley HA, Patterson-Brown S (1986) Pseudo-obstruction. Br Med J 292:1157–1158

Dudley HA, Sinclair IS, McLaren et al. (1958) Intestinal pseudo-obstruction. J R Coll Surg Edinb 3:206–217

Faber J, Fich A, Steinberg A et al. (1987) Familial intestinal pseudo-obstruction dominated by a progressive neurologic disease at a young age. Gastroenterology 92:786–790

Faulk DL, Anuras S, Christensen J (1978a) Chronic intestinal pseudo-obstruction. Gastroenterology 92:786–790

Faulk DL, Anuras S, Gardner GD, Mitros FA, Summers RW, Christensen JA (1978b) A familial visceral myopathy. Ann Intern Med 89:600–606

Gottlieb SH, Schuster MM (1986) Dermatoglyphic evidence of a congenital syndrome of early onset constipation and abdominal pain. Gastroenterology 91:428–432

Greydanus MP, Camilleri M (1989) Abnormal postcibal antral and small bowel motility due to neuropathy or myopathy in systemic sclerosis. Gastroenterology 96:110–115

Groff W (1983) Colonoscopic decompression and intubation of the caecum for Ogilvie's syndrome. Dis Colon Rectum 26:503–506

Hinton JM, Lennard-Jones JE, Young AC (1969) A new method for studying gut transit times using radioopaque markers. Gut 10:842–847

Horowitz M, Harding PE, Chatterton BE, Collins PJ, Shearman DJC (1985) Acute and chronic effects of domperidone on gastric emptying in diabetic autonomic neuropathy. Dig Dis Sci 30:1–9

Kluck P, ten Kate FJW, Schouten R et al. (1987) Efficacy of antibody NF2F11 staining in the investigation of severe long standing constipation. Gastroenterology 93:872–875

Koruth NM, Koruth A, Matheson NA (1985) The place of contrast enema in the management of large bowel obstruction. J R Coll Surg Edinb 30:258–260

Krishnamurthy S, Schuffler MD (1987) Pathology of neuromuscular disorders of the small intestine and colon. Gastroenterology 93:610–639

Kukora JS, Dent TL (1977) Colonoscopic decompression of massive nonobstructive caecal dilatation. Arch Surg 112:512–517

Leon SH, Schuffler MD, Kettler M et al. (1986) Chronic intestinal pseudo-obstruction as a complication of Duchenne's muscular dystrophy. Gastroenterology 90:455–459

Levien DH, Fiallos F, Barone R, Taffet S (1985) The use of cyclic home hyperalimentation for malabsorption in patients with scleroderma involving the small intestines. J Parent Ent Nut 9:623–625

Malagelada JR, Rees WDW, Mazzotta IJ, Go VLW (1981) Gastric motor abnormalities in diabetic and post vagotomy gastroparesis: effect of metoclopramide and bethanecol. Gastroenterology 78:286–293

Malagelada JR, Robertson JS, Brown ML et al. (1984) Intestinal transit of solid and liquid components of a meal in health. Gastroenterology 87:1255–1263

Maldonado JE, Gregg JA, Green PA et al. (1970) Chronic idiopathic intestinal pseudo-obstruction. Am J Med 49:203–212

Mayer EA, Schuffler MD, Rotter JI, Hanna P, Mogard M (1986) Familial visceral neuropathy with autosomal dominant transmission. Gastroenterology 91:1528–1535

Mayer EA, Elashoff J, Hawkins R, Berquist W, Taylor IL (1988) Gastric emptying of mixed solid–liquid meal in patients with intestinal pseudo-obstruction. Dig Dis Sci 33:10–18

Metcalf AM, Phillips SF, Zinsmeister AR, MacCarthy RL, Beart RW, Wolff BG (1987) Simplified assessment of segmental colonic transit. Gastroenterology 92:40–47

Milner G (1969) Gastrointestinal side effects of psychotrophic drugs. Med J Aust 2:153–155

Mitros F, Schuffler MD, Teja K, Anuras S (1982) Pathology of familial visceral myopathy. Hum Pathol 13:825–833

Mughal MM, Marples M, Bancewicz J (1986) Scintigraphic assessment of oesophageal motility: what does it show and how reliable is it? Gut 27:946–953

Murley RS (1959) Painful enteromegaly of unknown aetiology. Proc R Soc Med 52:479–480

Murphy JB (1896) Ileus. JAMA 26:15–22

Naish JM, Cooer WM, Brown NJ (1960) Intestinal pseudo-obstruction with steatorrhea. Gut 1:62–66

Nivatvongs S, Vermeulen FD, Fang DT (1982) Colonoscopic decompression of acute pseudo-obstruction of the colon. Ann Surg 196:598–600

O'Connell PR, O'Connor MK, Byrne PJ, Hennessy TPJ (1984) A simple screening test for achalasia. Br J Surg 71:378

Ogilvie H (1948) Large intestine colic due to sympathetic deprivation. Br Med J ii:671–673

Perino LE, Schuffler MD, Mehta SJ, Everson GT (1986) Radiation induced intestinal pseudo-obstruction. Gastroenterology 91:994–998

Pitt HA, Mann LL, Berquist WE, Ament ME, Fonkalsrud EW, DenBesten L (1985) Chronic idiopathic intestinal pseudo-obstruction. Arch Surg 120:614–618

Rodrigues CA, Shepherd NA, Lennard-Jones JE, Hawley PR, Thompson HH (1989) Familial visceral myopathy: a family with at least six involved members. Gut 30:1285–1292

Rohrmann CA, Ricci MT, Krishnamurthy S, Schuffler MD (1984) Radiologic and histologic differentiation of neuromuscular disorders of the gastrointestinal tract. Am J Radiol 143:933–941

Roy AD, Bharucha H, Nevin NC, Odling-Smee GW (1980) Idiopathic intestinal pseudo-obstruction: a familial visceral neuropathy. Clin Genet 18:291–297

Schuffler MD (1988) Chronic idiopathic intestinal pseudo-obstruction. In: Kumar D, Gustavsson S (eds) An illustrated guide to gastrointestinal motility. Wiley, Chichester, pp 383–399

Schuffler MD, Deitch EA (1980) Chronic idiopathic intestinal pseudo-obstruction: a surgical approach. Ann Surg 192:752–761

Schuffler MD, Jonak Z (1982) Chronic idiopathic intestinal pseudo-obstruction caused by a degenerative disorder of the myenteric plexus: The use of Smith's method to define the neuropathy. Gastroenterology 82:476–486

Schuffler MD, Pope CE (1977) Studies of idiopathic intestinal pseudo-obstruction II. Hereditary hollow visceral myopathy: family studies. Gastroenterology 73:339–344

Schuffler MD, Bird TD, Sumi SM, Cook A (1978) A familial neuronal disease presenting as intestinal pseudo-obstruction. Gastroenterology 75:889–898

Schuffler MD, Rohrmann CA, Chaffee RG, Brand DL, Delaney JH, Young JH (1981) Chronic intestinal pseudo-obstruction. Medicine 60:173–196

Schuffler MD, Pagon RA, Schwartz R, Bill AH (1988) Visceral myopathy of the gastrointestinal and genitourinary tracts in infants. Gastroenterology 94:892–898

Smith B (1973) Pathologic changes in the colon produced by anthroquinone purgatives. Dis Colon Rect 16:455–458

Stanghellini V, Camilleri M, Malagelada JR (1987) Chronic idiopathic intestinal pseudo-obstruction: clinical and manometric findings. Gut 28:5–12

Strodel WE, Nostrant TT, Eckhauser FE, Dent TL (1983) Therapeutic and diagnostic colonoscopy in nonobstructive colonic dilatation. Ann Surg 197:416–421

Summers RW, Anuras S, Green J (1983) Jejunal manometry patterns in health, partial intestinal obstruction and pseudo-obstruction. Gastroenterology 85:1290–1300

Tanner MS, Smith B, Lloyd JK (1976) Functional intestinal obstruction due to deficiency of argyrophyl neurones in the myenteric plexus. Familial syndrome presenting with short small bowel, malrotation, and pyloric hypertrophy. Arch Dis Child 51:837–841

Vanek VW, Al-Salti M (1985) Acute pseudo-obstruction of the colon. Dis Colon Rect 29:203–210

Wald A, Kichler J, Mendelow H (1981) Amyloidosis and chronic intestinal pseudo-obstruction. Dig Dis Sci 26:54–62

Wienbeck M, Korner MM (1981) Influence of opiates in colonic motility. Clin Res Rev 1:199–204

Wright RA, Thompson D, Syed I (1981) Simultaneous markers for fluid and solid gastric emptying: new variations on an old theme. J Nucl Med 22:772–776

Yoshida MM, Krishnamurthy S, Wattchow DA, Furness JB, Schuffler MD (1988) Megacolon in myotonic dystrophy caused by a degenerative neuropathy of the myenteric plexus. Gastroenterology 95:820–827

Zimmerman LM (1930) Spastic ileus. Surg Gynecol Obstet 50:721–732

ANORECTAL FUNCTION FOLLOWING SURGERY

This final section highlights the effect of low colorectal surgery on function of the residual proximal bowel and the continence mechanism. Extensive efforts to preserve the anal sphincter and pelvic diaphragm, with consequent low intestinal anastomosis, have increased the number of patients with intestinal continuity, but with resultant temporary or long-term problems with frequency of bowel habit or a degree of faecal incontinence. It is, therefore, incumbent on all surgeons offering this form of therapy to be aware of the possible functional consequences to the patient. While we can now be confident that the risk of disease recurrence is not increased, we must also strive to clarify what the patient can expect from a functional viewpoint, and be able to offer a reasonable, fully informed choice of treatment. Much work has already been reported in this important area and functional impairment does not seem to be a barrier to this form of surgery, but individuals who are likely to develop problems with postoperative function can be detected prior to surgery by means of the appropriate test. The next two chapters detail those investigations which play a role in the assessment of this expanding field of surgery and attempt to summarize relevant information which has come to light as a result. Without doubt, further work is required in units with a large referral practice in this area.

Finally, as an addendum in this section, the benefits of investigating and documenting indices of large bowel function in paediatric disorders have been described. This is a potentially interesting and informative area, not only for the problems in this age group but because many of the severe functional disorders of adulthood may have their source in childhood.

13 · Neorectum and Assessment of Anorectal Function Following Surgery

J. H. Pemberton

The goal of the ileal pouch–anal anastomosis (IPAA) operation is to preserve faecal continence in patients who require excision of the large intestine. In this operation, the abdominal colon and proximal two-thirds of the rectum are excised, but only the mucosa in the distal rectum is removed. Intestinal continuity is restored by anastomosing an ileal pouch to the mid-anal canal, thereby retaining, at least anatomically, the pathway for defaecation.

After IPAA, the great majority of patients do indeed achieve continence of stool and gas and eliminate content at will. This generally favourable functional outcome has both confirmed the importance of several established principles of enteric continence and challenged the validity of others; by assessing the function of patients after ileal pouch–anal anastomosis, advances have, in turn, been achieved in understanding the physiology of continence and of defaecation. The aim of this chapter is to outline the rationale, technique and clinical results of ileal pouch–anal anastomosis briefly and then to describe its impact on the several mechanisms of faecal continence and defaecation, as measured by newer quantative tests of anoneorectal function, illustrating how the operation recreates the physiological conditions necessary to achieve a satisfactory long-term outcome.

The Operation

The development and clinical application of ileo-anal anastomosis has been described by several authors (Pemberton et al. 1982; Stryker and Dozois 1985; Williams and Johnston 1985; Wong et al. 1985; Becker and Raymond 1986; Fonkalsrud 1982; Nicholls and Pezim 1985). The most significant developments in the history of ileo-anal anastomosis were undoubtedly Martin and colleagues' report (1977), which was responsible for the recent continuing surge of interest in the operation, and the reports by Parks et al. (1980) and Utsunomiya and colleagues (1980) that construction of an ileal pouch improved results. Currently, nearly all adult patients undergoing ileoanal anastomosis actually undergo ileal pouch–anal anastomosis using a "J" (Utsunomiya et al. 1980), "S" (Parks et al. 1980) or "W" (Nicholls and Pezim 1985; Harms et al. 1987) design.

Rationale

The rationale for the operation is that abdominal colectomy, proximal proctectomy and distal mucosal excision removes the disease, but preserves the muscles of the pelvic floor and anal sphincters, while the ileal pouch functions as a neorectum by restoring reservoir capacity. By preserving the anatomical barrier to outflow and restoring capacity, both continence and defaecation should be maintained. Moreover, because the mucosal dissection is performed endoanally, the nerves to the genitalia and bladder are preserved, thus minimizing sexual and urinary dysfunction. Finally, a persistent perineal wound, which often heals slowly and incompletely, is avoided.

Indications

Ileal pouch–anal anastomosis is performed most commonly for ulcerative colitis (CUC) and familial adenomatous polyposis (FAP). Recently, Nicholls and Kamm (1988) and Yoshioka and Keighley (1989) have reported its use in patients with constipation. Patients with Crohn's disease are not candidates for IPAA, but patients with indeterminate colitis determined at the time of operation are (Pezim et al. 1989). The operation should be performed electively, but patients who are bleeding acutely from chronic ulcerative colitis and who require emergency intervention can undergo IPAA with good results.

Patients

Children and adults up to approximately 65 years of age are candidates for the operation. Beyond 65 years there is a diminution of anal sphincter strength, particular in women who have borne children vaginally (McHugh and Diamant 1987); therefore patients older than 65 are not offered the operation at the Mayo Clinic. Relative contra-indications to IPAA include severe weight loss, use of Immuran and severe extra-intestinal manifestations. Whether steroids are a contra-indication to operation cannot be determined because nearly all of our patients are on steroids preoperatively. The only absolute contra-indication to IPAA is a dysfunctional anal sphincter mechanism. Furthermore, patients who are obese are not good candidates because excessive fat in the ileal mesentery and retroperitoneum prevents the pouch (either S, J or W) from reaching the anal canal without great tension.

Technique

Understandably, many technical approaches to the operation have been described. A detailed description of the techniques used at the Mayo Clinic is provided elsewhere (Pemberton 1987). The operative techniques described briefly below have been performed in approximately 1125 patients between 1981 and 1990.

The operation is performed in two stages. The abdominal colectomy and proximal proctectomy, distal rectal mucosal resection and diverting ileostomy comprise the first stage. The ileum is transected close to the caecum, even if "backwash ileitis" is present (Gustavsson et al. 1987). Mesenteric mobility is enhanced by dividing the attachments to the ileal mesentery to the level of the pancreas. When mobilizing the rectum, the sacral nerves of the sacral promontory are swept away from the superior haemorrhoidal vessels and an intramesenteric dissection is, therefore, unnecessary. The dissection is carried down close to the rectal wall to the coccyx posteriorly, to the mid vagina or mid prostate anteriorly and the levators laterally. The hypogastric plexuses are located on the investing pelvic fascia at the pelvic sidewalls bilaterally and are protected if the rectal "stalks" are gently mobilized and severed close to the rectum. Moreover, the prostatic plexus is protected by cutting through Denonvillier's fascia sharply and then bluntly sweeping the vessels and prostate away from the rectum anteriorly and laterally. The J pouch is constructed from the distal 24–30 cm of ileum using either the linear stapler or sutures. Usually the ileocolic artery is sacrificed to facilitate mobility of the pouch.

Beginning at the dentate line, a submucosal plane is developed for a distance of 4–6 cm (only 2–4 cm of which are *rectal* mucosa; the remainder is epithelium of the proximal anal canal or the anal transitional zone (ATZ)). The specimen is removed and the apex of the pouch delivered through the muscularis cuff to the mid-anal canal. The pouch is anchored to the puborectal muscle, the apex incised and a handsewn ileo-anal anastomosis performed. Figure 13.1 illustrates diagrammatically the construction and eventual anatomical location of the ileal pouch. The diverting ileostomy is placed in the right lower abdomen and immediately matured. At a second stage, 2–3 months later, the temporary ileostomy is closed.

Other Approaches

Pouch Design

The S design is favoured by some authors mainly because the outflow tract reaches to the anal canal

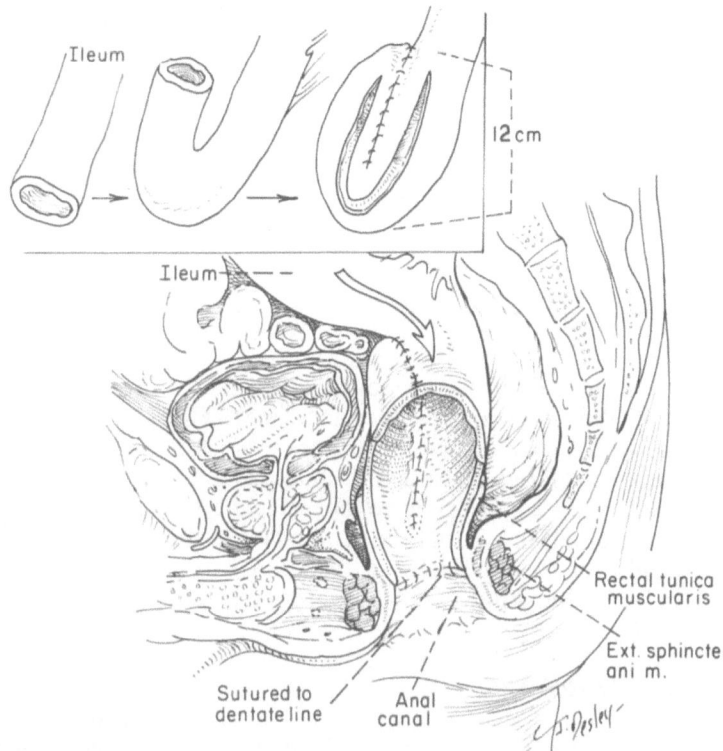

Fig. 13.1. Diagram of completed ileal J pouch anastomosed to the internal sphincter and the anoderm. (From B. M. Taylor et al. 1983 Straight ileoanal anastomosis vs ileal pouch–anal anastomosis. *Archives of Surgery* 118:696–701.)

more predictably and with less tension than does the apex of the J pouch. Since the first description of this pouch by Parks et al. (1980), the outflow tract has been shortened from 5 cm to nearly none at all, in order to avoid outflow obstruction and thus incomplete emptying of the pouch. Constructing the S pouch, however, is more time consuming than constructing a J pouch. The W pouch is appealing because it appears to offer the volume advantage of an S without its outflow problems (Nicholls and Pezim 1985; Harms et al. 1987). However, the W pouch is large and bulky and, unless constructed according to the design of Harms et al. (1987), may have difficulty fitting into the male pelvis. This pouch also requires hand suturing. The H design favoured by Fonkalsrud (1982) may reach the anal canal with less tension than the J or W, but unless the outflow segment is very short, the pouch empties poorly and as a consequence may dilate to great size.

If constructed properly, all the pouch designs provide adequate reservoir capacity and empty satisfactorily.

Distal Resection

An alternative approach to conventional endorectal mucosal resection, advocated with increasing frequency recently, employs no distal rectal mucosal resection at all (Johnston et al. 1987; Heald and Allen 1986; Brough and Schofield 1989; Williams 1989). Rather, the rectum is mobilized and divided near the levators leaving the proximal anal canal intact. The pouch is then anchored by hand or circular stapler to the top of the anal canal. The rationale for this approach is that the proximal 2 cm of the anal canal is lined by transitional epithelium but not columnar rectal mucosa. This region of the upper anal canal is the anal transitional zone (ATZ). Hypothetically, this zone does not participate in the inflammatory process in patients with CUC or in polyp formation in patients with FAP. Moreover, preserving the ATZ should enhance sensation and improve continence. While this approach is attractive theoretically, we have found the ATZ to be traversed by fingers of columnar mucosa in which changes of colitis *are* present (personal observation). Moreover, Emblem et al. (1988) found recurrent polyps in 10 of 13 patients with FAP in whom the ATZ had been preserved while Wolfstein et al. (1982) reported two of two patients experienced recurrence of polyps in the preserved ATZ. We therefore advise complete excision of the diseased mucosa, including the ATZ. If the ATZ is preserved, however, the operation should be more properly termed *low ileal rectal anastomosis*.

Table 13.1. Functional results of ileal pouch–anal anastomosis from 6 months to 5 years postoperatively in 389 patients

Parameter	Follow-up					
	6 months	1 year	2 years	3 years	4 years	5 years
Number of stools (mean±SD)						
Day	5±2	5±3	6±3	6±2	6±3	6±2
Night	1±1	1±1	2±2	2±1	1±1	2±1
Metamucil (% of patients)	43	36	40	38	30	27
Lomotil (% of patients)	26	19	17	25	6	4
Able to discriminate gas from stool (% of patients)	69	77	73	84	77	86

Some surgeons staple the pouch–anal anastomosis at the level of the dentate line. This approach is likewise attractive; the anal sphincters need not be dilated because the mucosa is not dissected. We, however, have not stapled the anastomosis, reasoning that the proximal internal anal sphincter would likely be included in the distal tissue "doughnut."

Clinical Outcome

The long-term results of ileal pouch–anal anastomosis in 390 patients with CUC who had a J pouch constructed and who were followed for a mean of 2.3 years (range 6 months to 5 years) was recently reported (Pemberton et al. 1987). In brief, the mortality was 0.2% and 29% of patients had a postoperative complication. Pelvic sepsis occurred in 5%. The principal late complications were anastomotic stricture (5%) and pouchitis (28%). Impotence and retrograde ejaculation occurred in 1.5% and 4% of men respectively while dyspareunia occurred in 7% of women. Figure 13.2 details the long-term outcome; in 6% of patients the operation failed. Table 13.1 and Fig. 13.3 detail the stool frequency and patterns of continence, ability to discriminate stool from gas and use of medication from 6 months to 5 years after operation. These data confirm that most patients after ileal pouch–anal anastomosis were continent, especially during the day, eliminated stool between five and seven times in 24 hours, had sensation and had few sexual or urinary problems.

Physiology of Ileal Pouch–Anal Anastomosis

Maintaining faecal continence *in health* requires the orchestration of several factors. These factors are: the anal canal high pressure zone (external anal sphincter (EAS); internal sphincter (IAS)); anorectal sensation and reflex mechanisms; the anorectal angle; rectal distensibility (compliance and capacity); rectal motility and evacuability; rapidity of transit through the more proximal bowel and the quality and quantity of enteric content.

Despite colectomy, rectal resection and mucosal stripping, patients after ileal pouch–anal anastomosis are continent of stool and gas and defaecate at will; clinically, therefore, patients do well. These good results prompted a series of investigations, the aims of which were to determine the impact of this operation upon the mechanisms which preserve continence and facilitate defaecation, to define the alterations of physiology that may have occurred and to attempt to define why the operation was successful.

Methodology

These series of investigations have employed several quantifying methodologies, some of which have been detailed in previous chapters, but several of which have not.

Anorectal Manometry

A low compliance, pneumohydraulic capillary perfusion system developed by Arndorfer et al. (1977) is the most reliable *perfused* manometry system. The pressures measured by this system are actually the yield pressures of the tissues of the anal canal. We have performed anorectal manometry using a 4-channel perfused Plexiglas probe (OD; 1.2 cm) (Heppell et al. 1982a; Taylor et al. 1983; O'Connell et al. 1988). The four 0.1 cm OD channels are oriented 90° apart and located 1 cm proximal to the tip. The channels were perfused with normal saline (37 °C) at the rate of 0.3

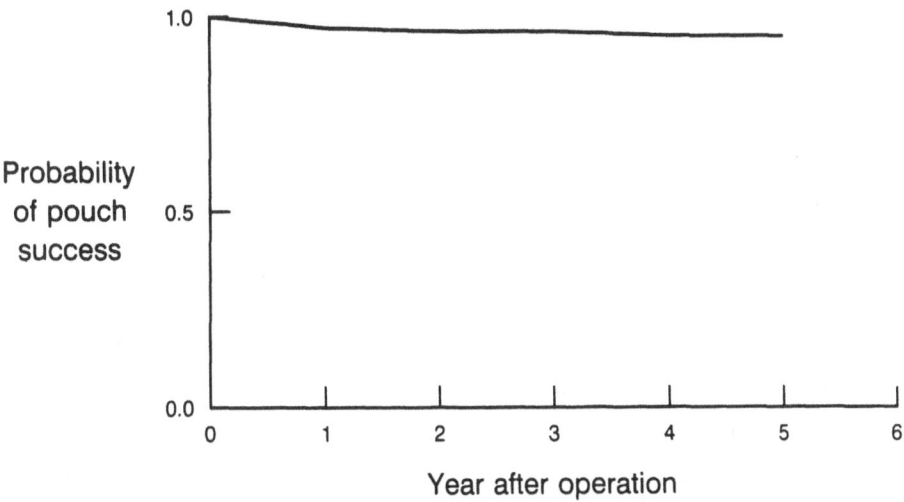

Fig. 13.2. The probability of a successful outcome with functioning pouch against year after operation. No patient failed after 3 years. (From J. H. Pemberton et al. (1987) Ileal pouch–anal anastomosis for chronic ulcerative colitis: long-term results. *Annals of Surgery* 206:504–512.

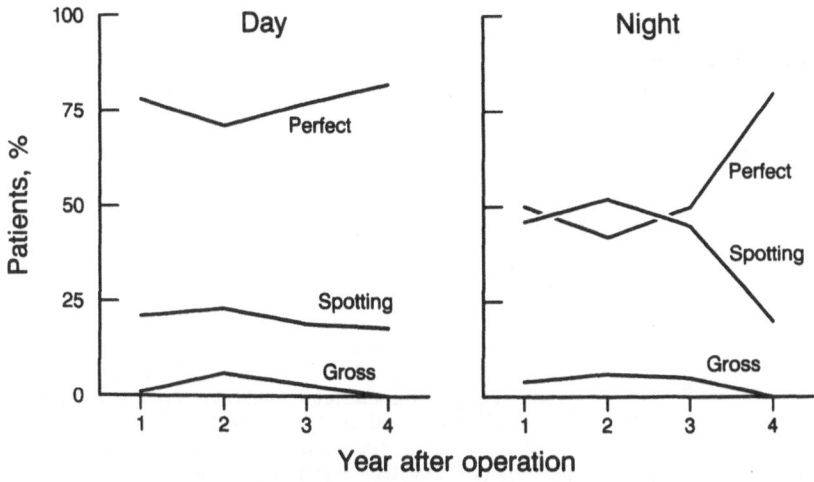

Fig. 13.3. Daytime and night-time continence after ileal pouch–anal anastomosis against the year after operation. *Perfect*, no faecal leakage; *Spotting*, faecal spotting of underclothes, 3 cm or less in diameter, twice or less per week; *Gross*, gross faecal incontinence more than twice per week. Data points are connected for illustrative purposes only. (From J. H. Pemberton et al. (1987) Ileal pouch–anal anastomosis for chronic ulcerative colitis: long-term results. *Annals of Surgery* 206:504–512.)

ml/min via a low compliance pneumohydraulic perfusion system connected to strain gauges and a multichannel recorder. A balloon attached to a catheter which traverses the middle of the probe allows assessment of rectal anal sphincter inhibitory response.

Subjects were placed in the left lateral decubitus position and the probe inserted through the anal canal until it rested in the rectum or pouch; the presence of the perfused ports in the rectum or pouch were confirmed by recording pressures of 5 mmHg or less. The anal canal accommodated easily for the presence of the probe in 3–4 min. A belt pneumograph recorded respiratory excursions. The probe was withdrawn 1 cm/min until the ports reached the anal verge and pressures dropped to zero. This technique provided a sequential pull-through resting pressure profile of the anal canal in four quadrants. The test was repeated and the subject asked to squeeze as long as possible with the probe positioned sequentially in the proximal, middle and distal anal canal. Finally, the probe was repositioned in the proximal anal canal and the rectal balloon inflated and immediately deflated in 5 ml increments in order to elicit proximal anal canal relaxation. The multiple data points obtained were, for simplicity, reduced to a single value for resting and squeeze pressures. Reflex anal canal relaxation was recorded as present or absent. Compliance and capacity of the rectum or ileal pouch was determined by placing a large, soft polyethylene bag connected to a small tube into the lumen of the rectum or pouch. The bag was infinitely compliant until an internal volume greater than 700 ml was reached.

Electromyography (EMG)

EMG of the external anal sphincter was performed using standard 37 mm concentric needle electrodes (Stryker et al. 1985a). Motor unit potentials were identified by separate insertion into the four quadrants of the external anal sphincter. The amplifier was set on a gain of 50 millivolts or 200 millivolts (low frequency filter 16 Hz, and high filter 16 000 Hz). Spontaneous resting activity was assessed for 20 or more motor unit potentials. In addition, motor unit potential activity during voluntary squeeze was assessed. Single fibre and pudendal nerve terminal motor latency studies, after ileo-anal anastomosis, have not been performed at the Mayo Clinic.

Scintigraphic Anorectal (Anopouch) Angle Analysis

This study (Barkel et al. 1988) utilized an "active" probe that consisted of a 8×2.4 cm Penrose drain filled with a 70 cc solution of water and 7 mCi of ^{99m}Tc 04. A 14 French Foley catheter was placed in the balloon for easy insertion. One end of the Penrose drain was permanently sealed while the other was sealed but for a three-way stopcock. This tube system was used for filling the Penrose drain with a radioactive solution prior to each examination (Fig. 13.4). This technique was modified after Lahr et al. (1986).

Subjects were placed in the left lateral decubitus position and the probe passed through the anal canal into the rectum or ileal pouch. Satisfactory placement provided an image of the probe lying within the rectum or neorectum, outside the anus and in the anal canal itself. A gamma camera scanning from the right lateral position was used for imaging. The camera was linked to a computer for ease of analysis. The subject's thighs were placed at right angles to the longitudinal axis of the body. Thirty-second images were then recorded

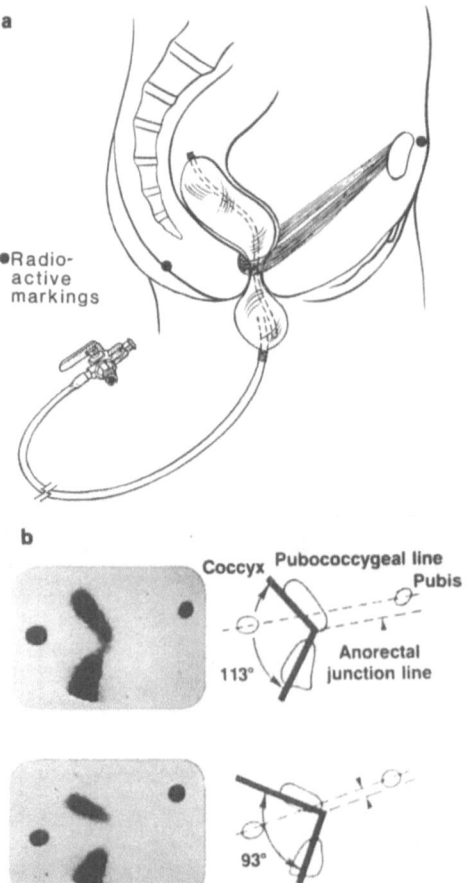

Fig. 13.4. a Diagram of the balloon device used to measure changes in the anorectal angle. A balloon was filled with ^{99m}Tc-labelled water. Radioactive markers were placed over the pubis anteriorly and coccyx posteriorly. b Hard-copy scintigraphic image of the anal rectal angle at rest (*above*) and during squeeze (*below*). To the right are diagrams of the same images. During squeeze, the angle narrows to 93° and the anorectal junction (level of the pelvic floor) ascends.

under the following conditions: rest, squeeze, Valsalva (in which the patient tried not to defaecate the balloon) and straining (in which the patient tried to defaecate the balloon). Each of these manouevres were repeated in the standing and sitting positions. The total radiation dose to the reproductive organs was 7% of that required for a conventional radiological examination of the pelvis.

Scintigraphic Assessment of Evacuation (O'Connell et al. 1986)

The scanning medium consisted of a 7.5% colloidal dispersion of aluminium magnesium silicate prepared by adding 1 mCi of a ^{99m}Tc sulphur colloid to 370 ml water, at 37 °C. Thirty grams of aluminium magnesium silicate powder were then slowly added while constantly stirring to produce a smooth thick paste. The gel was left stirring at 37 °C for 15 minutes prior to use. A 1 ml sample was taken and weighed and ^{99m}Tc activity counted in a well counter. The ^{99m}Tc/g of labelled aluminium magnesium silicate was then calculated. The material to be inserted into the patients was weighed.

The material was introduced to a predetermined maximum capacity using a 150 ml syringe connected to a soft 16 French tube 12 cm long, which was inserted 10 cm into the rectum or pouch. The subject was laid in the left lateral decubitus position. The residual uninserted material was weighed.

At 5 minute pre-evacuation anterior scan was obtained (Fig. 13.5). The subject was then seated on the radioluscent commode with a preweighed plastic bag lining the collection pan. The pre-evacuation right lateral scan was obtained in 5 minutes. The computer was set for dynamic acquisition of 2-second images in 4 minutes. Subjects were then asked to defaecate at will, but without moving. When this was completed, the subject was allowed to move about and, if possible, evacuate residual labelled material. The plastic liner containing the excreted aluminium magnesium silicate was removed and weighed. A 1 ml sample of the excreted material was weighed and its activity counted in a well counter. The activity per gram material excreted and the total activity excreted were calculated. The total activity excreted was divided by the total activity administered, and the percentage of instilled material that was evacuated was determined. The activity of the material evacuated was compared with the activity prior to instillation, following correction for decay, to determine if faecal material within the rectum had diluted the material.

Contrast Studies

A standard suspension of barium sulphate was used to delineate the anatomy of the ileal pouch and of the inflow tract to determine whether the anastomosis was intact or whether sinus tracts, fistulae or stenoses were present. This examination was performed transanally.

Contractile Activity

Intraluminal contractile activity of the small bowel was studied using perfused multilumen catheters placed orally so that the most distal of the nine perfused ports rested just proximal to the ileal pouch (Stryker et al. 1985b). The other ports spanned a distance of 125 cm above the pouch. A separate three-lumen catheter was used to record motility of the ileal pouch itself (Fig. 13.6). Both catheters were perfused by low compliance and pneumohydraulic perfusion systems and recordings were made on chart recorders.

Gastric Emptying and Small Bowel Transit

Scintigraphic techniques were used to study gastric emptying and transit through the small bowel after ileal pouch–anal anastomosis (Soper et al. 1989). Five hundred mCi of ^{99m}Tc DTPA was stabilized with 1.29 albumin and consumed as the liquid portion of a 300 kcal mixed meal. At the

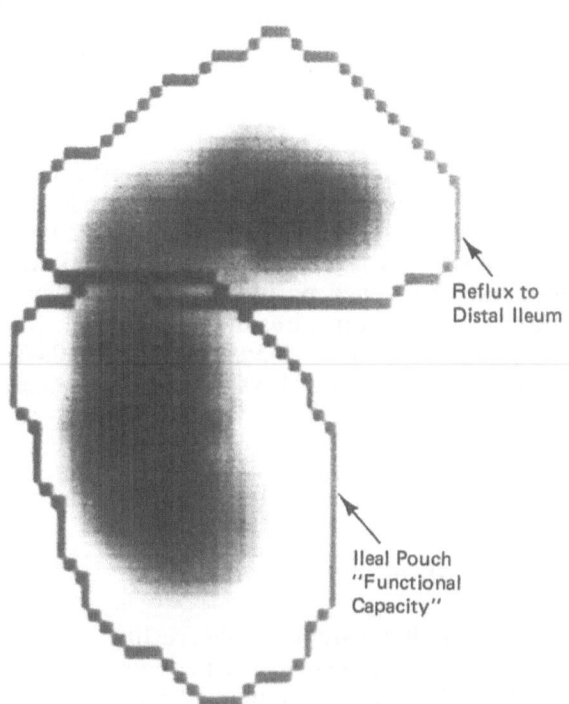

Fig. 13.5. Lateral scintigraphic scan of patient with ileal J pouch. Regions of interest outlined to show ileal pouch "functional volume" and reflux into distal ileum. (From P. R. O'Connell et al. (1987) Motor function of the ileal J pouch and its relation to clinical outcome after ileal pouch–anal anastomosis. *World Journal of Surgery* 11:735–741, by permission of Société Internationale de Chirurgie.)

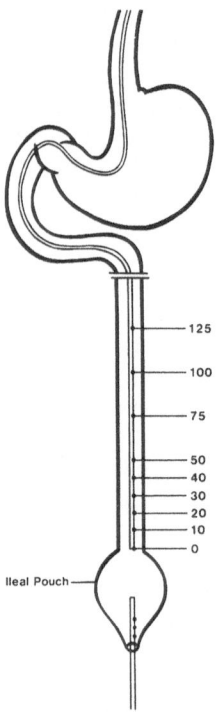

125
100
75
50
40
30
20
10
0

Ileal Pouch

Fig. 13.6. Position of manometric catheters in the two study groups used to monitor small intestinal motor events. (From S. J. Stryker et al. (1985) Motility of the small intestine after proctocolectomy and ileal pouch–anal anastomosis. *Annals of Surgery* 201:351–356.)

end of the meal, 250 mCi of ^{111}In-DTPA was instilled via an oroduodenal tube into the duodenum to study small bowel transit. Gamma camera imaging began 10 minutes after the intake of the meal and was performed every 10 minutes for 3 hours. Images were obtained every 20 minutes until all of the visible ^{111}In-DTPA had been passed.

Results

Anal Canal

Length

The mean length of the anal canal high pressure zone in healthy people is 4 cm. Women have shorter anal canals than men (3.7 vs 4.6 cm) Nivatvongs et al. 1981). During anal sphincter squeeze, the anal canal lengthens while during straining, it shortens. In 50 patients after ileal pouch–anal anastomosis and 30 healthy volun-

teers, the length of the anal canal did not differ (3.9±0.1 cm vs 3.8±0.1 cm; mean±SEM, P>0.05) (O'Connell et al. 1988). Moreover, there was no difference in the length of the anal canal of patients who had perfect continence and those who did not (3.9±0.1 cm vs 3.9±0.1 cm respectively, P>0.05).

Resting Pressure (Fig. 13.7)

After ileal pouch–anal anastomosis, global resting pressures were lower than control values (patients 56±3 mmHg vs control, 65±3 mmHg, P<0.05) (O'Connell et al. 1988). However, when mean resting pressures in the proximal, middle and distal anal canal were compared, only pressures within the *proximal* anal canal were lower than control values. When the resting pressures of patients with perfect continence were compared to those with episodes of incontinence, both the maximum mean resting pressure and the mean resting pressure in each third of the anal canal were less in patients with incontinence. Finally, the magnitude of radial variations in resting pressures were similar in patients and controls.

Squeeze Pressure

After ileal pouch–anal anastomosis, anal canal squeeze pressures were maintained (patients, 126±6 mmHg vs controls, 131±9 mmHg, P>0.01) (O'Connell et al. 1988). However, patients with impaired continence postoperatively had lower maximal squeeze pressures than patients who did not (104±7 mmHg vs 143±7 mmHg, P<0.05). Radial and longitudinal variations of squeeze pressure were similar in patients and controls and in patients who were fully continent and those who were not.

Motility of the Anal Canal

Slow phasic fluctuations of the resting pressure (slow waves) are noted in all patients after ileal pouch–anal anastomosis and in 80% of volunteers (O'Connell et al. 1988). Comparing the slow wave of patients and controls, the frequency was less and the amplitude greater in ileal pouch–anal anastomosis patients than in controls (frequency: patients 8.6±0.4 CPM vs controls 13.0±0.5 CPM, P<0.001; amplitude: patients 28±4 mmHg vs controls 7±1 mmHg, P<0.001) (Fig. 13.8). Forty-

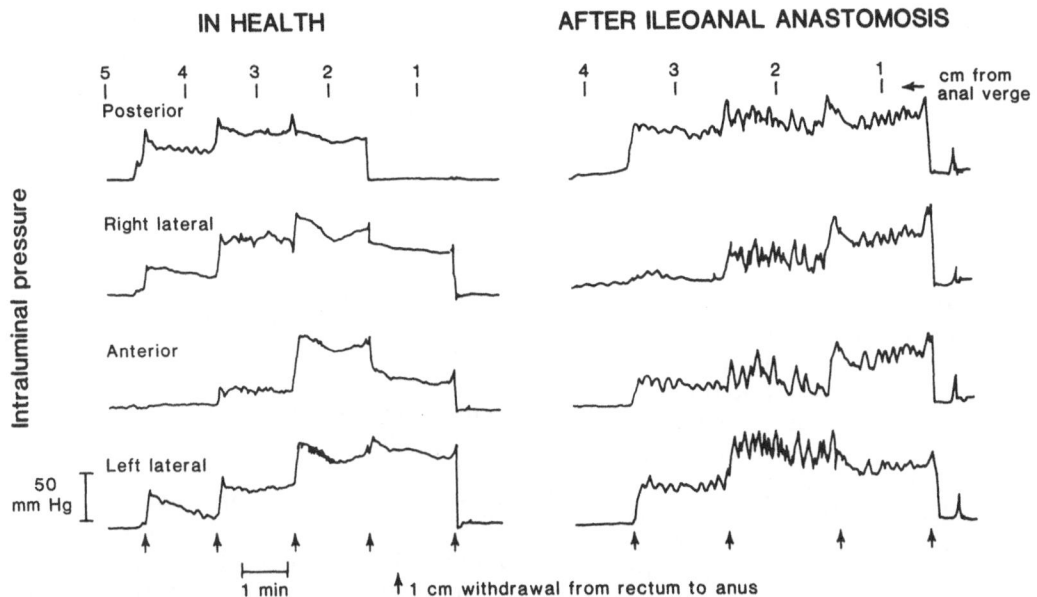

Fig. 13.7. Pressure recordings from the anal canal of a healthy volunteer (*left*) and a patient after ileo-anal anastomosis (*right*). A four-channel probe and a station pull-through technique were used. (From P. R. O'Connell, et al. (1988) Anal canal pressure and motility after ileoanal anastomosis. *Surgery, Gynecology and Obstetrics* 166:47–54, by permission of the journal.)

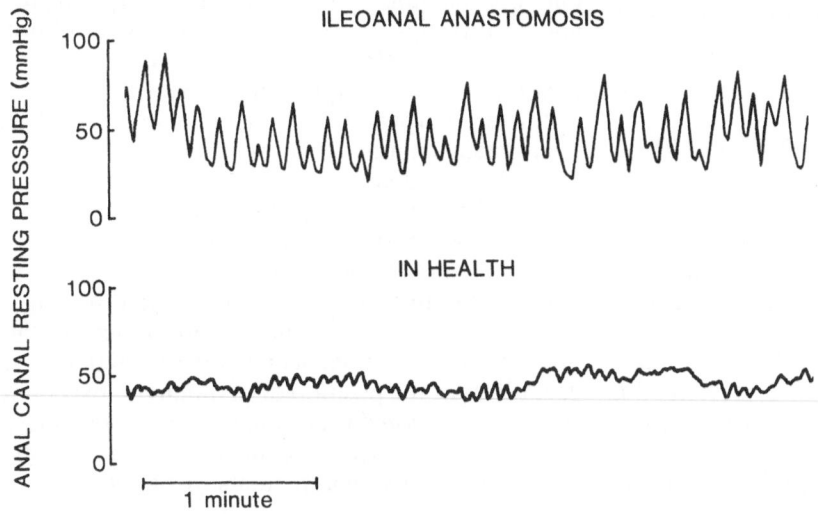

Fig. 13.8. Pattern of anal canal motility after ileo-anal anastomosis and in health as demonstrated by pressure recordings. (From P. R. O'Connell et al. (1988) Anal canal pressure and motility after ileoanal anastomosis. *Surgery, Gynecology and Obstetrics* 166:47–54, by permission of the journal.)

six per cent of the patients, but no volunteers, had "giant" slow waves. Ultra-slow waves were seen in 22% of patients and 17% of controls.

EMG

Electromyography using concentric needles was performed in 18 patients with normal continence and 9 patients with poor continence, a mean of 20 months after ileal pouch–anal anastomosis (Stryker et al. 1985b). Eighteen of the 27 patients had normal external anal sphincter motor unit potentials; that is, peak to peak amplitude of 200 millivolts to 3 microvolts, duration of 2–15 milliseconds and a biphasic or triphasic configuration. Sixteen of the 18 were continent. In contrast, nine patients had abnormal EMGs consisting of one or a combination of the following: high amplitude potentials, prolonged potentials or polyphasic potentials. Seven of the nine patients with EMG abormalities were incontinent ($\chi^2=12$; P<0.01). The mean duration of the motor unit potentials in incontinent patients was 6.4±1.3 microseconds vs 7.9±2.2 in the continent patients (P<0.05).

Summary: Anal Canal

Ileal pouch–anal anastomosis appears to preserve the length and longitudinal and radial integrity of the anal canal high pressure zone but in altered form; resting pressures were lower but squeeze pressures were not. Importantly, patients who had problems with continence after ileal pouch–anal anastomosis had lower resting *and* squeeze pressure than those who did not. Moreover, patients after ileal pouch–anal anastomosis exhibited a slower frequency and much greater amplitude of the slow wave compared to controls. These abnormal slow waves may reflect abormalities in contractility of the internal anal sphincter and be secondary to stretch injury. Alternately, slow waves recorded after ileal pouch–anal anastomosis may be produced by the segment of ileum which rests in the anal canal.

Anorectal Angle and Movements of the Pelvic Floor

An angulation exists between the anal canal and the rectum at the anorectal ring, which in healthy controls varies between 60° and 105° at rest (Barkel et al. 1988). The puborectalis muscle pulls the anorectal junction anteriorly, thus accentuating the anorectal angle. Parks (1975) described a "flap valve" function to the anorectal angle, but Bartolo et al. (1986) have asserted instead that the puborectalis muscle acts as a sphincter at the

anorectal junction. Whatever the mechanism, during times of rapidly increasing intra-abdominal pressure (cough, Valsalva, laughing), faecal content is kept from entering the anal canal by the action of the puborectalis muscle.

The angulation between the rectum and anal canal must be overcome in order to evacuate solid enteric content. This is accomplished by squatting; the angle is straightened to greater than 110° by flexing the hips 90°. This is augmented by straining, which usually causes the puborectalis muscle and EAS to become electrically silent in healthy people, although this does not always occur (Kerremans 1969). With the angle overcome, content passes into the anal canal.

In 13 volunteers and 6 patients after ileal pouch–anal anastomosis, we documented movements of the anorectal angle and pelvic floor using a real-time scintigraphic technique (Fig. 13.9) (Table 13.2). We found that for the left lateral decubitus position (at rest), the mean (±SD) anorectal angle in controls was 102±18°, whereas in patients after ileal pouch–anal anastomosis, the mean anopouch angle was 108±19° (P=0.3). Among controls and patients, moving to the sitting position straightened the resting angle; whereas standing did not have a similar effect. In controls, regardless of position, voluntary squeezing of the external anal sphincter sharpened the angle. In patients after ileal pouch–anal anastomosis, however, a voluntary squeeze sharpened the anal/pouch angle in the standing and sitting positions only. In controls, performing a Valsalva manoeuvre sharpened the anorectal angle in all positions. In patients, however, a Valsalva manoeuvre sharpened the angle only in the sitting position. No differences in the angle were present between controls and patients, regardless of the position or manoeuvre, except in the lying position during sphincter squeeze, where the angle was sharper in controls than in patients.

In controls as well as patients, the anorectal and

Table 13.2. Effect of position and of squeeze and Valsalva on the anorectal angle in health and on anopouch angle after ileal pouch–anal anastomosis (IPAA)

Manouevre	Anorectal/anopouch angle ($\bar{x}$±SD; degrees)		
	Decubitus (control/IPAA)	Sitting (control/IPAA)	Standing (control/IPAA)
Rest	102±18 /108±19	119±17[a]/116±16[b]	107±11 /105±8
Squeeze	81±19[c]/ 96±14[e]	87±15[c]/ 89± 9[d]	88± 6[c]/ 92±11[d]
Valsalva	87±23[c]/ 92±15	100±16[c]/ 96± 7[d]	95±17[c]/ 89±9

[a] Differs from control decubitus rest, P<0.02.
[b] Differs from IPAA decubitus rest, P<0.03.
[c] Differs from control resting *anorectal* angle of *same position*, P<0.03.
[d] Differs from IPAA resting *anopouch* angle of *same position*, P<0.02.
[e] Differs from decubitus control squeeze angle, P<0.05.

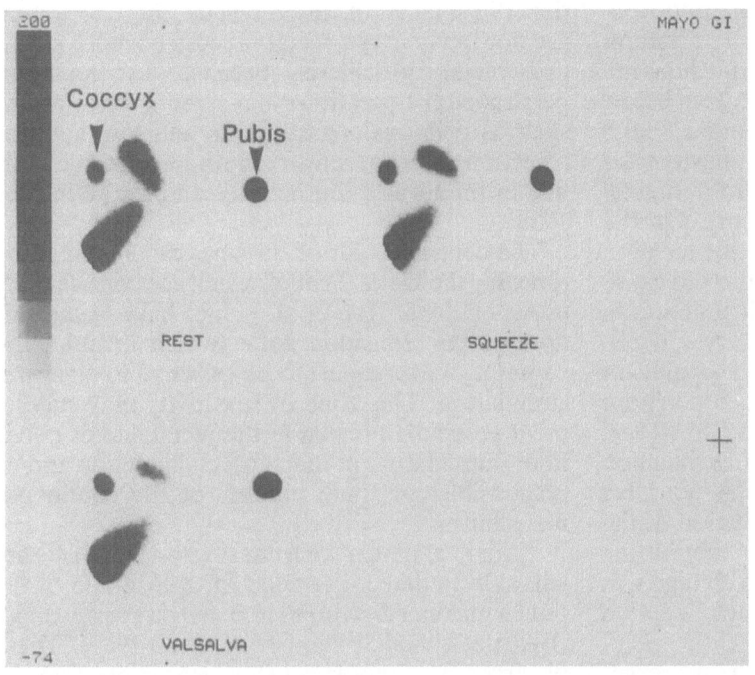

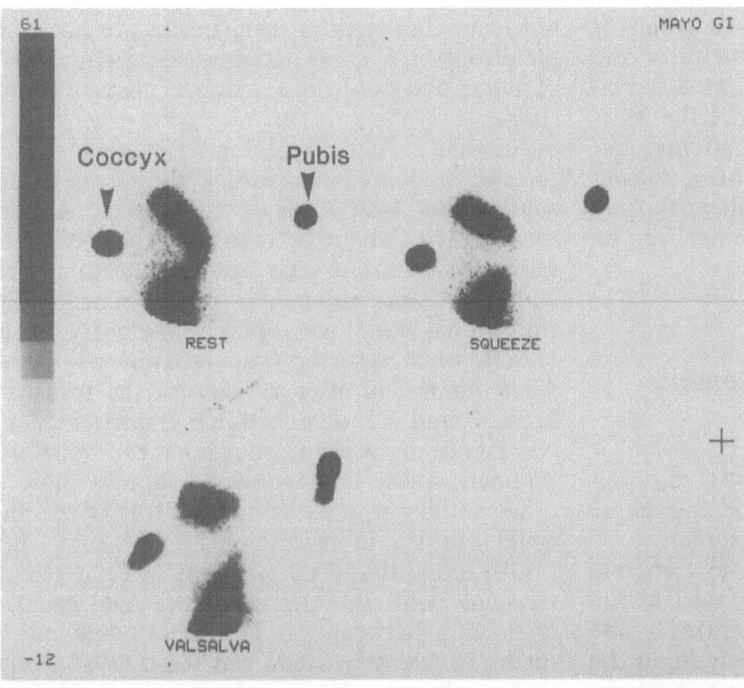

Fig. 13.9. a Scintigraphic image of balloon device in place in a healthy volunteer. During manoeuvres which facilitate continence (sphincter squeeze) or stress continence (Valsalva), the anorectal angle sharpens from its resting position. **b** Scintigraphic image of ballon device in place in a patient after ileal pouch–anal anastomosis. An angle is present between the pouch and the anal canal. As in health, this angle sharpens from its resting position during sphincter squeeze and the Valsalva manoeuvre. (From D. C. Barkel et al. (1988) Scintigraphic assessment of the anorectal angle in health and following ileal pouch–anal anastomosis. *Annals of Surgery* 208:42–49.)

anopouch junction remained below the pubococcygeal line in all positions. In the left lateral decubitus position at rest, the anorectal junction was located at a mean (±SD) of 2.8±1.7 cm below the pubococcygeal line in controls, and 1.8±0.8 cm in patients after ileal pouch–anal anastomosis (P=0.3). Sitting caused descent of the anorectal junction in controls, but not in patients. On the other hand, standing had no effect on the location of the anorectal junction in controls, but did cause significant elevation of the anopouch junction in patients. Among the controls, voluntary squeeze of the external anal sphincter caused significant ascent of the anorectal junction in each position. After ileal pouch–anal anastomosis, however, squeezing did not elevate the anopouch junction significantly, regardless of position. A Valsalva manoeuvre resulted in significant elevation of the anorectal junction in controls in the sitting position only, whereas in patients, no change was found in the position of the anopouch junction with Valsalva.

Ileal pouch–anal anastomosis, then, preserves the anatomical relationships of the pelvic floor such that an anoneorectal angle is restored which, in the main, functions as in health. Movements of the anoneorectal junction are altered, however, suggesting that in the patients we studied, the pelvic floor was tethered, either as a result of scarring or because of limited elasticity of the mesentery of the ileal pouch. Restricted movements of the pelvic floor may influence the functional outcome achieved by the patients, but whether or not the degree of continence achieved is directly related to the anal pouch angle and movements of the anopouch junction needs to be ascertained.

Anorectal and Anoneorectal Sensation and Reflex Mechanisms

Anorectal sensory mechanisms allow discrimination of the character of the enteric content as well as its presence within the rectal lumen.

Balloon distension of the rectal ampulla produces a sensation of pelvic fullness and the desire to defaecate (Akervall et al. 1989). The site of the receptors for this sensation may lie in the rectal muscularis and/or in the pelvic floor musculature surrounding the anorectal ring. Moreover, the ability to detect differential intrarectal pressures was hypothesized by Goligher and Hughes (1951) to be important in discriminating content character; flatus generated lower partial pressures

than did solid stool. Interestingly, these receptors are not likely in the rectal mucosa or more proximal rectal muscularis, because discrimination persists after operations that remove these areas, such as colo-anal anastomosis and low anterior resection. Indeed, sensory fibres have been identified in the levator ani muscle complex (Winckler 1958).

The cephalad half of the anal canal is lined by mucosa, the distal 2 cm of which contains sensory nerve endings. Roe et al. (1986) have found this area of the transition zone (which includes the columns of Morgagni) to be sensitive to electrical stimulation. This zone of sensitivity may supplement receptors present in the rectal and/or pelvic floor musculature at the anorectal junction and be responsible for "fine tuning" of the continence mechanism.

After ileal pouch–anal anastomosis, patients are still able to detect the need for evacuation of the pouch and can discriminate between gas and stool (Beart et al. 1985; Pemberton et al. 1987). These observations support previous suspicions that the rectal mucosa is not needed for rectal sensation. The 3–4 cm cuff of in situ rectal muscularis and the intact pelvic floor musculature must be responsible, therefore, for discrimination after ileal pouch–anal anastomosis. There is little question, however, that sensory mechanisms are not completely intact, as some patients leak small amounts of mucus and stool and sometimes mistake gas for stool.

An interesting physiological argument has recently appeared concerning the necessity for sparing the distal 2 cm of the transitional zone mucosa. It is claimed by Johnston et al. (1987) that improved sensation and better rates of perfect continence were obtained in patients in whom this transitional zone was spared. Keighley et al. (1987), while agreeing that sensation was somewhat diminished after excision of the transition zone, found no demonstrable improvement in continence in patients in whom the zone was retained. These findings would support those of other authors who examined the role of the anal canal mucosa in maintaining continence. Ihre (1974) found that if enteric content came in contact only with the tissues of the anal canal, a distinction between gas and stool could *not* be made. In addition, Read and Read (1982) found that continence to large volumes of saline infused into the rectum was unaffected when local anaesthesia was applied to the mucosa of the anal canal. It may be that retaining a perfectly intact distal sensory mechanism, after ileal pouch–anal anastomosis, will not be possible if extirpation of all mucosa at risk is to be assured. Nonetheless, although it is not perfect, sensation does persist after ileal pouch–anal anastomosis and complete rectal mucosa resection.

Rectal Anal Sphincter Inhibitory Response

The most readily identifiable and reproducible reflex present in the anorectum is the rectal anal sphincter inhibitory response (RASIR). Upon distending a balloon in the rectal ampulla acutely, the proximal portion of the anal canal relaxes while the distal portion contracts transiently. This response is present in all healthy adults (Gowers 1877; Duthie and Bennett 1963). The threshold response is about 5–10 ml of balloon distension. The hypothesized role of the RASIR is that it would allow rectal content to come into contact with the sensitive transitional zone mucosa transiently, while the contracted external anal sphincter would prevent leakage (Duthie and Bennett 1963).

After ileal pouch–anal anastomosis, the response is abolished (Fig. 13.10), but discrimination and recognition of the urge to evacuate are retained (Heppell et al. 1982a; Stryker et al. 1986). The response, however, has been demonstrated in some patients with long rectal muscular cuffs (Becker and Raymond 1986). The RASIR,

therefore, is probably mediated by receptors in the more proximal rectal muscular wall and carried intramurally or submucosally to the internal anal sphincter. Another reason why the response may not be demonstrable after operation is that the full thickness of the ileal pouch rests against the internal anal sphincter inside the anal canal; even if the internal anal sphincter relaxed, the relaxation would be dampened by the juxtaposed full thickness of the ileal wall and thus not recorded.

In summary, the RASIR cannot be demonstrated in most patients after ileal pouch–anal anastomosis, yet discrimination and the urge to defaecate remain intact. The role assigned traditionally to the reflex, therefore, may be in question.

Neorectal Compliance and Capacity

In healthy volunteers, the rectum accommodates passively to distension. Even at the maximum tolerable capacity (300–400 ml) (O'Connell et al. 1987a), intrarectal pressures rarely exceed 15–20 mmHg. Compliance of the rectum is calculated by plotting the slope of $\Delta P/\Delta V^{-1}$; in health compliance approximates $18 \text{ ml/cm } H_2O$ (O'Connell et al. 1987a). By comparison, the compliance of the terminal ileum in situ is $1.9 \pm 0.05 \text{ ml/cm } H_2O$ (Pemberton et al. 1983).

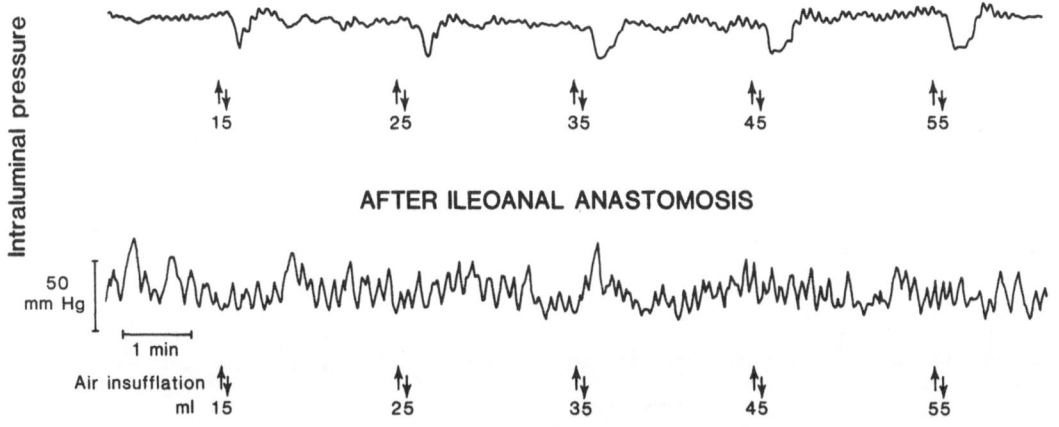

Fig. 13.10. Pressure recordings showing a transient decrease of proximal anal canal pressure in response to rectal distension in a healthy volunteer (the rectal anal sphincter inhibitory response), but not in a patient after ileo-anal anastomosis. (From P. R. O'Connell et al. (1988). Anal canal pressure and motility after ileoanal anastomosis. *Surgery, Gynecology and Obstetrics* 166:47–54, by permission of the journal.)

The capacity and compliance of the ileal pouches differ little from those of healthy rectums. In 23 patients, two years after ileal pouch–anal anastomosis, the maximum capacity was 320±36 ml while in six volunteers, the capacity was 330±29 ml (P>0.05) (O'Connell et al. 1987a). The compliance of ileal pouches, likewise, differed little from controls (pouches 14.7±1.4 ml/mmHg, control 18.6±2.0 ml/mmHg; P>0.05).

Patients with a good result postoperatively (less than six stools per day, perfect continence) had greater maximum capacities than those with a fair result (greater than six stools per day, episodic incontinence) (409±33 ml vs 290±27 ml) (P<0.05) (O'Connell et al. 1987a). However, compliance of the pouch was *not* related to outcome (good result 16.2±2.5 ml/mmHg vs fair result 13.4±1.6 ml/mmHg; P>0.01).

Importantly, ileal pouches appear to possess characteristics of true reservoirs – that is, passive accommodation to increasing volume with concomitant small increases in intraluminal pressure. Rectums and pouches, at least in these terms, behave similarly. This is not true, however, of intraluminal contractile activity.

Neorectal Motility

Patterns of intraluminal motility in the rectum contrast markedly with those of ileal pouches. The predominant contractile activity of the rectum consists of monotonous, infrequent (5–10 CPM),

small amplitude (<10 cm H_2O) contractions (Scharli and Kiesewetter 1970; Whitehead et al. 1980). This pattern does not change as intraluminal volume increases (Fig. 13.11, bottom). Also present are slower contractions (3 CPM) of amplitudes of up to 100 cm H_2O and slow contractions of high amplitude which appear to propagate. Kumar and colleagues (1988) have described several additional patterns of rectal contractions (isolated prolonged contractions, cluster contractions and phasic contractions). Whether *all* of these patterns are present is controversial and needs further study.

In contrast, the ileum displays different patterns of motility (Fig. 13.11, top; Fig. 13.12). Code et al. 1957), who studied motility in ileostomy patients, and Hepell et al. (1982b), who studied motility after straight ileo-anal anastomosis, described two types of ileal waves. One type was a wave of small amplitude (<10 mmHg) and short duration (3–6 s) and the other was a wave of large amplitude (>25 mmHg) and long duration (40–60 s). This latter wave has been termed a type 4 or high pressure wave (HPW). During a high pressure wave, pressures in the pouch may exceed resting anal canal pressure. The two types of waves sometimes occur together with the smaller wave superimposed on the larger. The stimulus for high pressure waves is luminal distension; construction of an ileal pouch increases the volume accommodated within the ileum before the onset of the waves (Akwari et al. 1980).

When high pressure waves occur, patients feel the need to evacuate. A series of investigations were performed in patients with J pouches to study

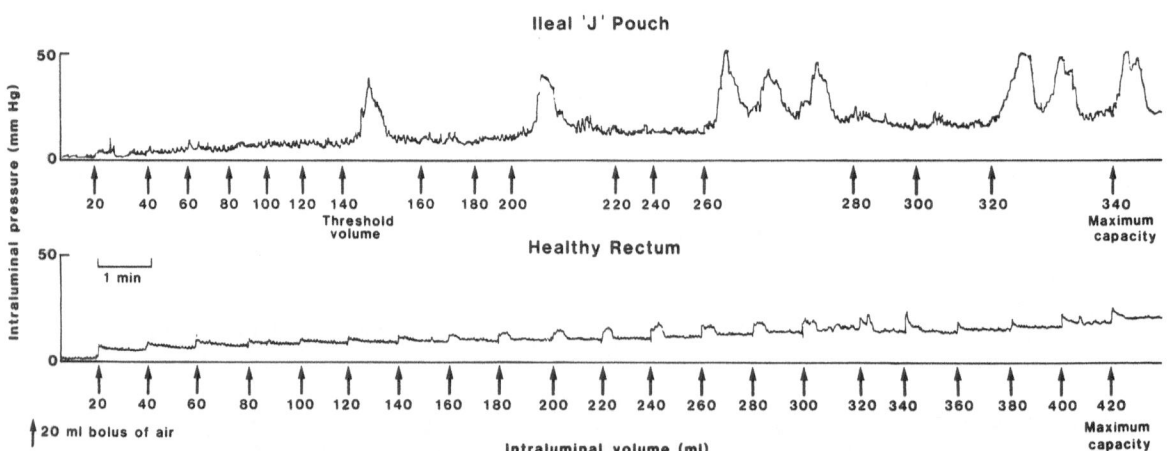

Fig. 13.11. Manometric tracing showing intraluminal pressure response to distension of the ileal pouch (*top*) and healthy rectum (*bottom*). Note the appearance of large pressure waves at the threshold volume of 140 ml distension in the pouch. (From P. R. O'Connell et al. (1987) Determinants of stool frequency after ileal pouch–anal anastomosis. *American Journal of Surgery* 153:157–164.)

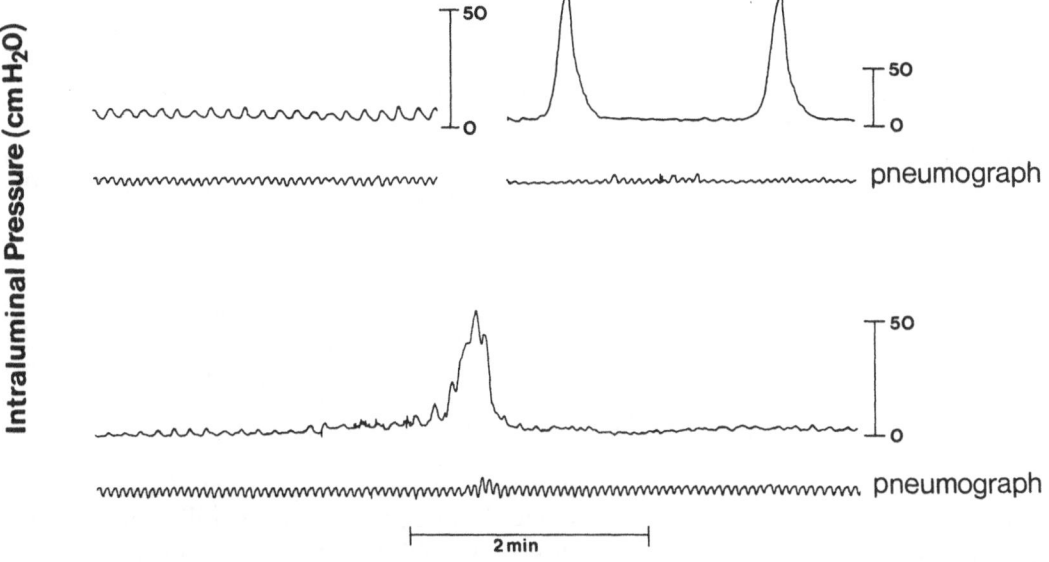

Fig. 13.12. Recordings of ileal motility 10 cm proximal to the anal sphincter after ileo-anal anastomosis. *Top left*: changes in intraluminal pressure of small amplitude and duration. *Top right*: changes in intraluminal pressure of large amplitude and duration. *Bottom*: changes in intraluminal pressure of both small and large amplitude. (From J. Heppell et al. (1982) Ileal motility after endorectal ileoanal anastomosis. *Surgical Gastroenterology* 1:123–127.)

the relationship between patterns of pouch motility and function.

Neorectal Filling

Patterns of motility in J shaped pouches are similar to those of Kock pouches. Gradual distension showed that the pouch accommodates well to distension. High pressure waves appeared in response to this distension, their amplitude being 49 ± 2 cm H_2O (mean$\pm$SEM) (O'Connell et al. 1987b). High pressure waves were associated with the urge to evacuate and occasionally, the pressure of a high pressure wave exceeded resting anal canal pressures. The frequency and amplitude of high pressure waves increased with time during fasting as the pouch filled (Fig. 13.13). High pressure waves occurred more frequently after feeding (Heppell et al. 1982b) and were abolished by evacuation of stool (Stryker et al. 1986). The interval to onset of high pressure waves was directly related to stool frequency (Stryker et al. 1986). The volume at which the onset of high pressure waves occurred was termed the threshold volume (TV) and was approximately $46\pm3\%$ of

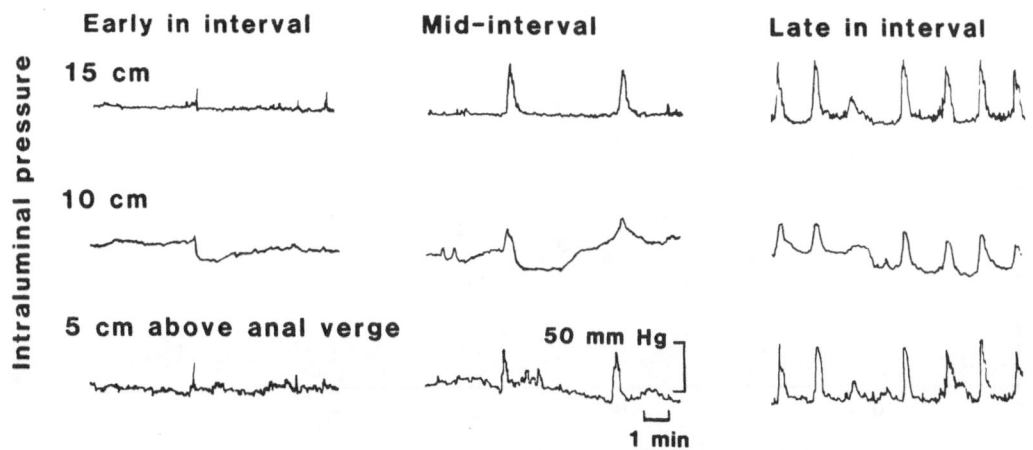

Fig. 13.13. Recordings of high-pressure waves from ileal pouch after ileal pouch–anal anastomosis. As the pouch fills (late in interval), the frequency of these waves increases. (From S. J. Stryker et al. (1986) Anal and neorectal function after ileal pouch–anal anastomosis. *Annals of Surgery* 203:55–61.)

the maximum pouch capacity. TV is a function of both maximum capacity and compliance. We have found that the motility parameter which best correlates to stool frequency is TV. If radiolabelled gel (described above) is instilled into the pouch to a predetermined maximum capacity, only about 60% remains in the pouch and the remainder refluxes into the proximal ileum (Fig 13.5). The volume of the gel remaining is termed the functional capacity and supports the findings of Rabau et al. (1982) and Neal et al. (1982). Furthermore, there is a direct correlation between functional capacity and threshold volumes, suggesting high pressure waves cause the reflux. This observation supports that of Berglund et al. (1985) in patients with Kock pouches.

Neorectal Emptying

Evacuation of ileal pouches is probably as important a parameter of function as is the ability to store content. Again using radiolabelled gel, J pouches were found to empty as rapidly and efficiently and completely as healthy rectums (Stryker et al. 1986; O'Connell et al. 1986). Ileal pouches generally evacuated with a 60%–70% rate of efficiency (Fig. 13.14). Although there was a direct correlation between evacuation efficiency and stool frequency, this was rarely clinically important except in patients with anastomotic strictures. The rate of evacuation of ileal pouches is approximately 11 ml/stool per second. This, combined with the observation that evacuation is initiated at will, suggests that intrinsic pouch motility is *not* responsible for neorectal evacuation.

In addition, although intuitively obvious, we examined the relationship between stool frequency and daily volume output, and found that the stool frequency and output were directly related (n=0.8) (O'Connell et al. 1987b).

In summary, the length of the interval between evacuations is determined by the timing of the high pressure waves; the longer the high pressure waves are delayed,the longer the interval between stools. This relationship is illustrated by the following: stool frequency is indirectly related to the threshold volume and maximum capacity (the larger the threshold volume and maximum capacity, the fewer the stools) and to the efficiency of evacuation (the more efficient the emptying, the fewer the stools per day). If the pouch capacity, threshold volume, or efficiency of evacuation is reduced, high pressure waves will appear prematurely, prompting frequent voiding of small amounts of stool.

If the normal efficiency of pouch emptying is about 50%–60% and the urge to defaecate occurs at a threshold volume which is approximately 45% of maximum pouch capacity, then the daily frequency of stooling can be calculated using the formula:

$$\text{Stool frequency} = \frac{\text{daily output}}{(\text{TV})\,(\%\ \text{evacuation})}$$

Because the daily output of normal ileostomies ranges between 400 and 800 ml, the calculated number of stools per day should vary between four and eight. This theoretical relationship is confirmed by the finding in our patients that the mean number of stools per day is six (Pemberton et al. 1987).

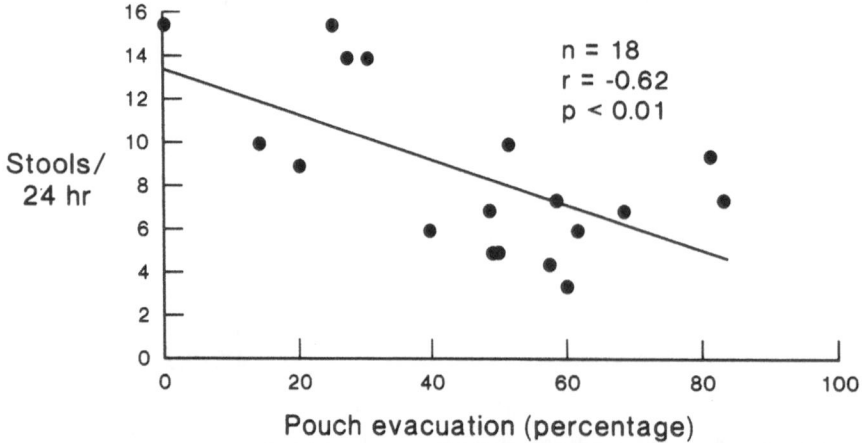

Fig. 13.14. Relationship of the completeness of ileal pouch evacuation to stool frequency after ileal pouch–anal anastomosis. (From S. J. Stryker et al. (1986) Anal and neorectal function after ileal pouch–anal anastomosis. *Annals of Surgery* 203:55–61.)

Proximal Small Bowel Motility

The ileal pouch does not disrupt patterns of proximal small bowel motility. Stryker et al. (1985b) found that the periodicity, appearance, duration and velocity of migrating motor complexes in patients after ileal pouch–anal anastomosis were similar to those found in healthy volunteers (Fig. 13.15). Interestingly, however, high pressure waves were recorded in the jejuno-ileum proximal to the pouch. These waves may be a response to distal occlusion of the small bowel by the anal canal. These waves may propel content aborally. Although reported to occur after ileal pouch–anal anastomosis by Chaussade et al. (1989), an obstructive motility pattern (clustered contractions within 2 hours of meal), such as that recorded by Summers et al. (1983), in patients with mechanical small bowel obstruction was not seen in patients after ileal pouch–anal anastomosis in Stryker et al's study (1985b).

The impact of ileal pouch–anal anastomosis upon proximal gut transit was addressed by Soper and colleagues (1989), who quantitated gastric emptying and transit through the small bowel in controls, in patients with a Brooke ileostomy and patients after ileo-anal anastomosis. They found that gastric emptying was similar in the three groups (T½ liquid phase: 51±10 min control, 57±7 min Brooke, 39±4 min IPAA; mean±SEM, P>0.05). Time to arrival of the radiolabelled material into the ileal pouch was much longer than in controls or Brooke ileostomy patients (control 75±15 min, Brooke 80±32 min, IPAA 178±26 min; P<0.01). Moreover, the interval to maximum filling of the caecum, ileostomy bag or pelvic pouch was much longer in Brooke and ileal pouch–anal anastomosis patients than in controls (control 243±32 min, Brooke 340±12 min, IPAA 341±19 min; P<0.01, IPAA and Brooke vs control). Among the ileal pouch–anal anastomosis patients, the mean interval to defaecation was 374±10 minutes (mean±SEM). In addition, the longer the interval to defaecation, the fewer stools per day (r=0.53).

These data suggest that the *effect of proctocolectomy* is to slow the transit of the bulk of chyme through the small bowel while the *effect of ileal pouch–anal anastomosis* is to slow the arrival of the head of chyme. However, there was no correlation between stool frequency and arrival time of either the head or bulk of the chyme at the pouch. Two of the ileal pouch–anal anastomosis patients had very frequent stools and these patients had very rapid transit. Finally, the ability of the pouch to accommodate chyme was not solely a function of volume because there was no correlation between maximal tolerable capacity and the amount of radiolabelled stool in the pouch; therefore, pouches may vary in their *sensitivity* to enteric content.

Neorectal Motor Function

In patients after ileal pouch–anal anastomosis, the rectum has been replaced by compliant, capacious reservoir with characteristics of motility distinctly different from those possessed by the rectum. The pelvic floor has been preserved, and its movements are largely similar to those in healthy people. The anal canal has also been preserved. However, the zone of sensation (ATZ) has been removed, the RASIR abolished and the resting tone weakened. Finally, the nature of enteric content which must be retained and, in turn, evacuated has been altered from firm and formed to a semiformed or frankly liquid consistency.

One hypothesis of neorectal motor function

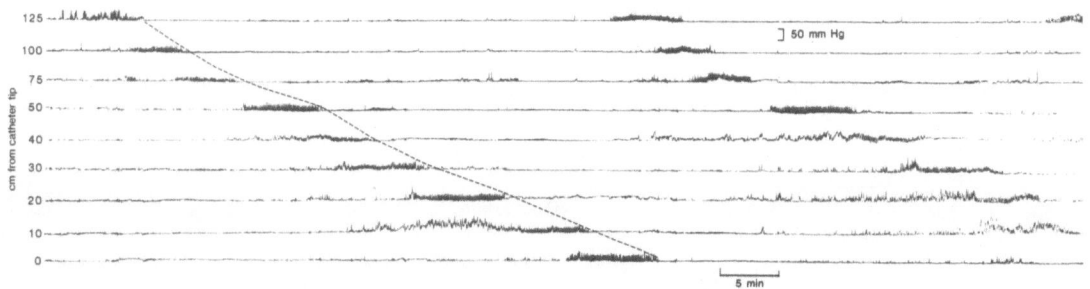

Fig. 13.15. Recording of interdigestive jejuno-fileal motility after ileal pouch–anal anastomosis. Two motor complexes are present which migrate distally (*dashed line*). Catheter tip was located approximately 10 cm orad to pouch. (From S. J. Stryker et al. (1985) Motility of the small intestine after proctocolectomy and ileal pouch–anal anastomosis. *Annals of Surgery* 201:351–356.)

after ileal pouch–anal anastomosis is shown in Fig. 13.16 (O'Connell et al. 1987b). After emptying, a residual volume of stool remains in the pouch. The pouch then begins to fill again with aboral movement of enteric content. As the pouch is filled to a threshold volume (determined by its maximal capacity) infrequent high pressure waves are evoked. These waves produce crampy abdominal discomfort and signal the call to stool. Although classic "sampling" of enteric content does not occur because the RASIR has been abolished, between 60%–80% of patients after ileal pouch–anal anastomosis distinguished between gas and enteric content (Pemberton et al. 1987). If defaecation is postponed by active contraction of the external anal sphincter, the pouch continues to fill with content until the functional capacity is reached. At this volume, more high pressure waves propel content proximally into the distal ileum so that the amount of content in the pouch does not exceed its functional capacity. As more content refluxes, high pressure waves are evoked in the distal ileum as well as in the pouch. Crampy discomfort then becomes more intense until evacuation occurs. Evacuation is initiated by straining and a Valsalva manouevre, and the anorectal angle is effaced by relaxation of the pelvic floor. Evacuation occurs rapidly and is about 80% complete.

Leakage of enteric content occurs most often at night, when resting anal canal tone is decreased (Orkin et al. 1989). Moreover, during the day, if high pressure waves generate pressures greater than resting anal canal tone and the external anal sphincter contracts weakly, leakage also occurs.

The ileal pouch–anal anastomosis operation is successful in the majority of the patients because the reservoir, which is compliant and capacious, is restored and the anal canal and pelvic floor are preserved. However, patients must learn to recognize different signals heralding the need for evacuation. Overall, neorectal function closely resembles that of the native rectum. Without question, however, motility patterns within the pouch reflect those characteristics of the small bowel from which they were constructed and these characteristics determine functional outcome. *Perhaps the principal problem is that in health, anal canal pressure nearly always exceeds rectal pressure but this relationship is abolished after ileal pouch–anal anastomosis.*

Clinical Usefulness of Physiological Measurements After Ileal Pouch–Anal Anastomosis

Several parameters of anoneorectal function are associated with specific functional outcomes. In an interesting discussion of parameters influencing function, Keighley et al. (1988) determined the number of abnormal physiological parameters which occurred in patients after ileal pouch–anal anastomosis. The parameters determined included resting pressure, squeeze pressure, compliance and threshold volume. The authors attempted to correlate physiological function with clinical function. They found that patients with an "imperfect result" had four abnormal parameters

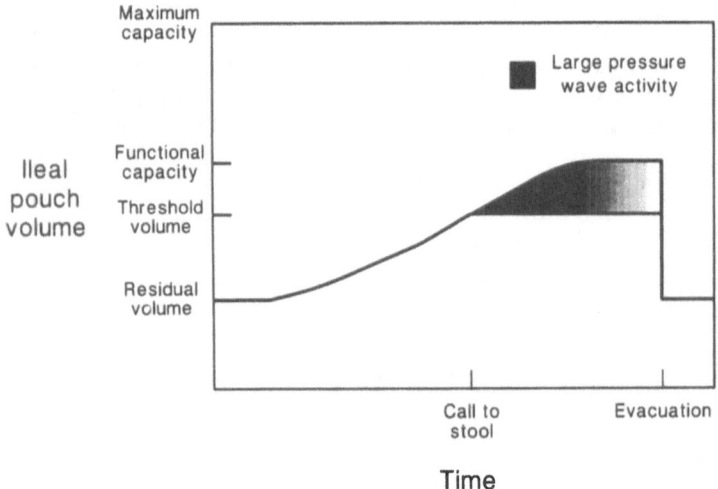

Fig. 13.16. Proposed model of relationship between neorectal motility parameters and neorectal function (see text for explanation). (From P. R. O'Connell et al. (1987) Motor function of the ileal J pouch and its relation to clinical outcome after ileal pouch–anal anastomosis. *World Journal of Surgery* 11:735–741, by permission of the Société Internationale de Chirurgie.)

present compared to one abnormal parameter in patients with a "good" result, implying that physiological defects in the internal anal sphincter, external anal sphincter or pouch capacity or compliance affected the *clinical* outcome dramatically.

Anal Canal Pressure

Low resting pressures are found in nearly all patients postoperatively. Indeed, it is the most frequently persistent abnormality found after ileal pouch–anal anastomosis. Therefore, relying on measurement of resting pressure *alone* to predict outcome is hazardous. Strikingly low resting pressures, however, are found most frequently in patients who had previous pelvic sepsis (Keighley et al. 1988).

In contrast, a poor squeeze effort *is* associated with an impaired functional result (O'Connell et al. 1988; Nasmyth et al. 1986).

Electromyography

EMG evidence of external anal sphincter denervation is associated with incontinence and, therefore, an impaired result (Stryker et al. 1985b; Emblem et al. 1989).

Neorectal Compliance

In general, the greater the compliance, the better the outcome in terms of stools per day (O'Connell et al. 1987a; Heppell et al. 1983) and episodes of incontinence. Interestingly, Keighley et al. (1988) could not link continence to the occurence of pelvic sepsis, which confirms our observations that pelvic sepsis had little effect on episodes of incontinence after ileal pouch–anal anastomosis (Pemberton et al. 1987).

Capacity

The greater the capacity, the greater the threshold volume and the longer the interval to the onset of HPWs. This, in turn, is associated with fewer stools and fewer episodes of incontinence. Harms et al. (unpublished observation) confirmed these observations in patients with W pouches; the larger the tolerated volume, the fewer the stools.

Sensation

The urge to evacuate after ileal pouch–anal anastomosis is signalled by the onset of HPWs, which in turn is related to the threshold volume; the longer the interval of time to reach the threshold volume, the more infrequent the call to stool. There is no doubt that sensation thresholds in the anal canal are very high in patients in whom the anal transition zone has been excised (Keighley et al. 1987). However, incontinence is not related to this loss of sensation (Keighley et al. 1987; Emblem et al. 1989).

Rectal Anal Inhibitory Response

This response is abolished in nearly all patients in whom a short anal canal and rectal mucosal dissection has been performed. The loss of the submucosal neural plexus and damage to the internal anal sphincter may be responsible for this abnormality. Alternatively, the internal anal sphincter may indeed relax, but the interposed ileum prevents recording the relaxation.

Integrity of the Pelvic Floor

Although movements of the anoneorectal angle are essentially preserved postoperatively, movements of the pelvic floor are not; tethering of the pelvic floor secondary to postoperative scarring or mesenteric immobility may affect continence adversely, but this has not been tested directly.

Predictors of Functional Outcome

In 22 patients, Heppell et al. (1983) correlated preclosure anal canal pressures and pouch compliance performed before closure of the ileostomy with functional outcome one month after closure. They found that low resting pressure and poor compliance correlated significantly with stool frequency and incontinence. Scott and colleagues (1989), expanding upon this report, correlated anal canal pressures and pouch compliance before ileostomy closure with functional results one year after closure. A low mean resting pressure was associated with subsequent nocturnal incontinence and the need to use constipating agents while low pouch compliance was associated with increased nocturnal stool frequency. Interestingly, in this study, low squeeze pressures were not associated with subsequent incontinence or stool frequency.

Usefulness of Physiological Measurements in Patients with Specific Problems

Preclosure

It is important that candidates for closure of the diverting ileostomy undergo pre-operative testing, including anorectal manometry and pouchography. Patients with low resting pressure (compared to normative values of patients after ileal pouch–anal anastomosis) but a normal squeeze increment may be closed safely. On the other hand, patients with low resting pressures *and* a poor squeeze effort should undergo EMG in order to determine whether the external anal sphincter has been denervated or traumatized. If motor unit potentials are normal, but pudendal nerve terminal motor latency prolonged, delay in closure is indicated in order to augment squeeze effort by biofeedback training. If EMG shows normal pudendal nerve terminal motor latency but abnormal motor unit potentials, trauma to the sphincter has occurred. If a specific defect is present, sphincteroplasty should be performed. If no defect is found, delay with biofeedback training is indicated.

Pouchography serves an important function by visualizing the anatomy of the pouch and the anastomosis. Sinus tracts and fistulae are easily identified by pouchography and should be corrected before closure of the diverting ileostomy.

In summary, preclosure testing will identify patients who may have problems with stool frequency and incontinence postoperatively, patients toward whom better education and sphincter training should be directed.

Pouchitis

Pouchitis, a clinical syndrome consisting of crampy abdominal discomfort, watery, often bloody diarrhoea, fever, malaise and weakness, occurs frequently after ileal pouch–anal anastomosis. Moreover, the mucosa is friable, oedematous and erythematous, and scattered ulcers may be present. The cause is unknown. The incidence ranges between 15% and 50% – the longer the follow-up, the higher the incidence (Lohmuller et al. 1990).

The problem which might be readily confused with pouchitis is inefficient emptying. Nearly all J shaped pouches empty spontaneously but some do not empty as completely or rapidly as others. In these patients, the time between emptying shortens as less content is required to distend the pouch to threshold volume. The shorter the interval, the greater the number of stools. Moreover, stool consistency changes to that of water.

In patients who manifest diarrhoea ($\pm$blood), crampy lower abdominal discomfort, frequency and incontinence, but who do not have acute inflammatory changes of the mucosa and in whom metronidazole is not efficacious, pouch emptying studies are indicated. In patients with poor emptying, dilatation of the anal canal, intubation of the pouch or pelvic floor retraining may be indicated to improve the efficiency of emptying.

Incontinence

Incontinence after ileal pouch–anal anastomosis during the day is caused by poor resting pressure, no squeeze effort or poor pouch capacity and compliance; if the threshold volume is reached after only 20%–25% of the pouch is filled, urgency incontinence is inevitable. At night, HPWs may overwhelm the low resting pressures common in patients after ileal pouch–anal anastomosis, causing incontinence. Capacity and compliance testing is rapidly performed and is safe. If a patient with incontinence has a small and poorly compliant pouch, biofeedback training aimed at desensitizing the pouch to HPWs is indicated.

Disturbed Defaecation

Although uncommon, patients after ileal pouch–anal anastomosis may be unable to empty their pouch completely and thus strain endlessly. Persistent straining might result in prolapse of the anterior wall of the pouch or, alternatively, cause the perineum to descend; perineal descent may in turn cause progressive sphincter denervation. Tests of pelvic floor function (defaecating proctogram, emptying studies, anorectal angle studies, balloon expulsion) identify such patients readily and facilitate instituting appropriate therapy early. This consists of repair of the pouch prolapse, pelvic floor retraining and biofeedback.

Conclusion

Enteric continence in health requires the orchestration of several factors, foremost being an ample and compliant reservoir, an intact and functioning pelvic floor and anal sphincters and a manageable form and volume of stool. Although each of these factors is adversely affected by ileal pouch–anal anastomosis, the operation nevertheless preserves critical mechanisms – perhaps, however, in altered form. The compliant capacious rectum is replaced by a less compliant, less voluminous ileal pouch. Intraluminal pressures in the rectum are nearly always lower than anal canal pressures and thus leakage rarely occurs. Intraluminal pressures in the ileal pouch, however, may be higher than the ileal resting pressures and indeed may even be higher than squeeze pressures; incontinence, particularly at night, therefore sometimes occurs.

The anal sphincters are largely preserved intact, but resting pressures are lower than in health and if squeeze pressures are likewise low, leakage occurs, particularly as the pouch fills to threshold levels. Movements of the pelvic floor are also abnormal after ileal pouch–anal anastomosis, but the significance of these findings are unclear.

Instead of small amounts of firm, formed stool presenting into the rectum each day, 600–1000 ml of semiformed or liquid stool empties into the pouch every 24 hours. This strains an already altered sphincter mechanism, and, in and of itself, may be responsible for leakage. Not surprisingly, stool frequency is directly related to the volume of stool produced each day.

Assessment of neorectal and anal canal function after ileal pouch–anal anastomosis has confirmed the importance of some principles of continence and questioned the importance of others, such as the requirement for a long rectal stump, preservation of the rectal anal inhibitory response and maintaining sensation in the upper half of the anal canal. Results, however, are not perfect and there is little doubt that altering these factors, while not important for maintaining gross faecal incontinence, results in subtle reductions of function compared to health.

Future efforts to improve functional outcome after IPAA will concentrate on increasing reservoir capacity while maintaining good emptying dynamics, increasing the threshold volume, decreasing ileal pouch contractility, increasing emptying efficiency, slowing transit, enhancing absorption and maintaining sensation in the anal canal.

References

Akervall S, Fasth S, Nordgren S, Oresland T, Hulten L (1989) Rectal reservoir and sensory function studied by graded isobaric distension in normal man. Gut 30:496–502

Akwari OE, Kelly KA, Phillips SF (1980) Myoelectrical and motor patterns of continent pouch and conventional ileostomy. Surg Gynecol Obstet 150:363–371

Arndorfer RC, Steff JJ, Dodds WJ, Linehan JH, Hogan WJ (1977) Improved infusion system for intraluminal esophageal manometry. Gastroenterology 73:23–27

Barkel DC, Pemberton JH, Pezim ME, Phillips SF, Kelly KA, Brown ML (1988) Scintigraphic assessment of the anorectal angle in health and after ileal pouch–anal anastomosis. Ann Surg 208:42–49

Bartolo DCC, Roe AM, Locke-Edmunds JC, Virjee J, Mortensen NJMcC (1986) Flap valve theory of anorectal continence. Br J Surg 73:1012–1014

Beart RW, Jr, Dozois RR, Wolff BG, Pemberton JH (1985) Mechanisms of rectal continence: lessons from the ileoanal procedure. Am J Surg 149:31–33

Becker JM, Raymond JL (1986) Ileal pouch–anal anastomosis: a single surgeon's experience with 100 consecutive cases. Ann Surg 204:375–381

Berglund B, Asztély M, Kock NG, Myrvild HE (1985) Reflux from the continent ileostomy reservoir: a radiologic evaluation combined with pressure recording. Dis Colon Rectum 28:502–505

Brough WA, Schofield PF (1989) An improved technique of J pouch construction and ileoanal anastomosis. Br J Surg 76:350–351

Chaussade S, Merite F, Hautefeuille M, Valleur P, Hautefeuille P, Courturier D (1989) Motility of the jejunum after proctocolectomy and ileal pouch anastomosis. Gut 30:371–375

Code CF, Rogers AG, Schlegel J, Hightower NC Jr, Bargen JA (1957) Motility patterns in the terminal ileum: studies on two patients with ulcerative colitis and ileal stomas. Gastroenterology 32:651–665

Duthie HL, Bennett RC (1963) The relation of sensation in the anal canal to the functional anal sphincter: a possible factor in anal continence. Gut 4:179–182

Emblem R, Bergan A, Larsen S (1988) Straight ileoanal anastomosis with preserved anal mucosa for ulcerative colitis and familial polyposis. Scand J Gastroenterol 23:913–919

Emblem R, Erichsen AA, Morkrid L, Ganes T, Stein R, Bergan A (1989) Failed ileoanal anastomosis: correlation between clinical function and anal canal neurophysiologic and histologic examinations. Scand J Gastroenterol 24:623–631

Fonkalsrud EW (1982) Endorectal ileal pullthrough with ileal reservoir for ulcerative colitis and polyposis. Am J Surg 144:81–86

Goligher JC, Hughes ESR (1951) Sensibility of the rectum and colon: role in the mechanism of anal continence. Lancet i:543–548

Gowers WR (1877) The automatic action of the sphincter ani. Proc R Soc London 26:77–84

Gustavsson S, Weiland LH, Kelly KA (1987) Relationship of backwash ileitis to ileal pouchitis after ileal pouch–anal anastomosis. Dis Colon Rectum 30:25–28

Harms BA, Hamilton JW, Yamamoto DT, Starling JR (1987) Quadruple-loop (W) ileal pouch reconstruction after proctocolectomy: analysis and functional results. Surgery 102:561–567

Heald RJ, Allen DR (1986) Stapled ileo-anal anastomosis: a

technique to avoid mucosal proctectomy in the ileal pouch operation. Br J Surg 73:571–572

Heppell J, Kelly KA, Phillips SF, Beart RW Jr, Telander RL, Perrault J (1982a) Physiologic aspects of continence after colectomy, mucosal proctectomy, and endorectal ileo-anal anastomosis. Ann Surg 195:435–443

Heppell J, Pemberton JH, Kelly KA et al. (1982b) Ileal motility after endorectal ileoanal anastomosis. Surg Gastroenterol 1:123–127

Heppell J, Taylor BM, Beart RW Jr, Dozois RR, Kelly KA (1983) Predicting outcome after endorectal ileoanal anastomosis. Can J Surg 26:132–134

Ihre T (1974) Studies on anal function in continent and incontinent patients. Thesis, Stockladen AAS and Wahl

Johnston D, Holdsworth PJ, Nasmyth DG, Primrose JN, Womack N, Axon ATR (1987) Preservation of the entire anal canal in conservative proctocolectomy for ulcerative colitis: a pilot study comparing end-to-end ileo-anal anastomosis without mucosal resection with mucosal proctectomy and endo-anal anastomosis. Br J Surg 74:940–944

Keighley MRB, Winslet MC, Yoshioka K, Lightwood R (1987) Discrimination is not impaired by excision of the anal transition zone after restorative proctocolectomy. Br J Surg 74:1118–1121

Keighley MR, Yoshioka K, Kmiot W, Heyen F (1988) Physiological parameters influencing function in restorative proctocolectomy and ileo-pouch-anal anastomosis. Br J Surg 75:997–1002

Kerremans R (1969) Morphological and physiological aspects of anal continence and defaecation. Arscia, Uigaven Brussel, Belgium

Kumar D, Williams NS, Waldron D, Hallan RI, Wingate DL (1988) Phasic and periodic motor activity in the human anorectum (abstract). Gastroenterology 94:A241

Lahr CJ, Rothenberger DA, Jensen LL, Goldberg SM (1986) Balloon topography: a single method of evaluating anal function. Dis Colon Rectum 29:1–5

Lohmuller JL, Pemberton JH, Dozois RR, Ilstrup D, Van Heerden J (1990) Pouchitis and extraintestinal manifestations of deflammatory bowel disease after ileal pouch–anal anastomosis. Ann Surg 211:622–629

Martin LW, LeCoultre C, Schubert WK (1977) Total colectomy and mucosal proctectomy with preservation of continence in ulcerative colitis. Ann Surg 186:477–479

McHugh SM, Diamant NE (1987) Effect of age, gender, and parity on anal canal pressures: contribution of impaired anal sphincter function to fecal incontinence. Dig Dis Sci 32:726–736

Nasmyth DG, Johnston D, Godwin PGR, Dixon MF, Smith A, Williams NS (1986) Factors influencing bowel function after ileal pouch–anal anastomosis. Br J Surg 73:469–473

Neal DE, Williams NS, Johnston D (1982) Rectal, bladder and sexual function after mucosal proctectomy with and without a pelvic reservoir for colitis and polyposis. Br J Surg 69:599–604

Nicholls RJ, Kamm MA (1988) Proctocolectomy with restorative ileoanal reservoir for severe idiopathic constipation: report of two cases. Dis Colon Rectum 31:968–969

Nicholls RJ, Pezim ME (1985) Restorative proctocolectomy with ileal reservoir for ulcerative colitis and familial adenomatous polyposis: a comparison of three reservoir designs. Br J Surg 72:470–474

Nivatvongs S, Stern HS, Fryd DS (1981) The length of the anal canal. Dis Colon Rectum 24:600–601

O'Connell PR, Kelly KA, Brown ML (1986) Scintigraphic assessment of neorectal motor function. J Nucl Med 27:460–464

O'Connell PR, Pemberton JH, Brown ML, Kelly KA (1987a) Determinants of stool frequency after ileal pouch–anal anastomosis. Am J Surg 153:157–163

O'Connell PR, Pemberton JH, Kelly KA (1987b) Motor function of the ileal J pouch and its relation to clinical outcome after ileal pouch–anal anastomosis. World J Surg 11:735–741

O'Connell PR, Stryker SJ, Metcalf AM, Pemberton JH, Kelly KA (1988) Anal canal pressure and motility after ileoanal anastomosis. Surg Gynecol Obstet 166:47–54

Orkin BA, Kelly KA, Dent J (1989) Influence of sleep on anal canal resting pressure (abstract). Gastroenterology 96:A378

Parks AG (1975) Anorectal incontinence. Proc R Soc Med 68:681–690

Parks AG, Nicholls RJ, Belliveau P (1980) Proctocolectomy with ileal reservoir and anal anastomosis. Br J Surg 67:533–538

Pemberton JH (1987) Surgery for ulcerative colitis. Surg Clin North Am 67(3):633–650

Pemberton JH, Heppell J, Beart RW Jr, Dozois RR, Telander RL (1982) Endorectal ileoanal anastomosis. Surg Gynecol Obstet 155:417–424

Pemberton JH, van Heerden JA, Beart RW Jr, Kelly KA, Phillips SF, Taylor BM (1983) A continent ileostomy device. Ann Surg 197:618–625

Pemberton JH, Kelly KA, Beart RW Jr, Dozois RR, Wolff BG, Ilstrup DM (1987) Ileal pouch–anal anastomosis for chronic ulcerative colitis: long-term results. Ann Surg 206:504–511

Pezim ME, Pemberton JH, Beart RW Jr et al. (1989) Outcome of "indeterminate" colitis following ileal pouch–anal anastomosis. Dis Colon Rectum 32:653–658

Rabau MY, Percy JP, Parks AG (1982) Ileal pelvic resevoir: a correlation between motor patterns and clinical behaviour. Br J Surg 69:391–395

Read MG, Read NW (1982) Role of anorectal sensation in preserving continence. Gut 23:345–347

Roe AM, Bartolo DCC, Mortensen NJMcC (1986) New method for assessment of anal sensation in various anorectal disorders. Br J Surg 73:310–312

Scharli AF, Kiesewetter WB (1970) Defecation and continence: some new concepts. Dis Colon Rectum 13:81–107

Scott NA, Pemberton JH, Barkel DC, Wolff BG (1989) Anal and ileal pouch manometric measurements before ileostomy closure are related to functional outcome after ileal pouch–anal anastomosis. Br J Surg 76:613–616

Soper NJ, Orkin BA, Kelly KA, Phillips SF, Brown ML (1989) Gastrointestinal transit after proctocolectomy with ileal pouch–anal anastomosis or ileostomy. J Surg Res 46:300–305

Stryker SJ, Dozois RR (1985) The ileoanal anastomosis: historical perspectives. In: Dozois RR (ed) Alternatives to conventional ileostomy. Year Book Medical, Chicago, pp 255–265

Stryker SJ, Borody TJ, Phillips SF, Kelly KA, Dozois RR, Beart RW Jr (1985a) Motility of the small intestine after proctocolectomy and ileal pouch–anal anastomosis. Ann Surg 201:351–356

Stryker SJ, Daube JR, Kelly KA et al. (1985b) Anal sphincter electromyography after colectomy, mucosal rectectomy, and ileoanal anastomosis. Arch Surg 120:713–716

Stryker SJ, Kelly KA, Phillips SF, Dozois RR, Beart RW Jr (1986) Anal and neorectal function after ileal pouch–anal anastomosis. Ann Surg 203:55–61

Summers RW, Anuras S, Green J (1983) Jejunal manometry patterns in health, partial intestinal obstruction, and pseudo-obstruction. Gastroenterology 85:1290–1300

Taylor BM, Cranley B, Kelly KA, Phillips SF, Beart RW Jr, Dozois RR (1983) Clinico-physiological comparison of ileal pouch–anal and straight ileoanal anastomoses. Ann Surg 198:462–468

Utsunomiya J, Iwama T, Imajo M et al. (1980) Total colectomy, mucosal proctectomy, and ileoanal anastomosis. Dis Colon Rectum 23:459–466

Whitehead WE, Engel BT, Schuster MM (1980) Irritable bowel syndrome: physiological and psychological differences between diarrhea-predominant and constipation-predominant patients. Dig Dis Sci 25:404–413

Williams NS (1989) Stapling technique for pouch–anal anastomosis without the need for purse-string sutures. Br J Surg 76:348–349

Williams NS, Johnston D (1985) The current status of mucosal proctectomy and ileo-anal anastomosis in the surgical treatment of ulcerative colitis and adenomatous polyposis. Br J Surg 72:159–168

Winckler G (1958) Remarques sur la morphologie et l'innervation du muscle releveur de l'anus. Arch Anat Histol Embryol (Strasb) 41:77–95

Wolfstein IH, Bat L, Neumann G (1982) Regeneration of rectal mucosa and recurrent polyposis coli after total colectomy and ileoanal anastomosis. Arch Surg 117:1241–1242

Wong WD, Rothenberger DA, Goldberg SM (1985) Ileoanal pouch procedures. Curr Prob Surg 22(3):1–78

Yoshioka K, Keighley MRB (1989) Clinical results of colectomy for severe constipation. Br J Surg 76:600–604

14 · Colo-anal Anastomosis

D. J. Waldron

Introduction

Sphincter-saving surgery is one of the major recent advances in the management of distal colorectal pathology. The technical developments include Parks' handsewn transanal technique of colo-anal anastomosis (Parks 1972), the pull-through colo-anal procedure (Goligher et al. 1979), the transsphincteric (Mason 1977) and transsacral approaches (Localio and Stahl 1969) and the transanal stapled technique of colorectal and colo-anal anastomosis (Goligher et al. 1979). Any misgivings as to the justification of sparing the anal sphincters in low rectal cancer were answered by the demonstration that distal intramural spread beyond 2 cm is extremely uncommon (Williams et al. 1983) and when it does occur, the more radical operation of abdomino-perineal excision would have provided no advantage with regard to survival as the disease is invariably widely disseminated (Pollett and Nicholls 1983). Attention to detail regarding total excision of the mesorectum (Heald et al. 1982) and the lateral ligaments of the rectum (Quirke et al. 1986) allows for as adequate a clearance of extramural microscopic cancer deposits as can be achieved with an abdomino-perineal excision. Having demonstrated, albeit by retrospective comparisons, that local recurrence and survival rates were not jeopardized by these new sphincter-saving resections, it remained to be

shown that the functional outcome for the patient was superior to that following a permanent colostomy. When these techniques were first introduced it was felt that patients would be left with no more than a perineal colostomy. These objections were based on the common belief that total removal of the rectum resulted in an inevitable loss of sensation of filling and the desire to defaecate (Goligher and Hughes 1951). Many workers began to investigate the functional aspects of restorative surgery. This work was also influenced by data highlighting the psychological morbidity of a colostomy (Prudden 1971; Devlin et al. 1971; Williams and Johnston 1983). This chapter reviews the information documented to date on the functional outcome following low colorectal or colo-anal anastomosis.

Considerations in Sphincter-Saving Surgery (for Rectal Cancer)

Major considerations are:

1. No detrimental effect on long-term survival
2. No detrimental effect on local pelvic recurrence rates
3. Adequate functional outcome

Factors Involved in the Recto-anal Continence Mechanism

1. Anal sphincter muscle function
2. Anorectal angle
3. Rectal and anal sensation
4. Rectal reservoir capacity/compliance
5. Stool volume and consistency
6. Rectal/distal colon propulsive effect

Each of the above, either individually or in common with the other factors, can influence the continence mechanism which in ideal circumstances should be able to:

1. Control defaecation voluntarily
2. Discriminate between various forms of rectal content
3. Maintain nocturnal control

The internal and external anal sphincter muscles can maintain continence as they are influenced by a variety of physiological neural reflexes. They have been shown to respond to rectal filling in a specific manner. The internal sphincter relaxes in response to rectal filling, a reflex known as the recto-anal inhibitory response (Denny-Brown and Robertson 1935). The external sphincter initially contracts in response to rectal filling and relaxes only at large intrarectal volumes (Parks et al. 1962). It also maintains continence during various postural changes and even during sleep (Taverner and Smiddy 1959; Parks et al. 1962; Kumar et al. 1988).

The influence of a normal anorectal angle was thought to be a crucial element of the mechanism of continence, in that it created a "flap-valve" effect during periods of stress on the sphincter, i.e. sneezing, coughing etc. (Bartolo et al. 1986). Some doubt has been cast on this theory by the demonstration of a lack of correlation between improved clinical symptoms in faecal incontinence following operative repair procedures and the measurement of this angle (Womack et al. 1988; Miller et al. 1988).

The rectal wall itself was formerly considered a necessary constituent for normal appreciation of filling prior to development of an urge to defaecate (Goligher and Hughes 1951; Parks et al. 1962). Balloon distension of the rectal reservoir has been shown to give the typical pre-defaecatory sensation of perineal discomfort, whereas similar distension above 15 cm from the anal verge produces a feeling of intestinal colic (Goligher and Hughes 1951). Early suggestions that the sensation of reservoir fullness may not be due to sensory modalities in the rectal wall were derived from studies in children, which showed that children with rectal agenesis who underwent pull-through operations retained the sense of rectal filling (Scharli and Kiesewetter 1970). These were followed by physiological evidence from the postoperative assessment of patients in whom the rectal cuff was almost totally removed in operations for low rectal cancer (Lane and Parks 1977; Williams et al. 1980). These patients seem to retain their awareness of reservoir filling. Similarly, anal sensation is felt to be necessary to allow discrimination with regard to the nature of rectal content. This discriminatory ability is thought to reside in the nerve-rich transitional zone in the upper anal canal, which is frequently exposed to rectal content as rectal filling occurs and the recto-anal inhibitory response induces a relaxation of the proximal anal canal by inhibition of internal sphincter tone (Duthie and Bennett 1963). Again, doubt is cast on the need for this sensory area in the maintenance of continence by recent findings of an absence of ill effects in patients undergoing restorative pouch surgery for ulcerative colitis in whom the anal transition zone was stripped off (Keighley et al. 1987).

Undoubtedly, the capacity of the rectum or neorectum will influence bowel function with possible influences on the sphincter mechanism, particularly if the stool volume or consistency changes. These factors will be discussed later with reference to individual operations. Very little work is available on the influence or even the existence of rectal propulsion contributing to defaecation. Contractile activity is present at rest and occurs in a periodic fashion (Kumar et al. 1989) but its exact function has not yet been established. Following defaecation, material from the descending colon is often evacuated (Halls 1965) and therefore the contractile activity in this area may also influence defaecation and continence. Indeed, recent work in the postoperative period following low anterior resection suggests that lack of activity in the descending colon may have a major influence on the frequency and consistency of stool (Catchpole 1988).

Surgical Procedures Associated with Low Pelvic Anastomoses

Surgical procedures include:

1. Ileo-anal anastomosis
2. Low anterior resection
3. Pull-through colorectal anastomosis
4. Colo-anal anastomosis
5. Colonic pouches

These operative procedures will be discussed with regard to functional outcome, with emphasis on the principles of anorectal continence.

Ileo-anal Anastomosis

This operation, which is performed following total proctocolectomy in cases of ulcerative colitis and adenomatous familial polyposis, allows for the total excision of all diseased tissue, the restoration of gastrointestinal continuity and therefore the avoidance of a permanent ileostomy. It was initially proposed by Ravitch and Sabiston (1947) but subsequently fell into disrepute owing to the frequent incidence of sepsis and incontinence. This was probably due to the extensive extrarectal mobilization and eversion of the anorectal stump to achieve mucosectomy, with resultant injury to the anal sphincter mechanism (Williams and John-

ston 1985). It was not until Martin's work (Martin et al. 1977), demonstrating that such side effects could be avoided by adopting Soave's combined abdominal and perineal approach to mucosectomy, and Parks' transanal approach to the anastomosis (Parks 1972), that the operation achieved popularity in the treatment of inflammatory bowel disease. Table 14.1 shows that the results of Martin et al. and others provided an outcome which was acceptable in terms of morbidity and continence. The only limiting factor to the operation soon became apparent – the relative frequency of bowel action which tended to persist with time. Initially, this was assumed to be due to loss of the rectal reservoir. Attempts to increase capacity by grafting the rectal muscular wall with ileal mucosa after mucosectomy failed (Peck 1980), while gradual balloon dilatation of the ileum above the anastomosis proved only slightly better (Tellander and Perrault 1981). The creation of a physiological valve 10 cm above the ileo-anal anastomosis was seen to prevent the rapid bowel transit which occurred after ileo-anal anastomosis in dogs and tended to reduce bowel motion frequency, but not to a significant degree (Williams and King 1985). The problem with excessive stool frequency stimulated the present vogue for ileal pouch formation (Parks and Nicholls 1978), and as this is the subject of another chapter it will not be discussed further, except to document its success in overcoming this problem as seen in Table 14.2.

Table 14.1. Functional outcome of ileo-anal anastomosis

Author	Number of patients	FU period (months)	Continence			BM frequency		Comments
			Perfect	Minor defects	Poor	24 hours	Night	
Tellander and Perrault (1981)	24	3–35 (av. 13.6)	22	2	0	3–10(5.4)	0.5(1.7)	
Martin et al. (1977)	13	up to 10 years	13			30% frequent stool	watery	
Beart et al. (1982)	39	12–48	–	majority	–	3–20 (8)	2 (av.)	1 reverted to ileostomy due to severe frequency
Johnston et al. (1981)	5	6–40 (28.6)	2	2	1	6–8		
Neal et al. (1982)	6	19±9	3	2	1	7.5±2	3±1	
Taylor et al. (1983a)	30	4–40(18) approx.	9	15	6	11±1		Main problem was nocturnal leakage
Heppell et al. (1982)	12	5–29 (11.4)	1	11	0	12±4	4±1	Minor incontinence difficulty due to nocturnal leakage

Table 14.2. Functional outcome of ileo-anal anastomosis with and without ileal pouch

	Number of patients	FU interval (months)	Continence			BM frequency		Comments
			Perfect	Minor defects	Major defects	24 hours	Night	
Neal et al. 1982								
IAA	6	19±9	3	2	1	7.5±2*	3±1*	2 of 7 with
RES	7	9.5±4	6	1	0	4.7±1	1±0.5	pouches are only ones without constipating drugs
Taylor et al. (1983a)								
IAA	30	4–40 approx. (18)	9	15	6	11±1		Nocturnal leak-
RES	33	(6.5)	12	21	0	7±1		age main problem in IAA (approx. 5% of both groups had major leakage during day)
Taylor et al. (1983b)								
IAA	11	10–45 (25)	2	3	6	–		Minor degrees
RES	14	4–12 (8)	2	6	6	–		of incontinence mainly due to nocturnal leakage

* P=0.05.

Low Anterior Resection

Since low sphincter-saving resection and abdominoperineal excision seem equally as good in eradicating rectal cancer, the former technique is now being more frequently offered to patients with cancer of the lower two-thirds of the rectum. While it is evident that anterior resection carried out for upper third or rectosigmoid lesions is associated with a relatively uncomplicated functional outcome (Mayo and Cullen 1960; Goligher et al. 1979; McDonald and Heald 1983), as the anastomosis approaches the anal canal the functional outcome deteriorates. How can this be avoided? What is its aetiology? Does it cause inconvenience for the patient, making a colostomy preferable, or does a postoperative functional deficit improve with time?

Table 14.3 tabulates some of the functional parameters measured in various studies during the follow-up of these patients. These reports relate to low anterior resection performed with an EEA stapling instrument. It might be expected that the loss of the rectum, with its reservoir and accommodative functions, would result in some frequency of defaecation. This is supported by the findings of a reduced maximum tolerable volume and rectal compliance in the early postoperative period which correlates well with a frequent bowel habit (Williams et al. 1980; Suzuki et al. 1980;

Pedersen et al. 1986). This, however, tends to improve with time. Continence may also be impaired to a slight degree in the immediate postoperative period with very little inconvenience to the patient. This again tends to improve with time and most minor problems occur within two years following operation (Williams et al. 1980). Any major problem with regard to continence tends to result from a documented intra-operative injury (Horgan et al. 1989). Imperfections in continence do not correlate directly with anal sphincter resting pressures (Suzuki et al. 1980; Pedersen et al. 1986) or the presence or absence of the recto-anal inhibitory response (Pedersen et al. 1986; Horgan et al. 1989). The former, indicating internal sphincter activity, is generally not significantly reduced by low anterior resection (Suzuki et al. 1980; Pedersen et al. 1986), although in some recent reports there have been significant effects noted (Williams et al. 1980; Horgan et al. 1989). These may indicate an increasing tendency to tackle very low lesions with consequential effects directly on the anal sphincter mechanism. However, such a drop in resting sphincter pressure or the loss of the recto-anal inhibitory response, which is an almost invariable initial consequence of the operation (Williams et al. 1980), has not been shown to have any marked effects on faecal continence. Most studies also do not indicate any deleterious effect on the external

Table 14.3. Functional outcome after low anterior resection

Author	Number of patients	FU (months)	Distance of tumour* or anastomosis from anal verge (cm)	Continence Perfect	Minor defects	Poor	BM frequency/ 24 hours	Comments
Cade et al. (1981)	50		8–13	48	–	2		
Goligher et al. (1979)	24		5–10	19	3	2		Minor and poor results re continence were in group of 10 with anastomosis below 7 cm
Heald (1980)	32	3	3–8 (includes some colo-anal)	30	2	0		
Williams and Johnston (1983)	40	39.6±18	5–12*	30	10	0	65% 3/day	Of 10 with minor incontinence 4 had problems with flatus only
Kirkegaard et al. (1981)	29	3	7–12*	29	0	0	86% 2/day (others had 3–4/day)	
Williams et al. (1980)	20	6–180	3–7	14	6 (all 2 years FU)	0	75% 3/day	10 patients had colo-anal (no distinction made)
Pedersen et al. (1986)	13	12	6–12*	Not specified (no major problems)			92% 3/day (2 3/day had colo-anal)	2 had endoanal colo-anal anastomosis
McDonald and Heald (1983)	22	3–34 (20.5)	10	20	2	0 ⎫		
	32	3–31 (19.5)	5–10	23	8	1 ⎬ Not specified		
	21	5–28 (16)	5	8	12	1 ⎭		
Horgan et al. (1989)	15	6	5–12*	12	2	1	Not specified	Poor outcome, had poor pre-op anal pressures

(i.e. * relates to heading above these parameters, not to comparisons of data)

sphincter musculature during this procedure, as the squeeze incremental pressure is generally unchanged following operation. An important aspect of the operation is the proper visualization and avoidance of damage to the levator ani muscles, which probably contain sensory nerves and pressure receptors which may play a role in neorectal sensation (Williams 1984). It is interesting to note from one study (McDonald and Heald 1983) the frequent incidence of anorectal functional abnormalities in a randomly selected group of patients who had rectal tumours but no rectal surgery. Such findings indicate the importance of prospective pre- and postoperative studies in order to determine the influence of low rectal anastomosis on anorectal function. Similarly in a recent study by Horgan et al. (1989), one of 20 patients could have been predicted to have poor function following surgery on the basis of a significantly diminished anal sphincter pressure pre-

operatively. This patient had the only functional failure and subsequently had a colostomy fashioned.

Pull-Through Colo-anal Anastomosis

Resection of rectal tumours using this technique has been well described (Goligher et al. 1965; Kirwan et al. 1978) but has fallen into disfavour owing to problems with necrosis of the distal bowel, pelvic sepsis and poor functional outcome in many cases (Kennedy et al. 1970; Mann 1972). Modifications in an attempt to overcome these problems – two stage resections (Cutait and Figlioni 1961; Turnbull and Cuthbertson 1961), sleeve anastomosis, shortening of the rectal cuff and performing the anastomosis at the level of the pectinate line (Castrini et al. 1985) – have decreased the former risk factors, but the functional

Table 14.4. Functional outcome after pull-through operations

Author	Number of patients	FU (months)	Continence			BM frequency/ 24 hours	Comments
			Perfect	Minor defects	Poor		
Kennedy et al. (1970)	80	Not stated	27	34	19	Not stated	1 of 19 poor outcome needed colostomy. Others had moderate soiling
Kirwan et al. (1978)	39	12	10	29	0	Not stated	
Mann (1972)	61	12–396 (approx.)	Not stated		6	Not stated	Serious postop. morbidity in 72%
Goligher et al. (1965)	28	12–18	11	9	8	Not stated	Poor results correlated with significant drop in anal pressures
Castrini et al. (1985)	17	22 (mean)	17	0	0	1	

outcome is still unpredictable in comparison with more recently devised procedures. Table 14.4 summarizes the functional outcome of patients who have undergone this procedure in recent years. The operative technique proposed by Castrini et al. (1985) does seem to give very satisfactory results both with regard to continence and frequency of bowel action. Perhaps this may offer a further alternative to surgeons in their approach to low sphincter-saving resections.

Transanal Colo-anal Anastomosis

Prior to the introduction and general acceptance of the stapling instrument for low colorectal and colo-anal anastomoses, distal rectal pathology had to be dealt with by handsewn anastomotic techniques if continuity was to be restored. Despite the present availability of stapling techniques, there may still be occasions when, either due to instrument failure or the physical build of the patient, a handsewn technique is preferable. The traditional approach to complete such an anastomosis involved either a transsacral (Localio and Stahl 1969) or a transsphincteric approach (Mason 1977). Both these techniques involve division of pelvic floor musculature. While outcome is satisfactory from a functional viewpoint (Table 14.5), a technique which would avoid such division would seem to have lesser risks in patients where advancing age and impaired healing may have detrimental effects. Sir Alan Parks' original description of the transanal method of performing a sutured colo-anal anastomosis therefore offered a potentially better alternative. This technique gained popularity in the treatment of a variety of rectal

abnormalities (Jeffrey et al. 1976; Parks et al. 1978; Varma and Smith 1986) but its main use was in the resection of low rectal cancer when it was possible to preserve the sphincter mechanism. Table 14.5 gives an overview of the functional outcome of this procedure as reported from a number of centres. Most reports suggest that frequency of bowel action combined with urgency and soiling may pose problems in the first 3–6 months following operation, although Parks himself reported 69 of 70 patients as having normal continence at the first out-patient visit with approximately half having a frequency of 4–5 stools/day, the other half being normal in this respect (Parks and Percy 1982). This may be influenced by the level of the anastomosis, as measured from the anal verge in different series (Keighley and Matheson 1980). Despite early problems, most patients seem to return to normal function within one year. The physiological findings in this group of patients suggest that while the internal sphincter may be weakened and the recto-anal inhibitory response lost, at least the latter returns to normal after one year (Lane and Parks 1977). Perhaps these imperfections in internal anal sphincter function account for some of the minor problems with continence in these patients. The potential for direct damage to the internal sphincter muscle during stretching by the retractor to allow for visualization of the anastomosis in a transanal approach was thought to be the cause of this damage, and this was supported by Keighley's finding (1988) of improved function following a totally abdominal mucosectomy without anal retraction. Attempts to show that the use of a stapling instrument would overcome this problem have not succeeded in demonstrating a beneficial

Table 14.5. Functional outcome after colo-anal anastomosis

Author	Number of patients	FU (months)	Continence			BM frequency/ 24 hours	Comments
			Perfect	Minor defects	Poor		
Parks and Percy (1982)	70	3	69	0	1	56% 3 (others had 4–5)	
Keighley and Matheson (1980)	6	12	4	1	1	3–4/day	Poor result associated with local recurrence
Castrini et al. (1985)	17	22 (mean)	17	0	0	1	
Enker et al. (1985)		12					
Drake et al. (1987)	25	20±3	21	4	0	3±1	
Lane and Parks (1977)	12	12	10	1	1	60% approx. "normal", others had 2–3/day	One poor outcome due to ascending colon used in anastomosis with overflow incontinence
Hautefeuille et al. (1988)	31		30			2	
Bernard et al. (1989)	30	6	26	2	2	63% 3 (mean 3.8)	

effect on the internal sphincter (Johnston et al. 1987; Williams et al. 1989), although the drop in basal sphincter pressure tends to be less following the latter technique. Low rectal transection, ligation of the inferior mesenteric artery or mobilization of the rectum itself have been shown not to cause a drop in sphincter pressure when using peroperative monitoring (Horgan et al. 1989). Therefore it seems likely that transanal anastomosis will result in some minor weakening of internal sphincter function, although stapled anastomoses seem to be associated with lesser degrees of nocturnal leakage (Williams et al. 1989). Problems with bowel frequency seem to correlate with the demonstration of reduced rectal compliance and capacity in the early months after operation (Varma and Smith 1986; Keighley and Matheson 1980) and therefore the concept of creating a neorectum with a greater storage capacity, i.e. a pouch from the residual colon, was introduced in a number of specialist centres. Poor functional results may also be related to pelvic sepsis (Lane and Parks 1977), the presence of extrarectal tumour infiltration (Keighley 1986) and the presence of radiation injury to the rectum (Varma and Smith 1986).

Colonic Pouch–Anal Anastomosis

As a result of the success achieved with the ileal pouch in the surgical treatment of inflammatory bowel disease and the relatively persistent problems with frequency of bowel habit even after one year following a colo-anal anastomotic procedure, there have recently been a number of reports on the use of a colonic J pouch fashioned from the proximal colon and anastomosed directly to the anal canal (Lazorthes et al. 1986; Parc et al. 1988; Nicholls et al. 1988). All three reports have concerned colo-anal anastomoses and, with the exception of two cases, involved the excision of a rectal neoplasm. One report used the transsphincteric approach (Lazorthes et al. 1986) while the other two utilized Parks' endoanal route. All three reports were able to demonstrate reduced bowel frequency (Table 14.6). Parc et al. (1988) noted a frequency of 1.1/day after 3 months but some problems with continence were present in up to 33% of patients at one month. These, however, as with the straight colo-anal technique, tended to resolve with time and all patients were completely continent at 3 months. Lazorthes et al. (1986) and Nicholls et al. (1988) were able to compare outcome with a parallel group who had undergone the straight colo-anal anastomosis, and included tests of anorectal function in their follow-up. The former group demonstrated a direct correlation between a much diminished frequency of bowel action and a significantly increased neorectal capacity. A significantly greater number of pouch patients had a stool frequency of less than two/day and an increased number fell within this range in the second postoperative year, as opposed to the

Table 14.6. Functional outcome after colonic pouch–anal anastomosis

Author	Number of patients	FU (months)	Continence			BM frequency/ 24 hours	Comments
			Perfect	Minor defects	Poor		
Lazorthes et al. (1986)							
colo-anal	15	20 (mean)	12	3	0	33%* 2 (mean 3±1.2)	No problems with
pouch	36	36 (mean)	28	8	0	87% 2 (mean 1.7±0.7)	evacuation of pouch
Nicholls et al. (1988)							
colo-anal	15	47±23	9	6	1	1–6.5 (mean 2.3)	All patients with a pouch
pouch	13	7±4	10	3	0	0.5–2 (mean 1.4)	had 2 BM/day. Only 1 patient had difficulty evacuating the pouch
Parc et al. (1988)	24	3	24	0	0	1–3 (mean 1.1)	All colonic pouches. 25% needed suppository to aid emptying every other day (no sense of desire to evacuate)

* p=0.01.

traditional colo-anal group where stool frequency did not improve with time. While the pouch group had slightly better continence levels in the first year, both groups were very satisfactory in this regard in the second year. In the study from Nicholls et al., estimates of neorectal evacuation were made using balloon and contrast proctography, in addition to anal and rectal pressure and sensitivity studies. Again, despite a follow-up bias in favour of the straight colo-anal group in terms of the mean duration of time since operation (47 months versus 7 months), a more favourable outcome with regard to frequency of bowel habit existed in the pouch patients. While the overall mean frequency was not significantly different, all pouch patients had less than two motions/day while 40% of straight colo-anal patients lay outside this range. Again, this was reflected in a significantly greater neorectal maximal tolerable volume in the pouch group without any difference in neorectal compliance. Anal sphincter pressures were not significantly different between groups and this was reflected in the lack of problems with continence, although minor abnormalities tended to be more prominent in the straight colo-anal group.

With regard to evacuation difficulties, some interesting findings have emerged from a recent study. Using dynamic proctography, Marzouk has been able to associate two aspects of colonic pouch design with problems in evacuation (Marzouk 1990). Firstly, the use of excessively long limbs (10–12 cm) leading to too large a pouch was more often noted in patients with evacuation problems. This association was also suggested by the earlier work of Lazorthes et al. (1986). Secondly, as with the ileal pouch, the presence of a residual rectal "spout" between the pouch and the anal canal was significantly associated with emptying abnormalities. It was felt that both of the above allowed the pouch, when full, to fall back into the sacral hollow and interfere with opening of the anoneorectal angle during attempted defaecation. It would therefore seem advisable at this time to recommend fashioning a colonic pouch from approximately 6 cm limbs of residual colon and re-establishing continuity at the level of the upper anal canal. Therefore, while transient problems with continence seem an inevitable outcome of low colo-anal anastomatic procedures, there would seem to be a definite benefit for stool frequency with a colonic pouch. All three reports to date show no increase in morbidity or mortality due to the fashioning of a pouch in this situation and the procedure itself is not complex, once attention is given to adequate mobilization and the avoidance of tension at the anastomosis.

Investigation of Poor Function Following Colo-anal Anastomosis

It is evident from the previous sections of this chapter that, while restoration of continuity following resection of the lower gut results in an acceptable functional outcome, nevertheless minor difficulties may persist or specific individuals may present with major functional problems. Management of such complaints can, without doubt, be facilitated by accurate definition of the source of the problem and measurement and calibration of the severity of the functional impairment. Ideally, a unit with a large commitment to surgical treatment of rectal pathology should have access to some or all of the following investigative techniques, both for the work up of potentially problem patients pre-operatively and in the assessment of those who develop functional problems postoperatively.

Anorectal Manometry

Measurement of maximum basal (resting) and maximum squeeze (incremental) anal sphincter pressure, reflecting the function of the internal and external sphincter respectively, is a relatively simple procedure to perform and ideally should be carried out in all patients prior to this form of surgery. Reference has already been made in this chapter to the pre-operative identification, using this technique, of a solitary functional failure in one series of low anterior resections (Horgan et al. 1989). In this way, advice based on objective grounds can be offered to the patient pre-operatively on the possibility of a poor functional outcome and the choice of an alternative procedure. Equally, regular follow-up examinations of sphincter strength may identify patients with post-operative problems who are most likely to improve spontaneously with the passage of time.

The length of the high pressure zone in the anal sphincter can also be easily assessed using this technique. While most reports on outcome of low colorectal resections have not made reference to this variable, it has been documented in a number of reports on the treatment of idiopathic faecal incontinence by postanal repair as being the only recurring factor associated with improvement in symptoms. Perhaps the length of the high pressure zone may also be found to influence function following rectal excision.

Proctometrogram

There can be no doubt that the loss of all or a significant portion of the rectal reservoir must influence frequency of defaecation and continence. Inflation of a balloon in the rectum or neorectum can give valuable information on the capacity of this area and has already been used successfully to associate improved bowel frequency with the fashioning of a pouch above the colo-anal anastomosis (Lazorthes et al. 1986; Nicholls et al. 1988). This investigation may also be of use in those patients without pouches and in whom severe frequency may be attributed to a spastic or stenosed neorectal segment.

Electromyography of the Pelvic Floor

While this investigative technique has not achieved obvious prominence in this area, when available it may be useful in the pre-operative selection of those patients who are clinically suspect with regard to postoperative continence problems. Electromyographic studies can give quantitative and qualitative information on the anal sphincter muscles, particularly the external component.

Proctography

Radiological visualization of the anoneorectum, especially during a dynamic study, can have a role in the elucidation of evacuation problems. This applies in particular to potential difficulties arising from the use of colonic pouches to improve postoperative frequency. The work of Marzouk (1990) has already been quoted, where the use of dynamic proctography highlighted the importance of pouch size and level of anastomosis to the incidence of evacuation difficulties. These features can therefore contribute to the success or failure of the operation and would have been difficult to identify without the aid of proctography. Anastomotic strictures are often more easily appreciated and appropriately treated on the basis of their appearances on proctography.

Conclusion

Sphincter-saving resections can now safely be performed for the treatment of rectal disorders at all levels. The problems of local recurrence and long-term survival in these patients do not now provide a barrier to this operation. The most significant problems are frequent bowel action and minor degrees of soiling and urgency. Problems with continence tend to improve within 3–6 months using the more up-to-date approach to rectal excision and the avoidance of eversion of the anorectal cuff. The functional outcome following handsewn endoanal anastomoses does not differ greatly from that achieved after stapled distal anastomosis. Problems with frequency of bowel action, which have obvious effects on the patients' lifestyle, may result from altered left-sided colonic activity following denervation at operation, in addition to reduced neorectal capacity and compliance. The use of a colonic pouch seems to have some advantages in this regard, without introducing additional morbidity. Any long-term evacuation problems due to the presence of the pouch can not be estimated as yet, but in the short term emptying is not impaired if attention is paid to the avoidance of an excessively long pouch and performing a direct pouch–anal anastomosis.

References

Bartolo DCC, Roe AM, Locke-Edmunds JC, Virjee J, Mortensen NJMcC (1986) Flap-valve theory of anorectal continence. Br J Surg 73:1012–1014

Beart RW, Dozois RR, Kelly KA (1982) Ileo-anal anastomosis in the adult. Surg Gynecol Obstet 154:826–828

Beart RW, Dozois RR, Wolff BG, Pemberton JH (1985) Mechanisms of rectal continence. Lessons from the ileo-anal procedure. Am J Surg 149:31–34

Bernard D, Morgan S, Tasse D, Wassef R (1989) Preliminary results of coloanal anastomosis. Dis Colon Rectum 32:580–584

Cade D, Gallagher P, Schofield PF, Turner L (1981) Complications of anterior resection of the rectum using the EEA stapling device. Br J Surg 68:339–340

Castrini G, Pappalardo G, Mobarhan S (1985) A new technique for ileoanal and coloanal anastomosis. Surgery 97:111–116

Catchpole BN (1988) Motor pattern of the left colon before and after surgery for rectal cancer: possible implications in other disorders. Gut 29:624–630

Cutait DE, Figlioni FJ (1961) A new method of colorectal anastomosis in abdominoperineal resection. Dis Colon Rectum 4:335–342

Denny-Brown D, Robertson EG (1935) An investigation of the nervous control of defaecation. Brain 58:256–310

Devlin HP, Plant JA, Griffin M (1971) Aftermath of surgery for anorectal cancer. Br Med J iii:413–418

Drake DB, Pemberton JH, Beart RW Jr, Dozois RR, Wolff BG (1987) Coloanal anastomosis in the management of benign and malignant rectal disease. Ann Surg 206:600–605

Duthie HL, Bennett RC (1963) The relation of sensation in the anal canal to the functional anal sphincter; a possible factor in anal incontinence. Gut 4:179–182

Enker WE, Stearns MW Jr, Janov AJ (1985) Peranal coloanal anastomosis following low anterior resection for rectal carcinoma. Dis Colon Rectum 28:576–581

Goligher JC, Hughes ESR (1951) Sensibility of the rectum and colon: its role in the mechanism of anal continence. Lancet i:543–548

Goligher JC, Duthie HL, Dedombal FT et al. (1965) Abdominal–anal pullthrough excision for tumours of the mid-third of the rectum. Br J Surg 52:323–325

Goligher JC, Lee PWR, Macfie J et al. (1979) Experience with the Russian model 249 suture gun for anastomosis of the rectum. Surg Gynecol Obstet 148:517–524

Halls J (1965) Bowel content shift during normal defaecation. Proc R Soc Med 58:859–860

Hautefeuille P, Valleur P, Perniceni T et al. (1988) Functional and oncological results after coloanal anastomosis for low rectal cancer. Ann Surg 207:61–64

Heald RJ (1980) Towards fewer colostomies – the impact of circular stapling devices on the surgery of rectal cancer in a district hospital. Br J Surg 60:198–200

Heald RJ, Husband EM, Ryall RDH (1982) The mesorectum in rectal cancer surgery – the clue to pelvic recurrence. Br J Surg 69:613–616

Heimann T, Gelernt I, Bauer J et al. (1983) Mucosal protectomy without reservoir. Am J Surg 145:674–677

Heppell J, Kelly KA, Phillips S et al. (1982) Physiological aspects of continence after colectomy, mucosal proctectomy and endo-rectal ileo-anal anastomosis. Ann Surg 195:435–440

Horgan PG, O'Connell PR, Shinkwin CA, Kirwan WO (1989) Effect of anterior resection on anal sphincter function. Br J Surg 76:783–786

Jeffrey PJ, Hawley PR, Parks AG (1976) Coloanal sleeve anastomosis in the treatment of diffuse cavernous haemangioma involving the rectum. Br J Surg 63:678–682

Johnston D, Williams NS, Neal DE, Axon ATR (1981) The value of preserving the anal sphincter in operations for ulcerative colitis and polyposis: a review of twenty-two mucosal proctectomies. Br J Surg 68:874–878

Johnston D, Holdsworth PJ, Nasmyth DG et al. (1987) Preservation of the entire anal canal in conservative proctocolectomy for ulcerative colitis: a pilot study comparing end-to-end ileo-anal anastomosis without mucosal resection with mucosal proctectomy and endo-anal anastomosis. Br J Surg 74:940–944

Keighley MRB (1986) Anal sphincter function and sphincter preserving surgery. Ann Chir Gynaecol 75:121–126

Keighley MRB (1988) Abdominal mucosectomy reduced the incidence of soiling and sphincter damage after restorative proctocolectomy and J pouch. Dis Colon Rectum 30 (supp):386–390

Keighley MRB, Matheson D (1980) Functional results of rectal excision and endo-anal anastomosis. Br J Surg 67:757–761

Keighley MRB, Winslet MC, Yoshioka K, Lightwood R (1987) Discrimination is not impaired by excision of the anal transition zone after restorative proctocolectomy. Br J Surg 74:1118–1121

Kennedy JT, McOmish D, Bennett RC et al. (1970) Abdomino-anal pullthrough resection of the rectum. Br J Surg 57:589–596

Kirkegaard P, Christiansen J, Hjartrup A (1981) Anterior resection for mid rectal cancer with the EEA stapling instrument. Am J Surg 140:312–314

Kirwan WO, Rupert B, Turnbull B Jr, Fazio VW, Weakley FL

(1978) Pullthrough operation with delayed anastomosis for rectal cancer. Br J Surg 65:695–699

Kumar D, Williams NS, Waldron DJ, Browning C, Hutton MRE, Wingate DL (1988) Prolonged anorectal manometry and external sphincter electromyography (EMG) in ambulant human subjects. Gastroenterology 94:A241

Kumar D, Williams NS, Waldron DJ, Wingate DL (1989) Prolonged manometric recording of anorectal motor activity in ambulant human subjects: evidence of periodic motor activity. Gut 30:1007–1011

Lane RHS, Parks AG (1977) Function of the anal sphincters following colo-anal anastomosis. Br J Surg 64:596–599

Lazorthes F, Fages P, Chiotasso P, Lemozy J, Bloom E (1986) Resection of the rectum with construction of a colonic reservoir and colo-anal anastomosis for carcinoma of the rectum. Br J Surg 73:136–138

Localio SA, Stahl WM (1969) Simultaneous abdominotranssacral resection and anastomosis for midrectal cancer. Am J Surg 117:282–289

Localio SA, Eng K, Coppa GF (1983) Abdominosacral resection for midrectal cancer: a fifteen year experience. Ann Surg 198:320–324

Mann C (1972) Results of "pull-through" operations for carcinoma of the rectum. Proc R Soc Med 65:976

Martin LW, LeCoultre C, Schubert WK (1977) Total colectomy and mucosal proctectomy with preservation of continence in ulcerative colitis. Ann Surg 186:477–480

Marzouk D (1990) Investigation of colonic and ileoanal pouch function. Thesis, University of Cairo, Egypt

Mason AY (1977) Trans-sphincteric surgery for lower rectal cancer. Surg Tech Illus 2:71–88

Mayo CW, Cullen PK Jr (1960) An evaluation of the one stage low anterior resection. Surg Gynecol Obstet 111:82–86

McDonald PJ, Heald RJ (1983) A survey of postoperative function after rectal anastomosis with circular stapling devices. Br J Surg 70:727–729

Miller R, Bartolo DCC, Locke-Edmunds JC, Mortensen NJMcC (1988) Prospective study of conservative and operative treatment for faecal incontinence. Br J Surg 75:101–105

Neal DE, Williams NS, Johnston D (1982) Rectal, bladder and sexual function after mucosal proctectomy with and without a pelvic reservoir for colitis and polyposis. Br J Surg 69:599–604

Nicholls RJ, Lubowski DZ, Donaldson DR (1988) Comparison of colonic reservoir and straight colo-anal reconstruction after rectal excision. Br J Surg 75:318–320

Parc R, Tiret E, Frileux P, Moszkowski E, Loygue J (1988) Resection and colo-anal anastomosis with colonic reservoir for rectal carcinoma. Br J Surg 73:139–141

Parks AG (1972) Trans-anal technique in low rectal anastomosis. Proc R Soc Med 65:975–976

Parks AG, Nicholls RJ (1978) Proctocolectomy without ileostomy for ulcerative colitis. Br Med J ii:85–88

Parks AG, Percy JP (1982) Resection and sutured colo-anal anastomosis for rectal carcinoma. Br J Surg 69:301–304

Parks AG, Porter NH, Melzak J (1962) Experimental study of the reflex mechanism controlling the muscles of the pelvic floor. Dis Colon Rectum 5:407–414

Parks AG, Allen CLO, Frank JD et al. (1978) A method of treating post-irradiation rectovaginal fistulas. Br J Surg 65:417–421

Peck DA (1980) Rectal mucosa replacement. Ann Surg 91:294–303

Pedersen IK, Hint K, Olsen J, Christiansen J, Jensen P, Mortensen PE (1986) Anorectal function after low anterior resection for carcinoma. Ann Surg 204:133–135

Pollett WG, Nicholls RJ (1983) The relationship between the extent of distal clearance and survival and local recurrence rates after curative anterior resection for carcinoma of the rectum. Ann Surg 198:159–163

Prudden JF (1971) Psychological problems following ileostomy and colostomy. Cancer 38:236–238

Quirke P, Durdey P, Dixon MF, Williams NS (1986) Local recurrance of rectal adenocarcinoma due to inadequate surgical resection: histopathological study of lateral tumour and surgical excision. Lancet ii:996–998

Ravitch MM, Sabiston DC (1947) Anal ileostomy with preservation of the sphincter. Surg Gynecol Obstet 84:1095–1109

Scharli AF, Kiesewetter WB (1970) Defaecation and continence: some new concepts. Dis Colon Rectum 13:81–107

Suzuki H, Matsumoto K, Amano S, Fujioka M, Honzumi M (1980) Anorectal pressure and rectal compliance after low anterior resection. Br J Surg 67:655–657

Taverner D, Smiddy FG (1959) An electromyographic study of the normal function of the external anal sphincter and pelvic diaphragm. Dis Colon Rectum 2:153–160

Taylor BM, Beart RW Jr, Dozois RR, Kelly KA, Phillips SF (1983a) Straight ileoanal anastomosis v. ileal pouch–anal anastomosis after colectomy and mucosal proctectomy. Arch Surg 118:696–701

Taylor BM, Cranley B, Kelly KA, Phillips SF, Beart RW Jr, Dozois RR (1983b) A clinico-physiological comparison of ileal pouch–anal and straight ileoanal anastomosis. Ann Surg 198:462–468

Tellander RL, Perrault J (1981) Colectomy and rectal mucosectomy and ileo-anal anastomosis in young patients: its use for ulcerative colitis and familial polyposis. Arch Surg 116:623–629

Turnbull RB, Cuthbertson AM (1961) Abdominorectal pull-through resection for cancer and for Hirschsprung's disease. Cleve Clin Q 28:109–115

Varma JS, Smith AN (1986) Anorectal function following colo-anal sleeve anastomosis for chronic radiation injury to the rectum. Br J Surg 73:285–289

Williams NS (1984) The rationale for preservation of the anal sphincter in patients with low rectal cancer. Br J Surg 71:575–581

Williams NS, Johnston D (1983) The quality of life after rectal excision for low rectal cancer. Br J Surg 70:460–462

Williams NS, Johnston D (1985) The current status of mucosal proctectomy and ileo-anal anastomosis in the surgical treatment of ulcerative colitis and adenomatous polyposis. Br J Surg 72:159–168

Williams NS, King RFGJ (1985) The effect of a reversed ileal segment and artificial valve on intestinal transit and absorption following colectomy and low ileo-rectal anastomosis in the dog. Br J Surg 72:169–174

Williams NS, Price R, Johnston D (1980) The long term effect of sphincter preserving operations for rectal carcinoma on function of the anal sphincter in man. Br J Surg 67:203–208

Williams NS, Dixon MF, Johnston D (1983) Reappraisal of the 5 centimetre rule of distal excision for carcinoma of the rectum: a study of distal intramural spread and of patients' survival. Br J Surg 70:150–154

Williams NS, Marzouk DEMM, Hallan RI, Waldron DJ (1989) Function after ileal pouch and stapled pouch–anal anastomosis for ulcerative colitis. Br J Surg 76:1168–1171

Womack NR, Morrison JFB, Williams NS (1988) Prospective study of the effects of postanal repair in neurogenic faecal incontinence. Br J Surg 75:48–52

15 · Assessment of the Paediatric Patient

V. Loening-Baucke

Introduction

In man, very special control mechanisms are developed to save the individual from the embarrassment of passage of wind, stool or urine. Unconscious regulation of bowel movements is the normal phenomenon at birth. Conscious regulation of bowel movement is achieved at an average age of 28 months. Anal malformation, spina bifida and some muscle disorders can interfere with bowel control. Constipation in infancy and the toddler years may inhibit or delay bowel control and in later childhood may disturb the mechanism for bowel control after normal control had been established. The purpose of this chapter is to review the techniques of anorectal manometry and their application in the investigation and management of disorders of the colon and anorectum in childhood.

Faecal continence is the ability to recognize rectal ampullary filling, to discriminate between formed stool, liquid and gas, and to retain the content until emptying is socially convenient. Defaecation is the planned voluntary action which combines intrinsic reflex forces with an increase in intra-abdominal pressure and relaxation of the anal sphincters.

Anatomy and Physiology

The major structures responsible for continence and defaecation are the external anal sphincter, the puborectalis muscle, the internal anal sphincter and the rectum. Continence requires a healthy motor sphincter system as well as an effective sensing mechanism. Faeces stimulate nerve terminals in the rectal wall and/or pelvic floor musculature. The pudendal nerve carries the sensory impulses, via lateral afferents, through the dorsal root ganglia to the respective spinal segments and the sensory cortex. Faecal material can be retained in the rectum by contraction of the external sphincter and puborectalis muscle. It can be expelled by increase in intra-abdominal pressure produced by closure of the glottis, fixation of the diaphragm, contractions of the abdominal, perineal, and hamstring muscles, by relaxation of the internal and external sphincters and by rectal contractions.

Equipment, Conduct and Results of Anorectal Physiological Tests

Equipment

At the University of Iowa, anorectal manometry is usually performed with a probe containing microtransducers but Dent's sleeve device (Dent 1976) is used for the saline continence tests, a self made perfused catheter assembly in premature infants, and Schuster's three-balloon system (Schuster et al. 1965) for biofeedback training in faecal incontinent patients. These different devices and their utilization in our laboratory will also be described.

The instrument used for the anorectal manometric evaluation is a commercially available probe (Model P31–D3, Sandhill Scientific, Littleton, Colorado, USA) (Loening-Baucke 1984a, b). This flexible, silicone rubber tube (5 mm in diameter) contains three intraluminal transducers which are staggered at 120° intervals around the probe and are spaced 5 cm apart at the distal end. The tube is marked in 1 cm increments to provide external reference for intraluminal transducer position in the anal canal and rectum. A latex balloon (2.5×3 cm when deflated) is attached to the end of a thin polyethylene tube and tied to the tip of the motility probe, 5 cm above the distal transducer (see Fig. 15.1). Pressure from the latex balloon is transmitted via the polyethylene tube to a pressure transducer. The outputs of all four transducers are fed into a recorder and graphed on running paper.

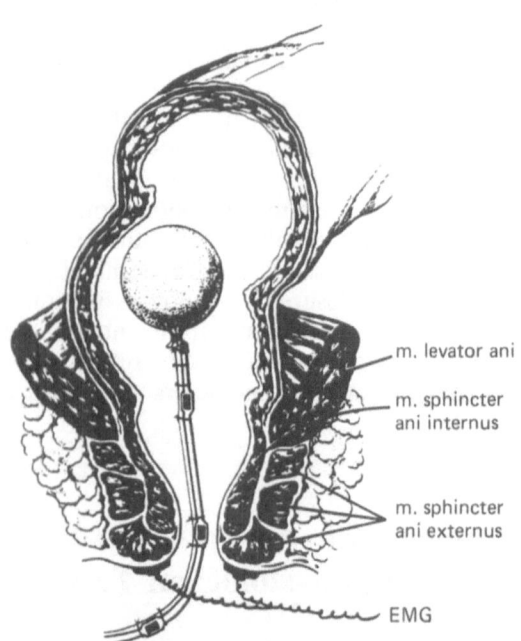

Fig. 15.1. Schematic diagram of the recording technique. One transducer of the motility probe is located in the lower part of the anal canal, one in the rectum. The balloon used for rectal distension is shown distended. The surface electrodes are placed as close as possible to the anal canal.

m. levator ani

m. sphincter ani internus

m. sphincter ani externus

EMG

Preparation of the Child for Testing

Anorectal manometry and the other studies are only performed after complete clearance of the lower bowel, except in sick newborns where no bowel preparation is used. Sedation of a child has never been necessary. A restless newborn or infant usually relaxes while sucking on a pacifier or drinking from a bottle, while some preschool children need to be distracted by having the parent read a story to them. Occasionally we had to wait until an infant fell asleep to perform manometry. The manometric studies were performed with the children in the left lateral position, with the hips and knees flexed.

Measurements

Studies of Anal Resting Pressure and Maximal Squeeze Pressure

Anal resting pressure and maximal squeeze pressure are determined during step-by-step retraction (0.5 cm/min) of one intraluminal pressure transducer of the motility probe from the rectum through the anal canal. Anal resting pressure is defined as the pressure (mmHg) at the troughs of the waves and is highest 1–2 cm above the anal verge. The maximum squeeze pressure (mmHg) is the highest pressure increase measured above anal resting pressure. Results in control children are given in Table 15.1. We use the station pull-through method and, like other centres a continuous withdrawal technique. Normal values will depend on the speed of withdrawal. Table 15.1 gives the pull-through pressures for a withdrawal speed of 1 cm/s.

Anal Canal Length

The anal canal is defined as the region with resting tone at least 5 mmHg higher than the tone in the rectum, showing a motor activity pattern different from in the rectum, and a reflex relaxation of anal pressure during rectal distension. The length of the anal canal is determined once by recording the resting pressure, motor activity pattern and reflex relaxation at each position during step-by-step retraction of 0.5 cm of the pressure transducer assembly from the rectum through the anal canal.

Table 15.1. Anal resting pressure, pull-through pressure and maximal anal squeeze pressure in healthy children, chronically constipated children and children with chronic constipation and faecal soiling, ages 4–12 years (means±SD)

	Controls (n=20)	Constipated children (n=12)	Constipated children with faecal soiling (n=20)
Anal resting pressure (mmHg)	53±12 range 25–72	62±12	37±10*
Anal pull-through pressure (mmHg)	133±14	143±37	103±28*
Maximal squeeze pressure (mmHg)	190±49	Not done	151±34*

* p<0.05 from healthy control children (Wilcoxon nonpaired rank sum test).

The mean length of the anal canal in healthy children over 4 years was 3 cm (range 2–5 cm).

Studies of the Effect of Rectal Distension

The internal anal sphincter provides most of the pressure in the anal canal, and is inhibited by rectal distension. This inhibition results in a fall in pressure in the anal canal (see Fig. 15.2a) and this phenomenon is referred to as the rectosphincteric reflex. The clinical significance of the fact that transient rectal distension produces a rectosphincteric reflex in healthy children and patients with chronic constipation but not in patients with Hirschsprung's disease (see Fig. 15.2b) was recognized by Callaghan and Nixon (1964) and Tobon et al. (1968). We evaluate response of the anal canal and rectum to rectal distension and rectal sensitivity with the base of the distending balloon 11 cm above the anal verge and one pressure transducer in the rectum and one in the anal canal, 6 cm and 1 cm above the anal verge (Fig. 15.1). We evaluate sigmoidal sensitivity with the base of the balloon placed 20 cm above the anal verge. We determine the minimal amounts of air (ml) required to elicit the thresholds of the rectosphincteric reflex (≥5 mmHg relaxation of anal pressure)

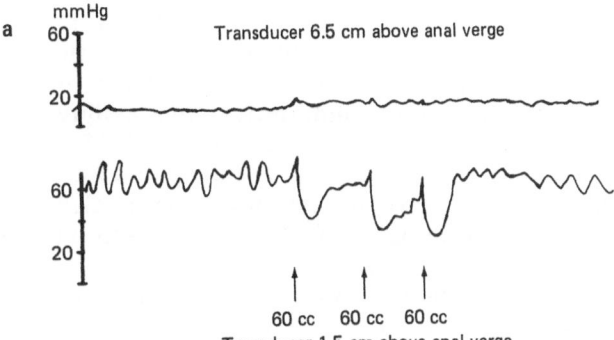

Fig. 15.2. a The *arrows* indicate distension of a rectal balloon with air for 1 second, which results in a decrease in anal pressure. The presence of the rectosphincteric reflex in this 10-year-old boy with severe constipation rules out Hirschsprung's disease. **b** Here distension of a rectal balloon with air for 1 second (*arrows*) produces no decrease in anal pressure. The absent rectosphincteric reflex in this 14-year-old male with chronic constipation and intermittent encopresis is due to Hirschsprung's disease.

Table 15.2. Measurements of anal responses to rectal distension and sigmoid and rectal sensations in controls and constipated children (means±SD)

Measurements in ml of air	Position of the balloon above the anal verge			
	20 cm		11 cm	
	Controls (n=15)	Constipated children (n=15)	Controls (n=15)	Constipated children (n=15)
Threshold of recto-sphincteric reflex	–	–	17± 7	14± 4
Volume of constant relaxation	–	–	122±46	172± 65*
Threshold of transient sensation	17± 7	18±10	19± 7	23± 16
Threshold of fullness	60±23	90±46*	58±27	110±111
Critical volume	110±27	224±95*	118±29	229± 98*

* p<0.05 as compared to controls by Student's t test for unpaired data.

and a transient sensation of rectal balloon distension by inflating the balloon two to three times transiently with volumes 60 and 5 ml in random order, starting each time at 0 ml. We determine the minimal amount of air required to produce a sensation of fullness, a lasting urge to defaecate (critical volume), a sustained complete relaxation of the internal and external sphincters (constant relaxation), and rectal contractility of ≥10 mmHg by adding step-by-step initially 10 ml air up to 60 ml and then 30 ml each 15 seconds into the rectal balloon. When the critical volume has been reached, but constant relaxation of rectal contractility of ≥10 mmHg has not occurred, the next higher volume is used as the volumes of constant relaxation and rectal contractility. Results in control children are given in Table 15.2.

In infants, the balloon lies in the rectum 6 cm above the anal verge, distension volumes to elicit the rectosphincteric reflex are smaller, 5–15 ml, and the critical volume is often <30 ml.

For the premature newborn our motility probe is too long. We place a three-lumen perfused catheter assembly with the three side holes starting 10 mm below its tip and spaced 2 mm apart into the anal canal and a small 1 cm by 1 cm balloon as far up into the rectum as possible – usually 4–5 cm. Volumes to elicit the rectosphincteric reflex are 2–5 ml air.

Studies of the External Sphincter and Pelvic Floor During Straining for Defaecation

Myoelectrical activity from the external sphincter is recorded at a speed of 10 mm/s with three surface electrodes (Andover Medical Supply, Bloomington, Minnesota, USA). Two electrodes are placed over the external sphincter and a third on the buttock (see Fig. 15.1). The area under the wave form of the action potentials, an index of total activity, is obtained by integrating the primary signal with an EMG averaging coupler (SensorMedics, Type 9852A, Anaheim, California, USA). We evaluate the combined function of the external and internal anal sphincters and rectal pressure changes simultaneously by placing one of the transducers of the motility probe into the rectum (6 cm) and a second into the anal canal (1 cm above the anal verge). The outputs of all transducers and surface electrodes are fed into amplifiers of the recorder and graphed on paper.

While lying on the left lateral position the child is asked to strain down as if defaecating and to squeeze (tighten up) in random order. During a normal defaecation attempt, the integrated EMG decreases and during an abnormal defaecation attempt the integrated EMG increases (Fig. 15.3). All healthy control children were able to relax the external sphincter during straining.

Studies of Balloon Defaecation

To stimulate defaecation of a stool from the rectum children were asked to expel while sitting on a toilet chair, rectal balloons filled with 30, 50 and 100 ml water, respectively, allowing 5 minutes for each balloon. Balloon defaecation for each size balloon is evaluated during the first minute and for 5 minutes. The intra-abdominal pressure exerted into the rectal balloon during attempts to defae-

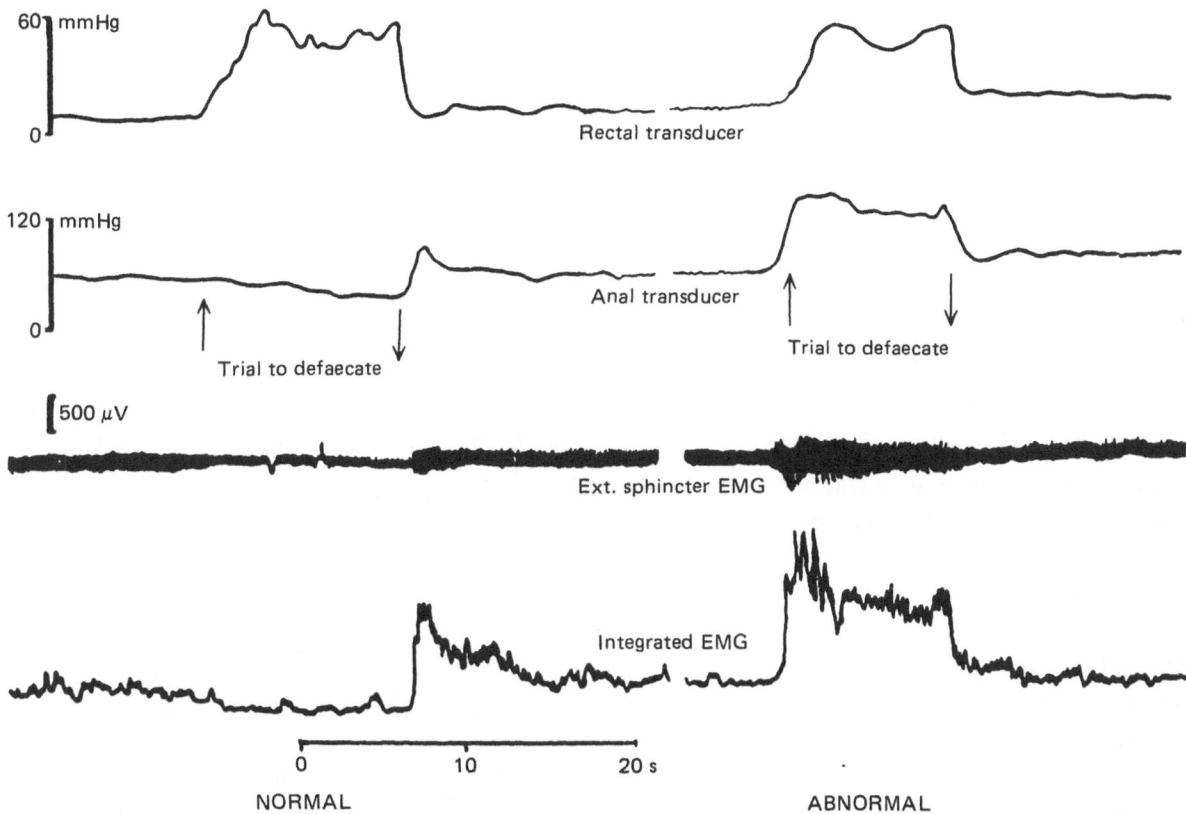

Fig. 15.3. The tracings depict the pressure changes in the rectum and anal canal, and the electromyographic changes from the external anal sphincter during a trial to defaecate. The duration of the defaecation trial is indicated with arrows. A normal defaecation consists of increased rectal (intra-abdominal) pressure, decreased anal pressure and decreased direct and integrated EMG activity. Abnormal defaecation consists of increased rectal (intra-abdominal) pressure, anal pressure, and direct and integrated EMG activity.

cate is transmitted via a polyethylene tube to a pressure transducer and recorded. The strongest and longest pressure changes are evaluated.

Eighty-eight per cent of healthy children aged 5 years and older could expel the 30 ml and 50 ml balloon and 100% could expel the 100 ml ballon in 1 minute (see Table 15.3). Different materials for the evaluation of the ability to defaecate, such as spheres, barium paste, slurs and saline, have been used by other investigators, mostly in adult patients.

Saline Continence

For objective measurement of continence we use the saline continence test immediately after the manometric evaluation (Haynes and Read 1982) in patients with weak sphincter pressure or poor voluntary squeeze (spina bifida, post repair of anal atresia, anal trauma, etc.). A small catheter is inserted into the rectum, with its tip positioned 10

Table 15.3. Ability to defaecate balloons in children ≥5 years of age

Balloon volume		Controls (n=16)	Constipated children with soiling (n=97)
30 ml:	≤1 minute	88%	23%*
	≤5 minute	88%	44%*
50 ml:	≤1 minute	88%	39%*
	≤5 minute	88%	48%*
100 ml:	≤1 minute	100%	47%*
	≤5 minute	100%	59%*

* $p < 0.05$ from controls (Fisher's exact test).

cm from the anal verge. Saline maintained at 37 °C is infused into the rectum at a rate of 60 ml/min up to 240 ml, while the child sits upright in a specially designed chair with a central round aperture. If no leakage occurs, the child is instructed to retain the 240 ml saline for 5 minutes. Any leakage is collected by means of a funnel and collecting cylinder which sits on top of a weight transducer. The volume infused into the rectum when leakage of ≥10 ml saline first occurrs is measured. Four of

12 healthy control children (aged 7–13 years) leaked saline prior to 240 ml (120, 125, 175 and 210 ml). The mean rectal volume when leakage of ≥10 ml occurred was 212±47 ml saline.

Indications for Anorectal Physiology Tests

Anorectal physiology is useful in all functional and organic disorders of anorectal continence:

Chronic constipation with or without faecal soiling
Segmental dilatation of the colon
Hirschsprung's disease
Chronic intestinal pseudo-obstruction
Myelomeningocoele
Anorectal anomalies
Anorectal trauma
Rectal prolapse
Neuromuscular diseases

Chronic Constipation With or Without Faecal Soiling

Constipation is an extremely common problem, with up to 10% of children suffering at times from constipation. Most often faecal soiling occurs in longstanding constipation. The faecal soiling is usually involuntary. Boys are affected three to four times more frequently than girls. Typically, the patient is a child, 3 years of age and older, with a history of constipation that started usually in the first or second year of life, occasionally at birth. The child will often assume certain characteristic postures, such as standing with the buttocks tightly clamped together and tiptoeing around (the "duty dance"). The parents frequently have to be specifically informed that these are stool withholding activities and not "attempts to defaecate".

The physician should monitor intervals, size and consistency of stools that are deposited into the toilet. Some children have daily bowel movements but apparently do not evacuate completely, as evidenced by periodic passage of very large amounts of stool (once every 3–30 days; occasionally the interval between huge bowel movements is 3–4 months). Many parents have not observed their child's stooling pattern, but when asked, they will remember stools which clogged the toilet. The intervals, size and consistency of stools that are deposited into the underwear are recorded. Faecal soiling may occur occasionally, once a day or many times a day. Often the leakage worsens when the child is in an upright position, especially during exercise or during the walk home from school. The frequency of faecal soiling varies among children as well as for a given child, and it is related to the severity of the faecal retention and the frequency and size of the stool deposited into the toilet. A period free of soiling may occur after a large bowel movement, and soiling will resume only after several days of stool retention. Usually the consistency of stool found in the underwear is loose or clay-like.

Visual study of the anus and perineum and simple neurological examination of the anus by determining perianal sensation should be part of a good physical examination. Loss of perianal skin sensation can be associated with various neurological diseases of the spinal cord and lumbosacral root lesions. For performing digital examination of the anus, the examining finger should be well lubricated. Anal pressure is normal to lax, and the examining finger usually enters into a huge faeces-filled rectum. A large, faeces-filled rectosigmoid may be palpated through the abdominal wall, often felt suprapubic and midline reaching up to the umbilicus. Sometimes the whole colon is distended with stool, giving rise to visible abdominal distension.

The principle of treatment is to keep the colon and rectum empty for a prolonged period of time so that colonic and rectal tone may increase as the patient undergoes retraining of bowel habits. The large rectal plug is removed with enemas, followed by sufficient laxatives to ensure that the child has at least one or two stools per day. A precise management plan can be found in Loening-Baucke (1987).

When a child presents with severe constipation, it is important to exclude Hirschsprung's disease and occult myelodysplasia. There are several extremely rare conditions that resemble Hirschsprung's disease but have a normal distribution of ganglion cells. These poorly understood conditions include the small left colon syndrome in infants (Berdon et al. 1976) and pseudo-Hirschsprung's disease in older children (Nixon 1966). In the vast majority of cases of childhood constipation no recognizable organic cause can be determined.

Anorectal manometry and electromyography and defaecation studies are helpful in the evaluation. We perform anorectal manometric tests, measure anal resting and squeeze pressures, and evaluate the presence of the rectosphincteric reflex (Fig. 15.3a) by rectal balloon distension as described above (p. 204). We also measure rectal sensation, critical volume, the volume for constant relaxation and rectal contractility in all children. Anal electromyography with surface electrodes and defaecation studies are performed in all children aged 4 years and older, and occasionally in younger co-operative children. We found the anal pressure to be normal or decreased in most chronically constipated children with faecal soiling (Table 15.1) (Loening-Baucke and Younoszai 1982; Loening-Baucke 1984b). Others have reported the anal pressure to be increased in some of these children with chronic idiopathic constipation (Meunier et al. 1984; Molnar et al. 1983; Mischalany and Wooley 1984), particularly in those without soiling. Results of maximal anal squeeze pressure and anal pull-through pressure (speed: 1 cm/s) are given in Table 15.1. The mean length of the anal canal was 3 cm (range 2–5 cm). Distension of the rectum with a balloon reveals an abnormally high rectal compliance (Loening-Baucke 1984a; Meunier et al. 1984) and blunted rectal sensation (Meunier et al. 1976, 1979, 1984; Molnar et al. 1983; Loening-Baucke 1984a), but causes normal relaxation of the internal anal sphincter in most patients. Most of those in whom no relaxation occurs have short segment Hirschsprung's disease. Many children with idiopathic constipation present with incontinence, probably because the internal anal sphincter is inhibited before the presence of faeces in the rectum is perceived and, therefore, no contraction of the external anal sphincter is initiated (Molnar et al. 1983; Meunier et al. 1984) or because both the internal and external sphincters are completely inhibited (Loening-Baucke 1984a) (see Table 15.2).

The air volumes required in the rectal balloon to inhibit both the external and internal anal sphincters are significantly larger than in control children (Table 15.2). In addition, the critical volume (air volume necessary to feel a persistent urge to defaecate, 178 ± 86 ml) and the volume to produce rectal contractility (106 ± 86 ml) were significantly increased in 97 chronically constipated children with faecal soiling as compared to 16 controls (104 ± 49 ml and 54 ± 28 ml; Loening-Baucke 1989). Studying constipated children during defaecation attempts showed that many had abnormal contraction of the pelvic floor and external anal sphincter making defaecation or balloon expulsion more difficult or impossible (Table 15.3) (Devroede 1985; Loening-Baucke

and Cruikshank 1986; Louis et al. 1985; Wald et al. 1987). The constipated children generated similar intra-abdominal pressures and were straining longer than healthy controls, but in spite of this were significantly less likely to expel rectal water-filled balloons (Loening-Baucke and Cruikshank 1986) or rectal infused saline (Loening-Baucke 1988).

We investigate the anorectal physiology in any child with constipation and/or faecal incontinence. Using the techniques described above gives information on the degree of rectal sensation abnormality, the degree of inhibition of the anal sphincter, and about normal and abnormal defaecation dynamics. It helps in explaining the problem to children and their parents. The anorectal physiology tests help the physician to plan effective management, either medical management, referral for biofeedback treatment or, rarely, surgical treatment. Patients with abnormal defaecation dynamics are often resistant to medical management but they can be taught normal defaecation dynamics through biofeedback training. For methods of biofeedback training see Loening-Baucke (1990), Louis et al. (1985) and Wald et al. (1987).

Segmental Dilatation of the Colon

Segmental dilatation of the colon is a rare condition causing severe constipation and abdominal distension from early infancy. The radiological appearance may resemble Hirschsprung's disease, but there is no aganglionic segment and the rectosphincteric reflex is present. Mischalany and Wooley (1984) found three cases in a group of 80 constipated children: two had dilatations of the sigmoid and in the third the transverse colon was dilated. These children do well following resection of the dilated segment and develop normal bowel habit.

Hirschsprung's Disease (Aganglionosis Coli)

This is a familial disorder that occurs in approximately 1 in 5000 live births. Most patients present with constipation or signs of intestinal obstruction in the immediate newborn period. Only 15% of patients are diagnosed within the first 30 days of life, two-thirds are identified by 3 months, and only a small number remain undetected after 5 years. The main features of Hirschsprung's disease are listed in Table 15.4.

Table 15.4. Major features of Hirschsprung's disease

Male to female ratio is 4:1
Genetics: 7% familial
Symptoms: meconium passage >48 hours
       severe constipation
       abdominal distension
       bilious vomiting
       bowel obstruction and perforation
       enterocolitis
       small-calibre stools
       faecal soiling is rare
       failure to thrive
Symptoms are usually present from birth
Diagnosis: manometry – no rectosphincteric reflex
      barium enema – transition zone, in 80% in the
      rectosigmoid area
      rectal biopsy – no ganglion cells

In older children, intractable constipation from birth is the main feature. There is often failure to thrive with palpable faeces in the abdomen. Stools are usually of small calibre. The rectum is typically empty of stool on digital examination. Occasionally the diagnosis of Hirschsprung's disease is made only in adult life (Anuras et al. 1984).

Anorectal manometry is characteristic in patients with Hirschsprung's disease. The rectosphincteric reflex is absent (see Fig. 15.2b) – no decrease of anal pressure occurs because of the absence of ganglion cells which would transmit this distension reflex (Callaghan and Nixon 1964; Loening-Baucke et al. 1985; Meunier et al. 1976; Tobon et al. 1968). We found that anorectal manometry is safe and non-invasive in the diagnosis of Hirschsprung's diseases in the neonate (Loening-Baucke et al. 1985), but the utmost care in performing manometry in the newborn is necessary, including an exact placement of the recording device and using the smallest distension volumes possible in order to avoid short-lasting displacement of the transducer out of the high pressure zone of the anal canal during rectal distension. Depending on age, the balloon volumes used for the rapid rectal distension range from 1–5 ml for the premature newborn, 5–15 ml for the newborn, 5–30 ml for the infant, ≤60 ml for the toddler, and 60 ml for children ≥4 years of age.

The use of anorectal manometry for diagnostic studies in the neonatal period is made more difficult when rhythmical activity is absent or the anal pressure is low. These findings have been encountered frequently in the stressed infant (Howard and Nixon 1968), and have led to the wrong diagnosis in about 26% of neonates suspected of having Hirschsprung's disease (McParland and Olness 1979; Meunier et al. 1978; Morikawa et al. 1979). We did not find that the maturity of the patient is a factor which influences the success or failure of manometry as a diagnostic method (Loening-Baucke et al. 1985).

Hirschsprung's disease is characterized by congenital absence of intrinsic nerve plexuses (absence of ganglion cells from the submucosa (Meissner's plexus) and muscular layers (Auerbach's plexus)) in the affected segment of bowel and by hypertrophy of the intrinsic nerve bundles. Rectal biopsy taken at least 2 cm from the dentate line will demonstrate absence of ganglion cells. The affected bowel is tonically contracted and may extend proximally from the rectum, involving the sigmoid or the whole colon. The absence of neurones results in spasticity and lack of propulsive activity in the affected segment, with hold up of faeces and dilatation of the colon proximally. Patients with involvement of the internal anal sphincter alone may present later in life with progressive constipation.

Barium enema is usually diagnostic and gives an estimation of the length of the aganglionic segment. This becomes evident as the barium flows into the large dilated ganglionic colon from the narrow aganglionic portion. Demonstration of the transition zone is easier if no effort is made to cleanse the bowel. In the newborn, dilatation of the proximal ganglionic bowel may not have developed and radiological diagnosis may be more difficult.

Surgery is the only effective therapy, but many children will have problems postoperatively: constipation (21%–42%), faecal soiling (19%–47%) and enterocolitis (15%–35%) (Holschneider 1983). Anorectal testing reveals that most continue with no rectosphincteric reflex, some will have an incomplete and 21% a normal rectosphincteric reflex. Therefore, these children are prone to develop secondary megarectum or megacolon. Anorectal manometry and defaecation studies (evaluating anal pressure, squeeze pressures, rectal sensation, rectal elasticity and rectal contractility in addition to the rectosphincteric reflex) help the physician in the evaluation and further planning of treatment.

Chronic Intestinal Pseudo-obstruction

Intestinal pseudo-obstruction occurs when there are signs and symptoms of bowel obstruction without evidence of an obstructive lesion. Colonic pseudo-obstruction often occurs as part of the more generalized chronic intestinal pseudo-obstruction syndrome (Falk et al. 1978). The disease may affect small or large areas of the gastrointestinal tract, from the oesophagus to the rectum. In isolated chronic colonic pseudo-obstruction the disease is limited to the colon. Symptoms include severe abdominal distension secondary to colonic dilatation, with elevation of the diaphragm, abdominal pain and often constipation, although diarrhoea may occur. Chronic intestinal pseudo-obstruction is an unusual but devastating disease that occurs in both sexes. In some cases, a specific myopathy is the problem (Falk et al. 1978; Anuras et al. 1983), degeneration of the ganglia or the nerves occurs in others (Schuffler and Jonak 1982), while in some cases no specific pathology has been detected. The disorder is occasionally familial.

The rectosphincteric reflex is present; larger distension volumes are necessary to sense rectal distension and to produce rectal contractility. The rectal wall elasticity is increased, particularly in those with colonic and rectal involvement. In adult patients with colonic involvement the normal postprandial increase in colonic spike activity and contractility was absent, suggesting a disruption in the mechanisms that link gastroduodenal receptors to the colonic myenteric plexus (Snape et al. 1980).

Onset is often in childhood. A particularly severe congenital variant in female infants is associated with an abnormally enlarged bladder: the megacystis–microcolon–intestinal hypoperistalsis syndrome (Berdon et al. 1976). Anorectal manometry in children with chronic intestinal pseudo-obstruction has been performed infrequently, therefore, no characteristic anorectal physiology has been described.

Myelomeningocoele

Myelomeningocoele is a congenital neural tube defect which occurs in approximately 0.1% of births. As a result of aggressive medical and surgical treatment, 80%–90% of the children survive, so rehabilitation is increasingly important in their management. Faecal incontinence because of neurological impairment occurs in 90% of the children. Many children suffer from severe constipation and overflow faecal incontinence, others have incontinence due to diarrhoea.

Varying degrees of nerve impairment exist in these patients, the most common being loss of anal and/or rectal sensation. Such patients are usually unable to differentiate sensation produced by gas from that produced by liquid or solid faeces. We found a significant increase in the threshold of rectal sensation in patients with myelomeningocoele compared to controls (Loening-Baucke et al. 1988). The level of the sensory motor deficit does not correlate to rectal sensation thresholds (Wald 1983; Loening-Baucke et al. 1988). We did not find an increased critical volume or rectal wall elasticity in patients with myelomeningocoele, therefore, the abnormal rectal sensation does not seem to be explained by a megarectum.

The second most common impairment in patients with myelomeningocoele produces loss of function of the external anal sphincter. The sphincter cannot be squeezed voluntarily (Meunier et al. 1976; Wald 1981, 1983; Whitehead et al. 1981; Arhan et al. 1984; Loening-Baucke et al. 1988). The absence of the external sphincter contraction and the reflex relaxation of the internal anal sphincter allow a rectal contraction to propel a bolus of faeces through the anal canal and prevent voluntary retention. Loss of external anal sphincter function results in a significant decrease in anal resting pressure and leakage during saline infusion. Leakage occurred at volumes of 25 ± 16 ml saline as compared to 212 ± 47 ml in controls. The rectosphincteric reflex is present (Arhan et al. 1972, 1984; Meunier et al. 1976; Loening-Baucke et al. 1988).

Results of the anorectal function evaluation help in the design of an appropriate treatment plan, e.g. medical therapy (stool softeners, laxatives, suppositories or enemas), frequent manual removal of faeces, a constipating diet or medication, behaviour modification and/or biofeedback training.

Methods for biofeedback training have been described by Wald (1981, 1983), Whitehead et al. (1981) and Loening-Baucke et al. (1988). More recent controlled studies did not show improvement in anorectal function after biofeedback training (Loening-Baucke et al. 1988) or better outcome in biofeedback treated children as compared to medical treatment and behaviour modification (Loening-Baucke et al. 1988; Whitehead et al. 1986).

Anorectal Anomalies

The reported overall incidence of anorectal anomalies (abnormalities in the formation of the anorectal canal or in the location of the anus within the perineum) varies from 1 in 3000 to 1 in 15 000 live births. These anomalies are 1.5 times more frequent in males than in females. Half of the affected males have the higher anomaly in contrast to only 19% of affected females. The classifications of anorectal anomalies have been revised several times. One of the more recent ones is by De Vries and Cox (1985), classifying anorectal anomalies into low, intermediate and high.

Anal stenosis represents about 10% of all anorectal anomalies. Digital examination may show a narrowed, tight area within the anus, or a fibrous ring. Normal anal size in premature and term infants were determined by El Haddad and Corkery (1985) through calibration, using Hegar's uterine sounds. Mean anal diameter was 8.6 mm in the 1–1.5 kg premature, 9.7 mm in the 2–2.5 kg newborn, 11.1 mm in the 3–3.5 kg newborn, and 12.8 mm in the 4–4.5 kg newborn.

Arhan et al. (1976) have demonstrated that continence after repair of anorectal malformations depends on many factors. Incontinence is associated with abnormal function of the rectum or the anal sphincters: absence of rectosphincteric reflex, abnormal low anal resting pressure, abnormally low squeeze pressure and abnormal anal sensation. Identification of the external anal sphincter and puborectalis muscle and their location should be done through electromyography using a needle electrode (Chantraine 1973; Swash and Snooks 1985). Taylor et al. (1973) reported that 24% of the patients in the high type group and 93% of patients in the low type group eventually gained good control (old classification).

Management depends on the cause and degree of incontinence, e.g. it may involve the patient cleaning the anal canal after defaecation or it may involve the surgical placement of the rectum through the puborectalis and the sphincters. Bowel training programmes consist of high fibre diet, stool softeners and lubricants. Resistant cases may require a treatment regimen designed to empty the rectum electively and regularly before spontaneous evacuation occurs or the rectum becomes overfilled. Biofeedback training may also be helpful. An abdominal colostomy is rarely necessary.

Anorectal Trauma

Anorectal trauma may be related to an impalement injury but child abuse should be considered. Presentations are rectovaginal tears, often extend-

ing through the anal sphincter, rectovaginal fistula, anorectal tears or even destruction of the rectum. Anorectal manometry to assess the external and internal anal sphincters should be performed. In addition, electromyographic mapping of the external anal sphincter with a needle electrode may be necessary (Pescatori and Ravo 1988; Swash and Snooks 1985).

Rectal Prolapse

Rectal prolapse involves all the layers of the rectal wall. It is rare in children, but usually occurs before 3 years of age, with its highest incidence in infants less than 1 year old. It occurs most often in children with constipation, cystic fibrosis and other diseases leading to malnutrition (e.g. coeliac disease). The anorectal physiology tests include measurement of anal resting pressure and squeeze pressure in the infant. The defaecation dynamics should be assessed in the older child (>4 years) to look for inappropriately increased intra-abdominal pressure and/or an abnormal contraction of the pelvic floor during defaecation attempts.

Since the sphincter muscles and the pelvic attachments are stretched with each successive prolapse, the primary goal of treatment is directed towards eliminating the primary disease, like treatment of constipation or enzyme replacement in cystic fibrosis. Surgery should be used only in the rare child who does not respond to conservative measures.

Neuromuscular Diseases

Occasionally we evaluate a child with faecal incontinence and myotonic dystrophy. The clinical evaluation of such a patient may reveal faecal impaction with incontinence. Most have low anal resting pressures and squeeze pressures. Treatment is often not very successful: the constipation is relieved with laxatives but faecal incontinence increases. Increasing dietary fibre and emptying the rectum electively and regularly can improve continence in some of these children.

Conclusion

The ability to investigate anorectal physiology has been advanced by technical improvements developed over the past decade. The new knowledge has clinical application in several areas as discussed in this chapter. Many inter-related mechanisms ensure continence and regulate normal bowel habits. Our knowledge of the pathophysiology of constipation and faecal soiling in children is rapidly increasing. This chapter should help physicians to distinguish several anorectal physiological abnormalities associated with these disorders and permit the selection of effective treatment.

References

Anuras S, Mitros FA, Novak RV et al. (1983) A familial visceral myopathy with external opthalmoplegia and autosomal recessive transmission. Gastroenterology 84:346–353

Anuras S, Hade J, Soffer E et al. (1984) Natural history of adult Hirschsprung's disease. J Clin Gastroenterol 6:205–210

Arhan P, Faverdin CL, Thouvenot J (1972) Anorectal motility in sick children. Scand J Gastroenterol 7:309–314

Arhan P, Faverdin C, Devroede G et al. (1976) Manometric assessment of continence after surgery for imperforate anus. J Pediatr Surg 11:157–166

Arhan P, Faverdin C, Devroede G et al. (1984) Anorectal motility after surgery for spina bifida. Dis Colon Rectum 27:159–163

Berdon WE, Baker DH, Blanc WA et al. (1976) Megacystis–microcolon intestinal hypoperistalsis syndrome: a new cause of intestinal obstruction in the newborn–report of radiologic findings in five newborn girls. Am J Roentgenol 126:957–964

Callaghan RP, Nixon HH (1964) Megarectum: physiological observations. Arch Dis Child 39:153–157

Chantraine A (1973) EMG examination of the anal and urethral sphincters. In: Desmedt JE (ed) New developments in electromyography and clinical neurophysiology, vol 2. Karger, Basle, pp 421–432

Dent JA (1976) A new technique for continuous sphincter pressure measurement. Gastroenterology 71:263–267

De Vries PA, Cox K (1985) Surgery of anorectal anomalies. Surg Clin North Am 65:1139–1168

Devroede G (1985) Mechanisms of constipation. In: Read NW (ed) Irritable bowel syndrome. Grune and Stratton, New York, pp 127–139

El Haddad M, Corkery JJ (1985) The anus in the newborn. Pediatrics 76:927–928

Falk DL, Anuras S, Christensen J (1978) Chronic intestinal pseudoobstruction. Gastroenterology 74:922–931

Haynes WG, Read NW (1982) Anorectal activity in man during rectal infusion of saline: a dynamic assessment of the anal continence mechanism. J Physiol 47:57–65

Holschneider AM (1983) Elektromanometrie des Enddarms. Diagnostik und Therapie der Inkontinenz und der chronischen Obstipation. Urban and Schwarzenberg, Vienna

Howard ER, Nixon HH (1968) Internal anal sphincter: observations on the development and mechanism of inhibitory responses in premature infants and children with Hirschsprung's disease. Arch Dis Child 43:569–578

Loening-Baucke V (1984a) Sensitivity of the sigmoid colon and rectum in children treated for chronic constipation. J Pediatr Gastroenterol Nutr 3:454–459

Loening-Baucke V (1984b) Abnormal rectoanal function in children recovered from chronic constipation and encopresis. Gastroenterology 87:1299–1304

Loening-Baucke V (1987) Encopresis and enuresis. In: Wolraich M (ed) Practical assessment and management of children with disorders of development and learning. Year Book Medical, Chicago, pp 352–378

Loening-Baucke V (1988) Emptying of rectal infused saline in children with chronic constipation. Gastroenterology 94:267A

Loening-Baucke V (1989) Factors determining outcome in children with chronic constipation and faecal soiling. Gut 30:999–1006

Loening-Baucke V (1990) Modulation of abnormal defecation dynamics by biofeedback treatment in chronically constipated children with encopresis. J Pediatr 116:214–222

Loening-Baucke V, Cruikshank B (1986) Abnormal defecation dynamics in chronically constipated children with encopresis. J Pediatr 108:562–566

Loening-Baucke V, Younoszai MK (1982) Abnormal anal sphincter response in chronically constipated children. J Pediatr 100:213–218

Loening-Baucke V, Pringle KC, Ekwo EE (1985) Anorectal manometry for the exclusion of Hirschsprung's disease in neonates. J Pediatr Gastroenterol Nutr 4:596–603

Loening-Baucke V, Desch L, Wolraich M (1988) Biofeedback training in patients with meningomyelocele and fecal incontinence. Develop Med Child Neurol 30:781–790

Louis D, Valancogne G, Loras O et al. (1985) Techniques et indications du bio-feedback dans les constipations chez l'enfant. Psychologie Medicale 17:1625–1627

McParland FA, Olness K (1979) Diagnostic uses of anorectal manometry in pediatrics. Minn Med 62:447–450

Meunier P, Mollard P, Jaubert de Beaujeu M (1976) Manometric studies of anorectal disorders in infancy and childhood: an investigation of pathophysiology of incontinence and defaecation. Br J Surg 63:402–407

Meunier P, Marechal JM, Mollard P (1978) Accuracy of the manometric diagnosis of Hirschsprung's disease. J Pediatr Surg 13:411–415

Meunier P, Marechal JM, Jaubert de Beaujeu M (1979) Rectoanal pressures and rectal sensitivity studies in chronic childhood constipation. Gastroenterology 77:330–336

Meunier P, Louis D, Jaubert de Beaujeu M (1984) Physiologic investigation of primary chronic constipation in children: Comparison with the barium enema study. Gastroenterology 87:1351–1357

Mischalany HG, Wooley MG (1984) Chronic constipation: manometric patterns and surgical considerations. Arch Surg 119:1257–1259

Molnar D, Taitz LS, Urwin OM et al. (1983) Anorectal manometry results in defecation disorders. Arch Dis Child 58:257–261

Morikawa Y, Donahoe PK, Hendren WH (1979) Manometry and histochemistry in the diagnosis of Hirschsprung's disease. Pediatrics 63:865–871

Nixon HH (1966) What is pseudo-Hirschsprung's disease? Arch Dis Child 41:147–149

Pescatori M, Ravo B (1988) Diagnostic anorectal functional studies: manometry, sphincter electromyography and defecography. Surg Clin N Am 68:1231–1248

Schuffler MD, Jonak Z (1982) Chronic idiopathic intestinal pseudoobstruction caused by a degenerative disorder of the myenteric plexus. The use of Smith's method to define the neuropathology. Gastroenterology 82:476–486

Schuster MM, Hookman P, Hendrix TR et al. (1965) Simultaneous manometric recording of internal and external anal sphincter reflexes. Bull Johns Hopkins Hosp 116:79–88

Snape WJ Jr, Sullivan MA, Cohen S (1980) Abnormal gastrocolonic response in patients with intestinal pseudo-obstruction. Arch Intern Med 140:386–387

Swash M, Snooks SJ (1985) Electromyography in pelvic floor disorders. In: Henry MM, Swash M (eds) Coloproctology and the pelvic floor. Butterworth, London, pp 88–103

Taylor I, Duthie HL, Zachary RB (1973) Anal continence following surgery for imperforate anus. J Pediatr Surg 8:497–503

Tobon F, Nigel C, Talbert J et al. (1968) Non-surgical test for the diagnosis of Hirschsprung's disease. N Engl J Med 278:188–194

Wald A (1981) Use of biofeedback in treatment of fecal incontinence in patients with meningomyelocele. Pediatrics 68:45–49

Wald A (1983) biofeedback for neurogenic fecal incontinence: rectal sensation is a determinant of outcome. J Pediatr Gastroenterol Nutr 2:302–306

Wald A, Chandra R, Gabel S et al. (1987) Evaluation of biofeedback in childhood encopresis. J Pediatr Gastroenterol Nutr 6:554–558

Whitehead WE, Parker LH, Masek BJ et al. (1981) Biofeedback treatment of fecal incontinence in patients with myelomeningocele. Develop Med Child Neurol 23:313–322

Whitehead WE, Parker LH, Basmajian L et al. (1986) Treatment of fecal incontinence in children with spina bifida: comparison of biofeedback and behavior modification. Arch Phys Med Rehabil 67:218–224

Subject Index